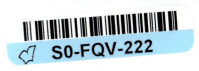

Natriuretic Peptides
The Hormones of the Heart

Aldo Clerico • Michele Emdin (Eds.)

Natriuretic Peptides

The Hormones of the Heart

Foreword by

Luigi Donato

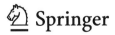 Springer

EDITORS

PROF. ALDO CLERICO
Department of Laboratory Medicine
Institute of Clinical Physiology
CNR – National Research Council
Pisa, Italy
clerico@ifc.cnr.it

DR. MICHELE EMDIN
Department of Cardiovascular Medicine
Institute of Clinical Physiology
CNR – National Research Council
Pisa, Italy
emdin@ifc.cnr.it

AUTHORS

ALDO CLERICO
MICHELE EMDIN
MAURO PANTEGHINI
CLAUDIO PASSINO
FABIO RECCHIA
SIMONA VITTORINI

ISBN-13   978-88-470-1556-2
e-ISBN-13   978-88-470-0498-6

Springer is a part of Springer Science+Business Media
springer.com
© Springer-Verlag Italia 2010
Printed in Italy

Cover image: Ursula Ferrara, Pisa, Italy
Cover design: eStudio Calamar, Girona, Spain

Foreword

Clinical progress is a complex resultant of the interaction between intelligent clinical observation, selected cohort studies, advances in the biophysiological understanding of regulatory mechanisms in health and disease, and technological innovation. In other words, it is through the interplay of clinical, epidemiological, biological and technological research that advances in disease understanding and treatment may be made.

While the above statement represents the philosophy that has inspired the Institute of Clinical Physiology of the Italian National Research Council since its foundation, this book, the work of Aldo Clerico and Michele Emdin, respectively chiefs of laboratory medicine and cardiovascular medicine at the institute, is an excellent demonstrator of the validity of this approach.

The pioneer work of de Bold and a few others would never have emerged from experimental medicine without the fantastic progress in immunometric methods, which has made it possible to move from bench to bedside.

In fact, the current and continuous progress in discovering, understanding and applying the emerging evidence on the endocrine function of the heart, not only represents a Copernican revolution in respect of the traditional mechanical conception, but it unveils entirely new and fascinating perspectives in the treatment and possibly prevention of cardiac failure.

Cardiology is increasingly obliged to enlarge its horizons to the vast regions upstream and downstream of the acute cardiac event. This new demand goes beyond the classical borders of cardiology, and justifies the birth and expansion of cardiology itself into a veritable cardiovascular medicine approach, mastering the multiple regulatory mechanisms and understanding the multiorgan concert coming into play in the long history of the cardiac patient.

Aldo Clerico comes from endocrinology and Michele Emdin from cardiology: they started working together some years ago, and their team was immediately very productive, both at laboratory and bedside level. It is my opinion that with this book they have done a very good job in presenting this complex matter first of all to cardiologists and endocrinologists.

Finally, I want to say that I am deeply convinced that, as far as its clinical relevance is concerned, this field is only at its early dawn.

Luigi Donato
Head of Institute of Clinical Physiology
CNR - National Research Council
Pisa, Italy

Contents

6 Clinical Applications in Extra-Cardiac Diseases 133
Aldo Clerico, Claudio Passino, Michele Emdin

**7 Cardiac Natriuretic Hormone System
as Target for Cardiovascular Therapy**. 161
Michele Emdin, Aldo Clerico

**8 "Inconclusive" Remarks:
Past, Present and Future of Natriuretic Peptides** . . . .

About the Authors

- **ALDO CLERICO** MD, is Director of the Laboratory of Cardiovascular Endocrinology 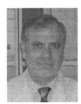 and Cell Biology, CNR Institute of Clinical Physiology, G Pasquinucci Hospital, Massa and Pisa. Prior to this position, he co-founded the Laboratory of Cardiovascular Endocrinology at the CNR Institute of Clinical Physiology. He is Associate Professor in Clinical Biochemistry at the Scuola Superiore S. Anna, Pisa. He has authored more than 600 scientific publications.

- **MICHELE EMDIN** MD, PhD in Cardiovascular Pathophysiology, is Head of the Cardiovascular Medicine Department, at the CNR Institute of Clinical 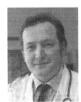 Physiology in Pisa. His field of expertise is neuro-hormonal control of cardiovascular system. He is widely published, and is a reviewer for numerous respected publications.

- **MAURO PANTEGHINI** MD, is Full Professor of Clinical Biochemistry and Clinical Molecular Biology and Director of the corresponding chair at the Medical School of the University of Milan, Italy. He also covers the di-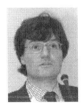 rection of the Laboratory of Clinical Biochemistry of the "Luigi Sacco" University Hospital in Milan. He has published over 265 manuscripts.

- **CLAUDIO PASSINO** MD, is Researcher at the Cardiovascular Medicine Department CNR Institute of Clinical Physiology in Pisa and at at the Scuola Superiore S. Anna, Pisa. He has authored more than 150 scientific publications.

- FABIO A. RECCHIA MD, PhD, is an Associate Professor of Physiology at the Scuola Superiore S. Anna, Pisa, and at the New York Medical College, Valhalla, NY. He is member of the American Physiological Society, of the Editorial Board of the American Journal of Physiology, and Fellow of the American Heart Association (FAHA). His field of expertise is hemodynamics, cardiac function and metabolism.

- SIMONA VITTORINI Ph.D., is Researcher at the Laboratory of Molecular Cardiology and Genetics, CNR Institute of Clinical Physiology, "G. Pasquinucci" Hospital, Massa. She has got her Ph. D. in Experimental Pathology and she is also specialized in Medical Genetics.

Abbreviations

ACE, angiotensin-converting enzyme
ACS, acute coronary syndrome
ADH, antidiuretic hormone
AMI, acute myocardial infarction
ANF, atrial natriuretic factor (another term for ANP)
ANP, atrial natriuretic peptide
ANS, autonomic nervous system
AUC, area under the curve
BMI, Body mass index
BNP, brain (B-type) natriuretic peptide
CNH, cardiac natriuretic hormones
CNP, C-type natriuretic peptide
CNS, central nervous system
COPD, chronic obstructive pulmonary disease
COX, cyclooxygenase
CRP, C-reactive protein
CV, coefficient of variation
cTnI, cardiac troponin I
cTnT, cardiac troponin T
DNP, dendroaspis (D-type) natriuretic peptide
ECE, endothelin-converting enzyme
ECG, electrocardiogram
ECLIA, electro-chemi-luminescence-immuno-assay
EDHF, endothelium-derived hyperpolarizing factor
EF, ejection fraction
EIA, enzyme-immuno-assay
ESRD, end-stage renal disease
GATA, zinc-finger proteins binding consensus sequence (A/T)GATA(A/G)
GC, guanylate cyclase
Gi protein, inhibitory guanine nucleodite regulatory (Gi) protein
HF, heart failure
HPLC, high pressure (performance) liquid chromatography
IFCC, International Federation of Clinical Chemistry and Laboratory Medicine
IL, interleukin
IRMA, immuno-radio-metric-assay
KO mice, knockout mice for some genes
LANP, long-acting natriuretic peptide

LDL, low density lipoprotein
LPS, lipopolysaccharide
LVEF, left ventricular ejection fraction
MAP, mean arterial pressure
MHC, myosin heavy chain
NEP, neutral endopeptidase
NO, nitric oxide
NOS, nitric oxide synthase (eNOS, endothelial NOS; iNOS, inducible NOS)
NPPA, human coding gene for ANP
NPPB, human coding gene for BNP
NPV, negative predictive value
NRP, natriuretic receptor peptide
NT-proANP, N-terminal fragment of proANP
NT-proBNP, N-terminal fragment of proBNP
NT-proCNP, N-terminal fragment of proCNP
NTS, nucleus of tractus solitarius
NYHA, New York Heart Association
PCR, polymerase chain reaction
PG, prostaglandin
PGI, prostaglandin I, prostacyclin (PGI_2)
PND, ANP gene
POCT, point-of-care testing
PPV, positive predictive value
ET-1, endothelin 1
PKG, cGMP-dependent protein kinase
PRA, plasma renin activity
RAAS, renin-angiotensin-aldosterone system
RIA, radio-immuno-assay
ROC, receiver operating characteristic
RT PCR, reverse transcription polymerase chain reaction
RVLM, rostral ventrolateral medulla
SAH, subarachnoid hemorrhage
T3, triiodothyronine
T4, tetraiodothyronine, thyroxine
TGF, transforming growth factor
TNF, tumor necrosis factor
VIP, vasoactive intestinal polypeptide
VLM, ventrolateral medulla
VNP, ventricular natriuretic peptide

Chapter 1

Historical Background and Book Aim

Aldo Clerico • Michele Emdin

OBERON
That very time I saw, but thou couldst not,
Flying between the cold moon and the earth,
Cupid all arm'd: a certain aim he took
At a fair vestal throned by the west,
And loosed his love-shaft smartly from his bow,
As it should pierce a hundred thousand hearts…

A Midsummer Night's Dream
William Shakespeare

1.1 Historical Background

As early as 1976, in the preface to the first edition of his popular monograph on the physiology of the heart, Arnold M. Katz pointed out:

"…Although it remains fashionable to consider the heart as a muscular pump, this organ is much more than a hollow viscus that provides mechanical energy to propel blood through the vasculature. It is an intricate biological machine that contains, within each cell, a complex of control and effector mechanisms…" [1].

Despite this prophetic observation, in the latter part of the past century the dynamics of circulation were stressed and cardiac disease was explained on a purely hemodynamic basis [2]. The discovery by de Bold [3] that the heart also has an endocrine function has made it necessary to revise completely the theoretical framework of heart function. At the dawn of the new century, we should not consider the heart simply as a pump, but rather as a multi-functional and interactive organ, part of a complex network, and an active component of the integrative systems of the body (including nervous, endocrine and immune systems) [4].

The possibility that low-pressure areas of the heart may be able to sense the fullness of the circulation has long intrigued the physiologist. However, the discovery of the cardiac endocrine function was difficult, probably because it contrasted with the general understanding of cardiac function. Indeed, in 1956, Kirsch and colleagues reported the presence of membrane-bound granules in atrial but not ventricular myocytes of guinea pigs [5]. In the same year, Henry and Pearce reported that balloon stretching of the left atrium produced increased urinary flow in dogs [6]. Poche, in 1957, described the same structure as membrane-bound granules, which he called "*dichte Körper*" [7].

In 1959, Bompiani and co-workers [8] reported the presence of "*corps denses*" in rat atrial cardiocytes and in the bundle of His of albino rats, while Jamieson and Palade named these "specific atrial granules" in 1964 [9] (Fig. 1.1).

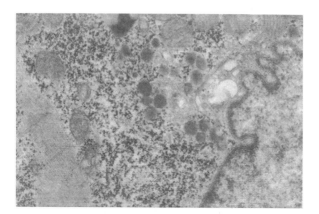

Fig. 1.1. Electron microscopic section through human atrial myocardium, showing atrial cardiomyocytes including some storage granules (i.e., the specific atrial granules containing cardiac natriuretic peptides)

Despite these findings, such a humoral link between atrial and renal sodium excretion received support only in 1976, when Marie et al. [10] reported that atrial granules could be modified by changes in hydro-electrolytic balance. The endocrine function of the heart was definitively established by de Bold et al. [11] in 1981, with the publication of findings regarding the diuretic and natriuretic properties of atrial muscle extracts using the non-diuretic rat bioassay. Injection of such extracts produced a very powerful natriuresis and accompanying diuresis with minimal effect on kaliuresis. The extracts also displayed blood pressure-lowering properties and increased hematocrit. Purification and sequencing of a peptide with the same biological properties as crude atrial extracts resulted in the discovery of a hormone peptide, named atrial natriuretic factor (ANF) by this group of investigators [3, 12].

These seminal studies paved the way for the isolation, purification and identification of a family of natriuretic and vasodilator peptides, now more commonly known as atrial natriuretic peptides (ANP). Furthermore, it was demonstrated that not only atrial but also ventricular cardiomyocytes can secrete peptides with natriuretic activity, in particular the brain natriuretic peptide (BNP), so called because it was first isolated from porcine brain [13].

More recently, C-type natriuretic peptide (CNP) [14], mainly produced and secreted by endothelial cells and by neurons of the central nervous system, and urodilatin [15], produced and secreted by renal cells (and present in urine, but not in plasma), were added to this peptide family. The "C" of CNP follows the fortuitous fact that the names of the first two natriuretic peptides use "A" and "B", respectively. For this reason, ANP is also called A-type natriuretic peptide and BNP is indicated as B-type natriuretic peptide. Finally, a new peptide, called DNP (dendroaspis natriuretic peptide or

D-type natriuretic peptide) was identified in mammal plasma, but its origin and pathophysiological importance are still unclear [16, 17].

On the other hand, several studies have indicated that natriuretic hormone-like peptides are present in the plant kingdom as well as in the animal kingdom; thus suggesting that this hormonal system, which has been shown to regulate solute transport in vertebrates, has evolved early in evolution [18]. These findings also suggest that natriuretic hormones are necessary for life.

Reliable immunoassays for the measurement of natriuretic peptides in blood and tissues of healthy subjects and patients with cardiovascular disease have been developed [19]. These methods have allowed a more comprehensive understanding of the relevant role played by cardiac natriuretic hormones in physiological conditions and disease [20].

The cultural impact of these studies was of paramount importance. We may consider this as a true "Copernican revolution" in the field of cardiovascular pathophysiology, whose effects can now be directly appreciated also in clinical practice [4, 20]. Cardiac endocrine function should be considered as closely related and integrated with other cardiomyocyte properties, such as excitability and contractility. Moreover, it should be evaluated and measured by means of classical methodological approaches and laboratory techniques commonly used for studying and measuring the activity of endocrine glands. Finally, the results of these investigations should be interpreted in the light of classical endocrinological concepts, such as hormone production, metabolism, peripheral action, and specific receptors [4, 20].

Reductionism, which has dominated biological research for over a century, has provided a wealth of knowledge about individual cellular components and their functions. Despite its enormous success, it is increasingly clear that a discrete biological function can only rarely be attributed to an individual molecule. Instead, most biological characteristics arise from complex interactions between the cell's numerous constituents, such as proteins, DNA, RNA and small molecules [21, 22]. Therefore, a key challenge for biology in the twenty-first century is to understand the structure and dynamics of the complex intercellular web of interactions that contribute to the structure and function of a living cell.

The behavior of most complex systems, including the biological system, emerges from the orchestrated activity of many components that interact with each other through pair-wise interactions [21]. The components of a biological network can be reduced to a series of nodes that are connected to each other by links, with each link representing the interactions between two components. According to this theory [21], cardiac natriuretic hormones (CNH) should represent highly connected nodes (hubs) in the complex network linking all the regulatory systems of the body (including nervous, endocrine and immune systems) [4].

1.2 Book Aim and Plan

The principal aim of this book is to demonstrate this assumption. It is important to note that this new theory, which considers the heart as a multi-functional and interactive organ that exchanges information with nervous, endocrine and immune systems, is more similar to the popular outlook on the heart. Indeed, some ancient peoples considered the heart as the seat of the soul, and also in modern times the heart is always related to courage, emotion and feeling in popular and artistic imagery.

In Chapter 2 we will summarize the "classical" view of heart physiology; the other chapters will be dedicated to biochemical characteristics and physiological actions (Chap. 3), measurement (Chap. 4), and pathophysiological and clinical relevance, including the cardiac (Chap. 5) and extra-cardiac (Chap. 6) diseases, of the CNH system, respectively. In Chapter 7, we will review the therapeutic applications of natriuretic peptides. Finally, in the last chapter (Chap. 8), we will report our conclusive remarks and also try to take a glance at the years to come.

As each chapter is an independent and self-sufficient unit, we have added a brief introduction at the start and a conclusion at the end of each chapter. For the same reason, the references have been listed at the end of each chapter.

The selection of references was a very serious problem. At the time of writing this manuscript (September 2005), a search for the key words "natriuretic peptides" gave more than 14,000 items, while "atrial natriuretic peptide" more than 13,600 and "B-type natriuretic peptide" more than 3,200 items on the website of the National Library of Medicine (Pub Med, *http://www.ncbi.nlm.nih.gov/*) (Figs. 1.2 and 1.3). It is interesting to note that the time-course seems to be different for articles concerning ANP- or BNP-related peptides. The publications including "atrial natriuretic peptide" seem to have a peak in the 1990s, while the number of articles on BNP and related peptides is still increasing (Fig. 1.3). This effect is clearly due to an explosion of clinical articles and trials concerning the routine use of BNP assays in the diagnosis and risk stratification of patients with cardiovascular diseases in the first years of the new century (see Chap. 5).

It is clearly impossible to cover all articles concerning the CNH; however, taking the reference sections of all the chapters as a whole, we have reported more than 800 references. In order to reduce the number of references, without missing the contribution of some important articles, we usually suggest some authoritative or systematic reviews to readers interested in examining particular topics more closely or in detail. Moreover, for each particular field, we have made every effort to report and discuss the contribution of all the most important scientific groups. We apologize in advance if we have not succeeded in some particular cases.

As demonstrated in Figures 1.2 and 1.3, the studies concerning the CNH (especially BNP) are still growing and expanding. The observations reported in this book are based on the scientific evidence published, judged as the most significant by consensus experts (when available), and should reflect the present knowledge in a topic that is enriched daily by novel methodological, pathophysiological, and clinical progress. This clearly implies a future re-evaluation of some (or even most) of the scientific data.

However, the findings reported in the literature are often conflicting, and consequently there is not a consensus. This is in part expected as a result of species-specific differences (especially between rodents and humans) or of different methods or experimental protocols used. As far as the clinical studies and trials are concerned, the diagnostic accuracy of the CNH assay depends not only on the type of peptide measured (ANP, NT-proANP, BNP or NT-proBNP) and on the respective assaying methods used [19, 20], but also on:

1. The gold (reference) standard used to classify the assay answers (positive/negative, true/false).
2. The clinical condition in which the diagnostic accuracy is tested.
3. The illness prevalence in the examined context.
4. The gravity and severity of the patient's pathology.
5. The type of statistical analysis or mathematical model used [20, 23].

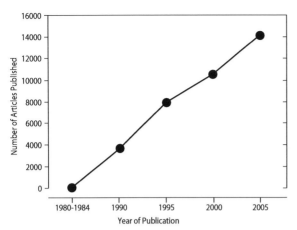

Fig. 1.2. Cumulative number of articles published and covered in the Pub Med website for the words "natriuretic peptides" from 1980 to 20 September 2005. The total number of items was 14,159

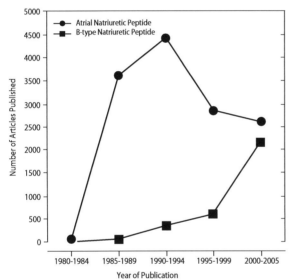

Fig. 1.3. Number of articles published and covered in the Pub Med website for the words "atrial natriuretic peptide" and "B-type natriuretic peptide" from 1980 to 27 September 2005. The articles are grouped in 5-year periods; i.e., each value indicates the total number of articles covered in the 5-year interval. The total number of items was 13,674 for "atrial natriuretic peptide" and 3,220 for "B-type natriuretic peptide", respectively

In the case of conflicting results, we have made every effort to report and discuss all scientific contributions. Of course, some subjective discretional power is possible in describing the scientific data and, especially, in their discussion and interpretation. We would be glad if the reader could point out to us possible omissions, mistakes or misleading sentences, so that we may improve our work in the future.

This work would not be possible without our Institute: set up in 1968 by Luigi Donato, it is still a unique multidisciplinary environment where clinical care of the patient, at the highest quality level, is accompanied by nearby research facilities. Finally, we would like to thank our co-workers, who in either the clinical setting or the laboratories allow us daily to look for the answer to our curiosity concerning the physiology and pathophysiology of the circulation and cardiovascular diseases.

References

1. Katz AM (2001) Physiology of the heart, 3rd edn. Lippincott Williams & Wilkins, Philadelphia
2. Bing RJ (1999) Preface. In: Cardiology - the evolution of the science and the art, 2nd edn. Harwood Academic Publishers GmbH, Chur (Switzerland), XIII-XIV
3. De Bold AJ (1985) Atrial natriuretic factor: a hormone produced by the heart. Science 230:767-770
4. Clerico A, Recchia FA, Passino C, Emdin M (2006) Cardiac endocrine function is an essential component of the homeostatic regulation network: physiological and clinical implications. Am J Physiol Heart Circ Physiol 290:H17-19
5. Kirsch B (1956) Electronmicroscopy of the atrium of the heart. I. Guinea pig. Exp Med Surg 14:99-112
6. Henry JP, Pearce JW (1956) The possible role of cardiac atrial stretch receptors in the induction of charge in urine flow. J Physiol 131:572-585
7. Poche R (1957) Elektronemikroskopische untersuchngen des lipofuscin in herzmuskel des menschen. Zentralbl Allg Pathol Pathol Anat 96:295
8. Bompiani GD, Rouiller C, Hatt PY (1959) Le tissu de conduction du cœur chez le rat. Etude au microscope électrique. I. Le tronc commun du fasceau de is et le cellules claires de l'oreillette droite. Arch Mal Coeur 52:1257-1274
9. Jamieson JD, Palade GE (1964) Specific granules in atrial muscle cell. J Cell Biol 23:151-162
10. Marie JP, Guillemont H, Hatt PY (1976) Le degré de granulation des cardiocytes auriculaires. Etude planimétriques au cours de differents apports d'eau et de sodium chez le rat. Pathol Biol 24:549-554
11. De Bold AJ, Borenstein HB, Veress AT, Sonnenberg H (1981) A rapid and important natriuretic response to intravenous injection of atrial myocardial extracts in rats. Life Sci 28:89-94
12. Flynn TG, Davies PL, Kennedy BP et al (1985) Alignment of rat cardionatrin sequences with the preprocardionatrin sequence from complementary DNA. Science 228:323-325
13. Sudoh T, Kangawa K, Minamino N, Matsuo H (1988) A new natriuretic peptide in porcine brain. Nature 332:78-81
14. Sudoh T, Minamino N, Kangawa K, Matsuo H (1990) C-type natriuretic peptide (CNP): a new member of natriuretic peptide family identified in porcine brain. Biochem Biophys Res Commun 168:863-870
15. Schulz-Knappe P, Forssmann K, Hock D et al (1988) Isolation and structural analysis of "urodilatin", a new peptide of the cardiodilatin-(ANP)-family, extracted from human urine. Klin Wochenschr 66:752-759
16. Schweitz H, Vigne P, Moinier D et al (1992) A new member of the natriuretic peptide family is present in the venom of the green mamba (Dendroaspis angusticeps). J Biol Chem 267:13928-13932
17. Richards AM, Lainchbury JG, Nicholls MG et al (2002) Dendroaspis natriuretic peptide: endogenous or dubious? Lancet 359:5-6
18. Takei Y (2001) Does the natriuretic peptide system exist throughout the animal and plant kingdom? Comp Biochem Physiol Part B 129:559-573
19. Clerico A, Del Ry S, Giannessi D (2000) Measurement of natriuretic cardiac hormones (ANP, BNP, and related peptides) in clinical practice: the need for a new generation of immunoassay methods. Clin Chem 46:1529-1534
20. Clerico A, Emdin M (2004) Diagnostic accuracy and prognostic relevance of the measurement of the cardiac natriuretic peptides: a review. Clin Chem 50:33-50
21. Barabasi AL, Oltvai ZN (2004) Network biology: understanding the cell's functional organization. Nat Rev Genet 5:101-113
22. Oltvai ZN, Barabasi AL (2002) Systems biology. Life's complexity pyramid. Science 298:763-764
23. Doust JA, Glasziou PP, Pietrzak E, Dobson AJ (2004) A systematic review of the diagnostic accuracy of natriuretic peptides for heart failure. Arch Intern Med 11:1978-1984

Chapter 2

The Heart Complexity
The Intrinsic Function (Intrinsic Regulation of Heart Rate and Mechanics)

Michele Emdin · Claudio Passino · Fabio Recchia

Knowledge is proud that it has learned so much,
wisdom is humble that it knows no more.

A. Cournand

2.1 Preamble

In classical physiology, the function of the heart is described as the target of autonomic nervous system modulation superimposed on a mechanistic regulation. The aim of this chapter is to remind us of the basic knowledge in this field, as a bridge to the thorough description of the physiological and clinical relevance of the discovery of cardiac endocrine function. An extensive review of the current physiological view of cardiovascular function is beyond the scope of this book and can be found in several excellent textbooks [1, 2].

2.2 Heart Physiology: the Classical View

The heart pumps blood into the pulmonary circulation for the exchange of oxygen and carbon dioxide, and into the systemic circulation to supply tissues with oxygen and nutritive substances, and to convey hormones and other regulatory molecules. The systemic blood flow also contributes to regulation of body temperature.

Respiratory activity is modulated in harmony with cardiovascular function to maintain blood oxygen, carbon dioxide and hydrogen ion concentration within a narrow physiological range.

A healthy heart pumps 3.5 liters of blood per square meter of body surface at rest, at a rate of between 60 and 100 beats per minute. Untrained subjects can increase blood flow up to 12 liters and athletes up to 20 liters during exercise, with the heart rate increasing up to 160 and 190 beats per minute. This shows the great adaptability of cardiac function in response to physiological stimuli.

Cardiac preload corresponds to the volume of blood in the ventricle in the end diastole: in the normal heart an increase in preload enhances the strength of ventricular contraction (Frank-Starling mechanism, or heterometric autoregulation, according to Sarnoff's definition). Cardiac afterload is the resistance against which the ventricle pumps, determined by the combination of aortic impedance and total vascular resistance: normal hearts are able to increase ejected blood volume despite augmented resistance (homeometric autoregulation or Anrep phenomenon). In the presence of a given preload or afterload, augmented cardiac contractility increases the amount of blood ejected with each beat of the heart (stroke volume).

The cardiac output (equal for the right and left ventricle) and the vascular resistance to blood flow are the main determinant factors in regulating tissue perfusion. The vascular resistances are distributed throughout the vascular bed, occurring mainly at the arterial sites (large arteries 19%, small arteries and arterioles 47%, versus capillaries 27% and veins 7%) and are influenced by the diameter of the precapillary arterioles. Most of the blood volume (64%) resides in the veins (lungs 9%, small arteries and arterioles 9%, large arteries 7%, heart in diastole 7%, capillaries 5%). The systemic circulation is arranged in a parallel fashion and is in series with the pulmonary circulation.

Cardiac rate and contractility, filling volume/pressure and vascular resistances are all influenced by neural control and hormonal agents, acting directly on the heart and vessels and by the regulation of circulating blood volume.

Nevertheless, the heart is not merely a target of a remote control, nor a simple mechanical pump modulated by hydrostatic forces, but because of its anatomy and histology, it holds an intrinsic capability to govern its function by itself. Therefore, the pacemaker cells of the sinoatrial node are able, even when denervated, to maintain the periodical spontaneous depolarization by the inward current of Na^+ ions during phase 4 of the action potential, which is spread through the conduction system and atrial and ventricular cardiomyocytes, forming the basis for electrical and mechanical systole and for the physiological repeat of cardiac cycles.

Moreover, two hearts (right and left) in one serve the two parallel vascular circuits, permitting the coupling of ventilation, blood supply and subsequent gas exchange within the lung, and distribution of oxygenated blood to the periphery of the body. The interventricular septum, simultaneously contributing to the contraction of both ventricles, is the key to this synchronism; its absence independently contributes to the development of heart dysfunction and failure.

The heart has many sensors to provide information about what is going on either within its chambers, concerning intracavitary pressure, or within its wall, with widespread chemo- and mechanoreceptors, evoking local as well as centrally mediated adaptive responses, or providing a painful sensation alerting the individual of pathological events, such as ischemia.

The heart is nourished through the coronary circulation: coronary blood flow varies with aortic pressure, and is influenced by the systolic mechanical compression of intramyocardial vessels, and by metabolic factors released by the myocytes. To adapt to increased metabolic needs, various stimuli, such as hypoxia, increased concentration of hydrogen ions, lactic acid, nitric oxide, carbon dioxide, and particularly adenosine may elicit vasodilatation and an increase in myocardial blood flow.

2.3 Neural Control of the Heart: Cardiac Receptors, Afferent/Efferent Neural Pathways, Baro- and Chemoreceptive Feedback

2.3.1 Premises on the Neuro-Humoral Control of the Cardiovascular System

Circulation is regulated by neural and humoral mechanisms, which, on a beat-to-beat basis, adapt heart rate and contractility, vascular pressures and cardiac output in order to provide an adequate perfusion of brain, myocardium, kidney, lungs and all the other tissues and organs whose viability and function allow the vegetative and relational life of the individual.

These neuro-hormonal mechanisms are continuously influenced by retroactive feedback signals, carrying information on hemodynamics (from arterial and cardiac baroreceptors), on gas exchange homeostasis (from peripheral and central chemoreceptors), as well as on muscle (from metaboreceptors) and visceral functions.

This informative flow from the "periphery" of the body, and from the cardiovascular system itself, is integrated by the medullary autonomic centers. In resting conditions, autonomic nervous outflow tonically inhibits the intrinsic heart rate activity via the predominant vagal control of sinus node pacemaker cells, and sustains via the sympathetic drive a tonic constriction of resistance and capacitance vessels [3].

The quick sudden response to endogenous and exogenous stimuli of various origins (defense reaction, response to pain, emotional stress and physical activity, external or body temperature changes, variations in body position, feeding) is achieved by the modulation of the autonomic outflow by changes in the sympatho-vagal balance.

Neural control allows the phasic (seconds to minutes) adaptation of heart and vessels to physiological stimuli, as for vagal control of heart rate and of sympathetic cardiac contractility and vasomotor control [3].

The autocrine and paracrine function of the endothelium, with the existence of a local balance between production of vasodilator (i.e. nitric oxide, bradykinin, prostaglandins, C-type natriuretic peptide) and vasoconstrictor (i.e. endothelin, serotonin, thromboxane) molecules, implies the possibility of the autoregulation of single-organ vascularization and perfusion in response either to local (e.g. metabolic, shear-stress) or systemic (e.g. temperature, neuro-hormones) stimuli [8].

The endocrine function regulates slower, plastic responses affecting the circulation in the longer term (minutes to hours) by the control of vasomotion and circulating blood volume. This includes the modulation of renal water/salt excretion by the adrenal glands via catecholamine and aldosterone secretion, by the hypothalamus-neurohypophyseal gland via secretion of vasopressin (antidiuretic hormone, ADH), and by the kidney, through renin-activated angiotensin production [1]. The thyroid, too, has a relevant role, through the cardiac inotrope and vasodilator effect of thyroid hormone [4].

The cardiovascular system is modulated by neuro-hormonal agents on a circadian basis, related to the wake/sleep cycle, whereas ultradian secretory cycles of some hormones, such as growth hormone, exert effects on cardiomyocytes [1, 2].

2.3.2 Autonomic Control of Heart Rate

Heart rate is determined by the pacemaker activity of the sinoatrial node in the posterior wall of the right atrium, which shows automaticity due to spontaneous changes in calcium, potassium and sodium ion conductances. This intrinsic automaticity has a spontaneous firing rate of about 110 beats per minute, which tends to decrease with age. Heart rate is decreased below the intrinsic rate primarily by activation of the vagus nerve, innervating the sinoatrial node, while it is increased above the intrinsic rate, both by withdrawal of vagal tone and by activation of sympathetic nerves innervating the pacemaker cells. Heart rate is also modified by circulating catecholamines acting via beta$_1$-adrenoceptors located on sinoatrial nodal cells, and by changes in circulating thyroxin (thyrotoxicosis causes tachycardia) or in body core temperature (hyperthermia increases heart rate) (Fig. 2.1).

The neural control of cardiovascular and respiratory systems is maintained by a medullary anatomical and functional network, generating an efferent outflow towards the spinal cord, and by structures permitting a reflex control of the network activity, via inhibitory and excitatory afferents [6].

On the whole, this network is represented by the vegetative (Reil, 1857) or autonomic nervous system (ANS), as defined by Langley and Dickinson [7], with the sympathetic and parasympathetic arms (Langley, 1901) regulating all body structures not subjected to voluntary control, whose function is usually kept under the level of consciousness [3].

The sympathetic nervous system sustains body mobilization and activity by adequate cardiovascular and respiratory adjustments, producing an increase in metabolic expenditure. On the other hand, the aim of the parasympathetic system is to conserve energy, supporting the physiologic responses related to rest, digestion, and recovery of body reserves. Parasympathetic predominance, such as in athletes, makes the cardiovascular response to exercise less expensive in energy loss and more effective.

The ANS activity is independent of, if not completely free from, voluntary influence, as well as from modulation by other medullary (respiratory) centers, or by other neural structures (hypothalamus, amygdala and cerebral cortex), which may modify or abolish the reflex activity and coordinate the autonomic outflow with cognitive and emotional functions [6].

Both autonomic branches consist of pre- and postganglionic neurons, acting mostly as functional antagonists (as is the case for their effect on sinoatrial and cardiac con-

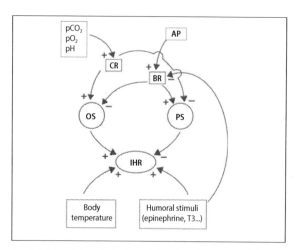

Fig. 2.1. Intrinsic heart rate is modulated by the autonomic balance, i.e. the interaction between the effect upon sinus node activity either of sympathetic or parasympathetic outflow, influenced by the activity of autonomic medullary centers, whose intrinsic activity is beat-to-beat modulated by chemo- and baroreflex feedback. Physical stimuli, such as body temperature, or humoral stimuli, act on heart rate both at the sinus node and at a central level. *IHR* intrinsic heart rate, *AP* arterial pressure, *CR* chemoreflex, *BR* baroreflex, *OS* orthosympathetic, *PS* parasympathetic, *T3* tri-iodothyronine

duction system cells), while their functions are rarely synergistic, or anatomically/functionally prevailing (as for the sympathetic control of vasomotor tone) [6].

Acetylcholine is the preganglionic neurotransmitter for both autonomic arms and the postganglionic mediator for the parasympathetic system, whereas norepinephrine is the neurotransmitter for almost all sympathetic postganglionic cells. Epinephrine is produced and secreted directly into the bloodstream by chromaffin cells in the medullary portion of the adrenal glands (which may be considered as postganglionic neurons of the sympathetic system, though they act as endocrine cells), with an endocrine effect mediated by the same peripheral receptors as norepinephrine, with a variable affinity [1, 2].

Sympathetic-mediated vasoconstriction is mediated by the agonism of norepinephrine on the alpha-1 postsynaptic receptors, whereas alpha-2 receptors mediate the presynaptic inhibition of norepinephrine release. Stimulation of beta-1 receptors by both epinephrine and norepinephrine induces an increase in heart rate and contractility, whereas epinephrine is more effective on beta-2 receptors, where it mediates vasodilatation, bronchodilatation and lypolysis, and on beta-3 receptors, inducing effects on lypolysis and thermogenesis [1, 2].

The effect of acetylcholine is associated with nicotinic receptors at autonomic ganglia level and with muscarinic receptors at postganglionic and effector cells. The muscarinic receptors are subgrouped as M1 (mainly present within the central nervous system [CNS] and in postganglionic vagal and sympathetic neurons), M2 (on smooth muscle cells, cardiomyocytes and endocrine cells), M3 and M4 (on smooth muscle cells and secretory gland cells), and M5 (in CNS cells). Other substances coexist with acetylcholine or norepinephrine and may act as co-transmitters, such as purines (adenosine, ATP), enkephalins, substance P, VIP, neuropeptide Y, and other molecules, and non-adrenergic, non-cholinergic neurons have been described [1, 2].

2.3.3 Afferent Stimuli

2.3.3.1 Baroreceptors

Two types of arterial baroreceptors have been characterized: a) carotid baroreceptors localized within the adventitial layer of the vascular wall of the coronary sinus (at the junction between each internal and external carotid artery) originating in myelinated fibers, which through the glossopharyngeal nerve reach the nucleus of tractus solitarius (NTS), and via the NTS the caudal ventrolateral medulla (VLM) and thereafter the rostral ventrolateral medulla (RVLM), projecting to the preganglionic sympathetic neurons; b) aortic baroreceptors located within the wall of the aortic arch, of the common carotid arteries and of the subclavian arteries, with amyelinated afferent fibers within the vagus nerve.

The role of the baroreceptors is the quick, beat-to-beat adjustment of arterial blood pressure around a mean value, achieved by evoking reflex changes in heart rate, stroke volume, cardiac inotropic state, systemic vascular resistance and venous capacitance.

These receptors respond, increasing their firing rate by as much as 7-fold, sensing changes in mean arterial pressure and in pulse pressure within the range 60-180 mmHg. Aortic baroreceptors recognize a higher threshold level of activation, being somehow less sensitive than the carotid receptors. Thus, aortic receptors are thought to play a more important role in the prevention of hypertension, while carotid receptors may prevent hypotension.

An increase in arterial pressure evokes, at every cardiac cycle, namely during the expiratory phase, a very fast (within less than one second) increment of the vagal drive to the heart, and an inhibition of the sympathetic discharge to vascular smooth cells [8]. On the other hand, a drop in arterial pressure is sensed and transformed by the barore-flex into withdrawal of vagal outflow and increase in adrenergic outflow, which persist independently of the respiratory phase, leading to increased heart rate and contractil-ity, and arterial resistances.

The maximum carotid sinus sensitivity occurs near the normal mean arterial pres-sure. This "set point" changes either transiently during physiological stimuli such as exercise (due to a change in the coupling of afferent nervous input to efferent nerve activity occurring within the central nervous system), or chronically such as during hypertension, heart failure, and other disease states (due to a local change in receptor response, characterized by a long-term change in mean pressure value, provoking an adaptive variation of the range of receptor response ("baroreceptor resetting") [9].

2.3.3.2 Venous, Cardiopulmonary and Renal Baroreceptors

Stretch receptors similar to aortic and carotid receptors are located within lung ves-sels, at the atrial junction with vene cavae or pulmonary veins and, to a lesser extent, with-in ventricles, coronary arteries and coronary sinus. They are able to modulate the blood volume (acting by inhibiting cortisol, ADH, and angiotensin-aldosterone secretion, and probably cardiac natriuretic peptide secretion) and to influence sympathetic outflow by decreasing it in response to low values of central venous pressure, and by increasing it in response to higher values [10].

A positive chronotropic reflex, stimulated by an increase in atrial pressure, and like-ly evoked by atrial receptors connected to myelinated vagal fibers, was described by Bainbridge in 1915, reproducible with rapid infusion of saline into the right atrium, and not inducing any effect on cardiac contractility or systemic vascular resistances. An increment in renal flow (by decreasing local vascular resistances), diuresis, with a decrease in plasma levels of vasopressin, cortisol and renin occurs in response to this stimulus, possibly elicited by natriuretic peptide secretion.

Atrial and ventricular receptors connected to amyelinated vagal fibers are spread within the cardiac walls, and respond to a greater degree of distension than receptors attached to myelinated nerves. They mediate bradycardia and a decrease in cardiac contractility (this mechanism being the basis of the "vaso-vagal response") [11].

Renal baroreceptors are excited by increases in renal arterial pressure, venous pres-sure or interstitial pressure [12].

Baroreceptor impulses from the carotid-aortic sinus regions and the kidney are important pathways involved in the neuro-endocrine control of ANP release. ANP release in response to volume expansion is mediated by afferent baroreceptor input to the anteroventral third ventricle region, which mediates the increased ANP release via activation of the hypothalamic ANP neuronal system [13].

2.3.3.3 Peripheral Central and Cardiac Chemoreceptors

Peripheral chemoreceptors are located within small "bodies", close to the carotid sinus-es (while others are located close to the aortic arch and the pulmonary artery), con-taining a vascular sinusoid network, contiguous to the receptors. The receptors respond to chemical stimuli, mainly hypoxia, evoking, via the glossopharyngeal nerve (and the vagus nerve, respectively) an increase in respiratory rate and depth. They possibly influence heart rate, though this effect might be masked by the respiratory response. If respiration is stopped, it is possible to observe that stimulated carotid chemoreceptors decrease, while aortic chemoreceptors increase heart rate [14].

The central chemoreceptors located on the ventral surface of the medulla respond mostly to hypercapnia and acidemia.

Atrial and (mainly left) ventricular chemoreceptors with vagal afferent innervation cause marked reflex bradycardia, vasodilatation and hypotension, in relation to the effect of various substances (both endogenous such as prostaglandin, serotonin, bradykinin, adenosine, and exogenous - coronary Bezold-Jarisch reflex after the administration of veratrum alkaloids). Whereas their physiological role is still unclear, they might be activated during tachycardia or myocardial ischemia. Other ventricular chemoreceptors or mechanoreceptors with both myelinated and unmyelinated neural afferent fibers discharge rhythmically during the cardiac cycle and induce tachycardia and vasoconstriction: some may be involved in cardiac pain perception.

Renal chemoreceptors are excited by renal ischemia, backflow of urine into the renal pelvis and pelvic perfusion with solutions of KCl. Injections of bradykinin and capsaicin also activate these receptors [12].

It is worthwhile noting that endogenous nNOS activity in the carotid body plays an important role in the activity of the carotid body chemoreceptors and peripheral chemoreflex function in experimental models [15].

2.3.3.4 Respiratory Mechanoreceptors

Several mechanoreceptors are located within the bronchial tree, which are sensitive to the cyclical tension by respiratory activity: some are responsible for the Hering-Breuer reflex, inducing a decrement in the firing rate of cardio-inhibitory neurons within the brainstem, thus increasing heart rate during inspiration and contributing to respiratory sinus arrhythmia.

2.3.3.5 Ergoreceptors

Isometric exercise and the rhythmic contraction of skeletal muscles induce an increase in heart rate, arterial blood pressure and tidal respiratory volume, opposing the decrease in muscle perfusion due to the mechanical compression.

This is due to a peripheral neural drive originating in the skeletal muscle that likewise activates brainstem cardiovascular control areas during physical activity. During exercise, activation of this reflex is mediated by stimulation of group III (predominantly mechanically sensitive Aδ fibers) and IV (predominantly metabolically sensitive C fibers) primary afferent neurons, which augment blood pressure and minute ventilation primarily via increase in sympathetic nerve activity and reduction in parasympathetic nerve activity. There is a degree of polymorphism in these afferents since some group III fibers respond to metabolic changes and a minority of group IV fibers respond to mechanical distortion.

These afferents project to the dorsal horn of the spinal cord, specifically to laminate I, II, V and X and following the spinal pathway reach the brainstem in the cuneate nucleus, NTS and the lateral reticular nucleus. These reflexes are proportional to the muscle mass, and initiated by muscle metabolism products, which excite muscle chemoreceptors and are mediated by changes in the sympathetic outflow to the vessels. These effects on blood pressure are not buffered by either arterial or cardiopulmonary mechanoreceptors, while arterial baroreceptors maintain their ability to modulate the blood pressure around the increased level [16].

Chemoceptive stimuli favor the cardiorespiratory coupling with muscle metabolic demand during dynamic exercise.

2.3.3.6 Other Reflexes
Relevant vasomotor, chronotropic, and respiration modulator reflexes are elicited by mostly amyelinated fibers, which reach the brainstem through the vagus, cranial pelvic, splanchnic and other autonomic nerves, while some fibers arising from skin and vessels are located within somatic nerves. Their stimulus is not associated with a sensory perception; substance P and glutamate have been indicated among their neurotransmitters. Vestibular stimuli during upright position evoke a sympatho-mediated vasoconstriction [17].

2.3.3.7 Cardiorespiratory Coupling
Respiration is supported by the automatic generation of a rhythm within the brainstem, probably in a region of the RVLM, the "preBoetzinger complex", where the activity of specialized pacemaker neurons controls periodic diaphragmatic, chest and abdominal respiratory muscles. These neural centers are modulated by both central inputs and peripheral feedback and are connected with medullary autonomic centers in order to couple respiration with cardiac and vasomotor activity. A role for NAD(P)H oxidase-derived reactive oxygen species as mediators of angiotensin II via AT1 receptors signaling in the modulation of sympathetic activity and arterial baroreflex function has been claimed in experimental heart failure at the RVLM level [18].

2.3.4 Efferent Neural Connections

2.3.4.1 Cardiac Connections
The efferent cardiac innervation is mediated by mixed sympatho-vagal nerves, which join via the aorta, pulmonary artery and vene cavae the cardiac muscle, the specific system and the coronary arteries. The preganglionic sympathetic fibers through the spinal cord form synapses with postganglionic neurons within the sympathetic chain, then innervating atria, ventricles, sinoatrial and atrioventricular nodes.

Cardiac parasympathetic control is mediated by cholinergic fibers, which connect with postganglionic neurons within cardiac ganglia innervating sinoatrial and atrioventricular nodes, and, to a lesser extent, cardiomyocytes, decreasing the spontaneous sinoatrial depolarization rate, inducing bradycardia and inhibiting the conduction rate at the atrial and atrioventricular node level.

2.3.4.2 Connections with Peripheral Circulation
The efferent connections responsible for vasomotor tone consist of sympathetic vasoconstrictive preganglionic fibers originating from neurons located within intermediolateral and medial columns of the spinal cord (through the first thoracic segment to the second-third lumbar segment). Neurons with cardiac chronotropic and inotropic influence are located within the upper thoracic segments (T1-T4) of the spinal cord [19]. The preganglionic fibers leave the spinal cord with the spinal nerves from the ven-

tral roots, forming the white rami communicantes, and have synapses with postganglionic neurons within the 22 pairs of sympathetic ganglia of the paravertebral chain, and within the intermediate ganglia (stellate, middle and superior dorsal ganglia). The axons of postganglionic neurons leave the paravertebral chain through the gray rami communicantes and through the peripheral nerves end at the small arterial and arteriolar level; fewer end at the precapillary level, and there are no endings at the capillary level. Veins and venulae have a small number of sympathetic endings, compared to precapillary sphincters. The vasoconstrictor fibers to the arms and limbs are located within somatic nerves, those to the head and neck within cervical and cranial nerves.

These fibers control either the resistance or the capacitance vessels, thus varying venous return to the heart by acting on the venulae within the superficial and deep venous system, as well as within the splanchnic system (e.g. in response to reflex sympathetic stimuli such as cold or emotion). The parasympathetic innervation may influence peripheral vascular resistances by inhibiting norepinephrine release from the postganglionic fibers, via M1 muscarinic receptors at the presynaptic level.

2.3.4.3 Vasodilator Fibers
Cholinergic sympathetic fibers originating from the thoracic-lumbar level innervate the skeletal muscles and are activated by the hypothalamus and motor cortex, while parasympathetic vasodilator fibers innervate cerebral vessels, the tongue, the salivary glands, external genitalia and rectum. The fibers are not tonically active, neither are they controlled by baro- and chemoreflexes.

2.3.4.4 Control of Arteriolar Tone:
Interaction Between Autonomic, Endocrine and Paracrine Actions
Small arterioles are the major determinants of systemic vascular resistances. Release of norepinephrine by sympathetic endings contributes to the resting tone, and with increased sympathetic outflow, further increase tone. Circulating hormones such as ANP, aldosterone, angiotensin II, and vasopressin (ADH) also act on the arterial smooth muscle and influence their tone. Paracrine molecules secreted by the endothelial cells (in response to shear stress, to acetylcholine released by parasympathetic nerves, which also inhibit at the presynaptic level the release of norepinephrine by adrenergic endings), such as endothelins, nitric oxide (NO), prostaglandins, and CNP act on the adjacent smooth muscle to modulate its tone. The angiotensin-converting enzyme on the surface of the endothelial cell is also able to convert circulating AI to AII.

2.3.5 Spinal Cord

The preganglionic sympathetic neurons may sometimes (e.g. after an inferior cervical section) exhibit spontaneous activity, which, after a transient subacute period characterized by vasodilatation and hypotension, permits constant pressure values to be maintained, independently of reflex stimuli of central nervous modulation. Thermal or nociceptive skin stimuli may induce splanchnic vasoconstriction, whereas visceral stimuli may induce significant changes in arterial pressure (skin vasoconstriction after a deep breath or posture changes; bladder filling with endovesical pressure increase is accompanied in spinal patients by increase in arterial pressure, sweating and vasoconstriction).

Axonal reflexes may take place in response to thermal or traumatic stimuli to the skin, inducing a vasodilator response, which increases local perfusion, contributing to defense and repair processes [20].

2.3.6 Medullary Centers

The NTS is the main site of integration of afferent impulses from peripheral baro-, chemo- and cardiopulmonary receptors within the CNS [10]. Its importance is evident since it is connected with various main stem regions (nucleus ambiguous and RVLM), mainly with two respiratory neuronal groups, the dorsal one close to the NTS and the ventral one close to the nucleus ambiguous, which innervate the spinal motor neurons of frenicus (cervical and intercostal thoracic nerves), with the pons (in particular nuclei for cardiorespiratory control), with spinal cord and anterior brain.

Both the nucleus ambiguous and the dorsal vagal motor nucleus are innervated by NTS: this permits a rapid activation of vagi and simultaneously a reduction in sympathetic outflow to the heart vessels and adrenal medulla. This neural network generates a baseline activity pattern towards the spinal cord, influenced by excitatory and inhibitory afferent inputs, by supramedullary influences and by medullary respiratory centers.

This activity is inherent, persisting after the elimination of all afferent neural inputs. Supramedullary centers are fundamental in modulating medullary activity dynamics, without dominating them: medullary brainstem section does not alter the arterial pressure levels.

2.3.6.1 Sympathetic Centers

The modulation of intrinsic heart activity and of vasomotor tone is ensured by the activity of the preganglionic autonomic motor neurons.

The preganglionic sympathetic neurons within the intermediate cell column are innervated by some brainstem neuronal groups, namely neurons in the RVLM [21, 22], raphe (which exert a serotonin-mediated inhibitory and excitatory influence), pontine reticular formation, NTS, reticulospinal neurons, and from the medial frontal cortex.

The RVLM neurons have an intrinsic "pacemaker" activity [23], which is related to cardiac activity and the level of arterial pressure. This medullary center is the "vasomotor center" [23], characterized by intrinsic rhythmicities, which are also present at the hypothalamic level and within the sympathetic efferent outflow, even in the absence of the baroceptive stimulus [22].

The activity of the RVLM neurons is markedly influenced by inhibitory baroceptive and excitatory chemoceptive inputs, increasing during inspiration (in response to pulmonary stretch afferent inputs) and is influenced by cortical and subcortical afferents [23]. The activity pattern of the respiratory neurons is recognizable at RVML neuron level, and in the sympathetic and parasympathetic preganglionic neuronal activity, with a postinspiratory depressed activity, variable during the expiratory phase, so demonstrating the high level of integration of the cardiovascular and respiratory activity.

Furthermore, the activity of the RVLM neurons is augmented by central or peripheral inputs such as during pain, wakefulness, emotional stress, and physical exercise.

Pre- and postganglionic sympathetic nerve activity shows respiratory and cardiac rhythms with a different pattern, which is related to the physiological condition. The respiratory rhythm of the sympathetic efferent outflow is determined by a brainstem source, by pulmonary stretching reflex stimuli, and by baroreflex stimuli sensing changes in arterial pressure determined by respiration.

The vasoconstrictive efferent traffic to the muscle vascular bed is inhibited by baroreflex stimuli and excited by chemoceptive and cutaneous nociceptive stimuli, by systemic hypoxia and hypercapnia, recognizing a respiratory fluctuation. The vasoconstrictive efferent traffic to the skin vascular bed is less influenced by baroreflex stimuli, variously modulated by chemoceptive stimuli and always inhibited by cutaneous nociceptive stimuli.

Postganglionic sympathetic fibers innervate the whole heart, including the pacemaker tissues and the ventricular myocardium. Their stimulation induces an increase in heart rate (mostly by the right sympathetic nerves), cardiac contractility (mostly by the left sympathetic nerves), and atrioventricular conduction rate. The delay in response to the sympathetic system is longer with respect to the response to parasympathetic one: 5 seconds, with a maximum after 30 seconds [24].

2.3.6.2 Parasympathetic Centers
The chronotropic regulation is mainly associated with vagal control [10], which affects the intrinsic heart rate of 100-120 beats per minute, determined by spontaneous depolarization of the sinoatrial node pacemaker cells, resulting in lower values.

The stimulation of both vagi decreases the heart rate (though the right vagus nerve seems more powerful) [25], with a shorter delay (400 milliseconds) [26], and slightly slower recovery (5 seconds) to an extent that is proportional to the frequency of stimulation, with a hyperbolic relationship [27].

The heart rate is beat-to-beat determined, as the result of the modulation of the intrinsic sinus node rhythm by sympatho-vagal innervation, which is, on its own, modulated by the complex integration of peripheral and central inputs.

The preganglionic vagal innervation originates from four distinct medullary regions: the dorsal motor nucleus, an intermediate zone, the nucleus ambiguous, and the ventrolateral section of the nucleus ambiguous, which receive afferent input from several brain regions, particularly from the NTS [6], which has a fundamental role in processing all kinds of reflex inputs from heart vessels and lungs [28]. Destruction of the NTS leads acutely to hypertension and pulmonary edema, and chronically to sustained hypertension [29]. The NTS is connected both with the lower brainstem (including the nucleus ambiguous and RVLM), with pontine nuclei implicated in cardiorespiratory control, and with the forebrain. Finally, the ascending NTS connections mediate baroreceptor and other reflexes and regulate the neuro-endocrine function [30].

The parasympathetic centers are close to the rostral RVLM where the preganglionic sympathetic neurons are, so indicating the high level of interconnection between the two branches of the ANS.

The chronotropic influence is mediated by B fiber neurons, mostly located within the nucleus ambiguous, whose activity is a major determinant of heart rate and cardiac output. These neurons have a firing rate synchronous with the cardiac cycle and with the systolic increase in arterial pressure, as the result of a phasic excitatory afferent input from arterial baroreceptors, followed by a diastolic silence.

The cervical vagal efferent activity and the vagal cardiac rami have an expiratory (particularly postinspiratory) pattern with an aspiratory silence. This originates the sinus respiratory arrhythmia, which is characterized by an aspiratory increase in cardiac output simultaneous to pulmonary distension. All stimuli enhancing inspiration increase heart rate, whereas peripheral or central stimuli inhibiting ventilation, or prolonging expiration induce bradycardia.

During the expiratory phase, systemic and regional (e.g. laryngeal) baro- and chemoceptive stimuli, processed at the NTS level, facilitate bradycardia mediated by vagi.

2.3.7 Supramedullary Control

2.3.7.1 Centrally Evoked Cardiorespiratory Responses

The central nervous system is able to modulate the cardiovascular and respiratory activity, supporting the behavioral response in relation to different degrees of physical activity and consciousness (from sleep to active wakefulness), and in response to emotional stimuli, or as a part of the defense reaction (characterized by concomitant increase in heart rate, in cardiac output and in arterial blood pressure due to a widespread - cutaneous, renal and mesenteric - vasoconstriction, with the exception of the skeletal muscle vascular bed, which is enhanced by the secretion of catecholamines from the adrenal gland).

The central nucleus of the amygdala [31] and the perifornical and paraventricular areas of the hypothalamus play a fundamental role in the definition of the autonomic cardiovascular and respiratory response patterns, associated with the alert reaction.

The defense reaction is associated with a central blockade of baroreceptors through a GABAergic mechanism and a facilitation of the chemoceptive feedback at the NTS level [32]. Furthermore, the vagal cardiac efferent outflow is inhibited as a consequence of an increased respiratory activity, because of an excitatory influence upon the inspiratory neurons.

This pattern of response may be obtained by stimulation in the experimental model of the central nucleus of amygdala [28], which influences different areas within the brainstem, such as the NTS, the vagal dorsal nucleus, the nucleus ambiguous, and the rostral RVLM. The activation of rostral hypothalamic regions has a vasodilator and vagomimetic effect; moreover, it supports, together with the preoptical area, the control of body temperature, through the modulation of vasoconstrictor fibers to the skin vasculature.

2.3.7.2 Cerebral Cortex

The stimulation of the prefrontal and posterior preorbital motor cortex results in a marked increase in arterial pressure associated with vasoconstriction of skin, splanchnic and kidney vasculature, cholinergic vasodilatation of skeletal muscles, increase in heart rate and cardiac output, also with an influence on respiratory activity. These centers are thought to govern the pressor response to pain, anxiety, and exercise, through the modulation of hypothalamic and brainstem areas.

2.4 The Integrated Neuro-Hormonal Response: Short- and Long-Term Response

Control of blood pressure and cardiac output is dependent on the beat-to-beat balance between the sympathetic and vagal arms of the ANS, modulated by high-pressure arterial and low-pressure venous baroreceptors. This interaction maintains the circulatory homeostasis in response to phasic stimuli, via vagal withdrawal and sympathetic predominance, e.g. while rising from sitting or supine to a standing position, or during physical exercise: the net effect is an increase in heart rate and contractility, as well as in arteriolar tone, which supports arterial pressure and cardiac output.

Slower pressor responses are due to the renal secretion of renin, a proteolytic enzyme, which acts on angiotensinogen, of hepatic origin, resulting in production of the powerful vasoconstrictor angiotensin II, which further activates the adrenal secretion of aldosterone. Moreover, sympathetic activation leads to vasopressin (ADH) release from the neurohypophysis. All these vasoconstrictor molecules have a sodium/water retentive effect, which tends to increase the intravascular volume.

2.5 Heart Physiology: What is New?

The heart is a regulatory organ, too: cardiomyocytes, fibroblasts and endothelial cells of the coronary circulation are able to produce and secrete several substances with complex regulatory auto-, para-, and endocrine biological effects, part of the neurohormonal network regulating homeostasis of the cardiovascular system, as well as other vital physiological functions.

Cardiac endocrine function, namely the secretion of cardiac natriuretic peptides, is essential to protect the integrity of the "milieu interieur", regulating blood volume, cardiac and renal function, growth and repair tissue processes, neuronal activities within the brain, and immune-inflammatory responses.

References

1. Opie LH (1998) Heart physiology, from cell to circulation, 3rd edn., Lippincott Williams & Wilkins, Philadelphia
2. Katz AM (2001) Physiology of the heart, 3rd edn. Lippincott Williams & Wilkins, Philadelphia
3. Appenzeller O (1997) Neurogenic control of the circulation, In: Appenzeller O, Oribe E (eds) The autonomic nervous system. Elsevier, Amsterdam, pp 65-183
4. Yang Z, Luescher TF (2002) Vascular endothelium. In: Lanzer P, Topol EJ (eds) Panvascular medicine. Springer Verlag, Berlin, Heidelberg, pp 190-204
5. Klein I, Ojamaa K (2001) Thyroid hormone and the cardiovascular system. N Engl J Med 15:501-509
6. Spyer KM (1994) Central nervous mechanism contributing to cardiovascular control. J Physiol 474:1-19
7. Langley JN (1898) On the union of cranial autonomic (visceral) fibres with the nerve cells of the superior cervical ganglion. J Physiol (London) 23:240-270
8. Eckberg DL (1978) Temporal response patterns of the human sinus node to brief carotid baroreceptors stimuli. J Physiol 258:769-782
9. Sleight P, Robinson JL, Brooks DE, Rees PM (1975) Carotid baroreceptor re-setting in the hypertensive dog. Clin Sci 2(suppl):261-263
10. Hainsworth R (1991) Reflexes from the heart. Physiol Rev 71:617-658
11. Van Lieshout JJ, Wieling W, Karemaker JM, Eckberg DW (1991) The vasovagal response. Clin Sci 81:575-586
12. Moss NG (1989) Electrophysiological characteristics of renal sensory receptors and afferent renal nerves. Miner Electrolyte Metab 15:59-65
13. Antunes-Rodrigues J, Machado BH, Andrade HA et al (1992) Carotid-aortic and renal barore-

ceptors mediate the atrial natriuretic peptide release induced by blood volume expansion. Proc Natl Acad Sci USA 89:6828-6831

14. Karim F, Hainsworth R, Sofola OA, Wood LM (1980) Responses of the heart to stimulation of aortic body chemoreceptors in dogs. Circ Res 46:77-83

15. Li YL, Li YF, Liu D et al (2005) Gene transfer of neuronal nitric oxide synthase to carotid body reverses enhanced chemoreceptor function in heart failure rabbits. Circ Res 5:260-267

16. Shepherd JT, Mancia G (1986) Reflex control of the human cardiovascular system. Rev Physiol Biochem Exp Pharmacol 105:1-99

17. Yates BJ (1992) Vestibular influences on the sympathetic nervous system. Brain Res Rev 17:51-59

18. Gao L, Wang W, Li YL et al (2005) Sympathoexcitation by central ANG II: roles for AT1 receptor upregulation and NAD(P)H oxidase in RVLM. Am J Physiol Heart Circ Physiol 288:H2271-2279

19. Cabot JB (1990) Sympathetic preganglionic neurones: cytoarchitecture, ultrastructure and biophysical properties. In: Loewy AD, Spyer KM (eds) Central regulation of autonomic functions. Oxford University Press, New York, pp 44-67

20. Henriksen O (1977) Local sympathetic reflex mechanism in regulation of blood flow in human subcutaneous tissue. Acta Physiol Scand 450(Suppl):1-48

21. Milner TA, Morrison SF, Abate C, Reis DJ (1988) Phenylethanolamine N-metiltransferase containing terminals synapse directly on sympathetic preganglionic neurones in the rat. Brain Res 448:205-222

22. Gebber GL (1990) Central determinants of sympathetic nerve discharge. In: Loewy AD, Spyer KM (eds) Central regulation of autonomic functions. Oxford University Press, New York, pp 126-144

23. Guyenet PS (1990) Role of the ventral medulla oblongata in blood pressure regulation. In: Loewy D, Spyer KM (eds) Central regulation of autonomic functions. Oxford University Press, New York, pp 145-160

24. Furnival CM, Linden RJ, Snow HM (1973) Chronotropic and inotropic effects on the dog heart of stimulating the efferent cardiac sympathetic nerves. J Physiol 230:137-153

25. Levy MN, Martin PJ (1979) Neural control of the heart. In: Berne RM (ed) Handbook of physiology. American Physiological Society, Bethesda, pp 581-620

26. Pickering TG, Davies JD (1973) Estimation of the conduction time of the baroreceptor-cardiac reflex in man. Cardiovasc Res 7:213-219

27. Rosenblueth A, Simeone FA (1934) The interrelations of vagal and accelerator effects on the cardiac rate. Am J Physiol 110:42-55

28. Jordan D, Spyer KM (1986) Brainstem integration of cardiovascular and pulmonary afferent activity. Progr Brain Res 67:295-314

29. Spyer KM (1981) Neural organisation and control of the baroreceptor reflex. Rev Physiol Biochem Exp Pharmacol 88:23-124

30. Harris MC, Loewy AD (1990) Neural regulation of vasopressin-containing hypothalamic neurones and the role of vasopressin in cardiovascular function. In: Loewy AD, Spyer KM (eds) Central regulation of autonomic functions. Oxford University Press, New York, pp 224-246

31. Jordan D (1990) Autonomic changes in affective behaviour. In: Loewy AD, Spyer KM (eds) Central regulation of autonomic functions. Oxford University Press, New York, pp 349-366

32. Mifflin SW, Spyer KM, Withington-Wray DJ (1988) Baroreceptor inputs to the nucleus tractus solitarius in the cat: modulation of the hypothalamus. J Physiol 399:369-387

Chapter 3

The Cardiac Natriuretic Hormone System

Aldo Clerico • Simona Vittorini

The aim of this Chapter is to summarize the most recent issues on the production, secretion, biological activity and metabolism of CNH. The hypotheisis that natriuretic peptides constitute a family sharing endocrine, paracrine and autocrine actions and neurotransmitter and immunomodulator functions closely related to the other regulatory systems (nervous, endocrine and immunological) in a biological hierarchical network will be discussed with particular emphasis. Finally, such as an example to support this hypothesis, the integrated action of CNH system during pregnancy and fetal life as well as in the regulation of vascuar system wil be illustrated in detail.

3.1 Chemical Structure and Gene Evolution of Cardiac Natriuretic Hormones

All natriuretic peptides share a similar structural conformation, characterized by a peptide ring with a cysteine bridge (Fig. 3.1). This ring is well preserved throughout the phylogenetic evolution, since it constitutes the portion of the peptide hormone that binds to its specific receptor (Fig. 3.2). Conversely, the two terminal amino acid chains (i.e., NH_2- and COOH-terminus) show a high degree of variability among the natriuretic peptides, in terms of both length and amino acidic composition [1].

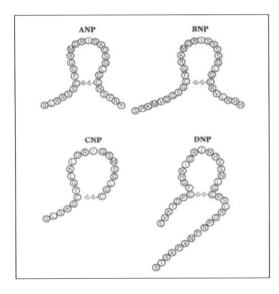

Fig. 3.1. Peptide chain of natriuretic peptide hormones ANP, BNP, CNP and DNP. The CNH share the same structure characterized by a cysteine bridge

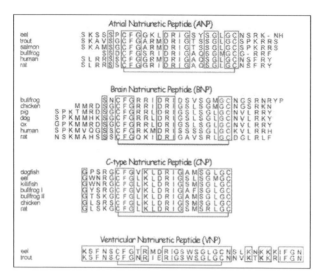

Fig. 3.2. Amino acid sequences of ANP, BNP, CNP and VNP in vertebrates. The identical amino acid residues in the same group are shaded. The C-terminus of eel ANP is amidated. The intramolecular ring is connected with a line (modified from Takei [1])

Natriuretic hormone-like peptides seem to be present in the plant kingdom as well as in the animal kingdom [1-3]; thus indicating that this hormonal system, which has been shown to regulate solute transport in vertebrates, has evolved early in evolution [1-6].

ANP-, BNP- and CNP-like peptides have been identified in tetrapods, ranging from amphibians to mammals [1]. Natriuretic peptides also exist in fish as a family of structurally related iso-hormones, including ANP, CNP and ventricular natriuretic peptide (VNP) (Fig. 3.2) [1]. A recent study has indicated that BNP is also present in some fish [6]. In vertebrates, ANP, BNP and VNP are endocrine hormones secreted from the heart, while CNP is principally a paracrine factor in the brain and periphery. In elasmobranches, only CNP is present in the heart and brain, and it functions as a circulating hormone as well as a paracrine factor [1]. Immunoreactive ANP-like peptide has also been detected in the unicellular *Paramecium* and in various species of plants [1].

CNP is the most structurally conserved member of the natriuretic peptide family (Fig. 3.3) [1,4]. The ANP sequence is conserved in mammals; however, the identity across different groups (e.g. between mammals and frogs) is rather low (about 50%) (Fig. 3.4). BNP is highly variable even in mammalian species (Fig. 3.5) [1, 4].

It is noteworthy that the complete pro-hormone sequences of ANP (proANP) and CNP (proCNP) are more conserved within mammals, but they are highly variable across different classes of vertebrates, except at the C-terminal mature ANP and CNP sequences. Thus, the N-terminal part of pro-hormones ANP (NT-proANP) and CNP may not have common biological function throughout vertebrate species [1]. The NT-proBNP is not well conserved even in mammals, as observed for BNP as well [1].

Studies in fish, based on nucleotide and amino acid sequence similarity, suggest that the natriuretic peptide family of iso-hormones may have evolved from a neuromodulatory CNP-like brain peptide (Fig. 3.6) [4]. However, caution should be exercised in identification and comparison of vertebrate hormones from phylogenetically distant organisms [1].

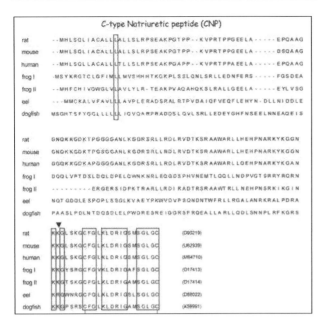

Fig. 3.3. Amino acid sequences of C-type natriuretic peptide precursors in selected species of mammals and in non-mammalian vertebrates. The C-terminal mature CNP is cleaved at the arrowhead. The identical amino acid residues within CNP precursors are shadowed.
The intramolecular ring is connected with a line.
The accession number to each molecule is noted in the figure (modified from Takei [1])

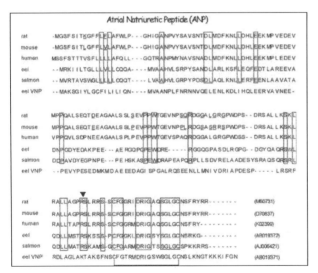

Fig. 3.4. Amino acid sequences of ANP precursors in selected species of mammals and in teleost fish. The sequence of eel ventricular natriuretic peptide VNP precursor is also given. The C-terminal mature ANP is cleaved at the position of the arrowhead. The identical amino acid residues within ANP precursors are shadowed. The intramolecular ring is connected with a line. The N-terminal prosegments are similar in three species of mammals, but several amino acid substitutions occur even between rat and mouse, as marked with an underline. The identity of prosegments between eel and salmon is 40.6%. No apparent homology was observed in the prosegments of teleost fish and mammals. The accession number to each molecule is noted in the figure (modified from Takei [1])

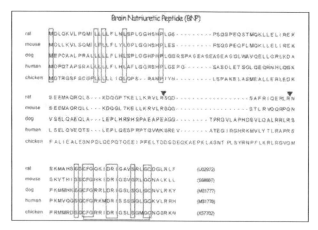

Fig. 3.5. Amino acid sequences of BNP precursors in selected species of mammals and chicken. The C-terminal mature BNP is cleaved at the right arrowhead except in rat and mouse BNP where the cleavage occurs at the left arrowhead. The identical amino acid residues within BNP precursors are shadowed. The intramolecular ring is connected with a line. Compared with ANP and CNP (Figs. 3.2 and 3.3), not only the N-terminal prosegments but also the C-terminal mature BNP sequence is highly variable even in mammals. The accession number to each molecule is noted in the figure (modified from Takei [1])

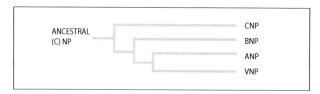

Fig. 3.6. Proposed evolutionary derivation of the vertebrate natriuretic peptide family from an ancestral CNP-like peptide (modified from Loretz and Pollina [4])

3.2 Genes Encoding for Cardiac Natriuretic Hormones

The ANP and BNP coding genes, named NPPA and NPPB, are tightly linked on human chromosome 1 and mouse chromosome 4 [7, 8]. Arden et al. [7] confirmed the assignment to the 1 p 36 region by FISH and Southern blot analysis. Moreover, pulsed-field gel electrophoresis placed NPPA and NPPB within 50 kb of each other.

The Gene Cards Data Base reports that NPPA maps on 1p36.2 and that it is less than 10 kb more telomeric than the BNP coding gene. NPPA spans 2,075 bp and constitutes three exons and two introns (Fig. 3.7). The splicing produces an mRNA of 840 bp that is translated in the ANP precursor of 153 amino acids.

NPPB is also organized in three exons and two introns that span 1,466 bp. The mRNA is 691 bp and the relative primary product is a peptide of 134 amino acids (Fig. 3.7).

The NPPA and NPPB genes are expressed in almost all tissues but, for both, the heart is the organ in which the expression is higher (Figs. 3.8 and 3.9).

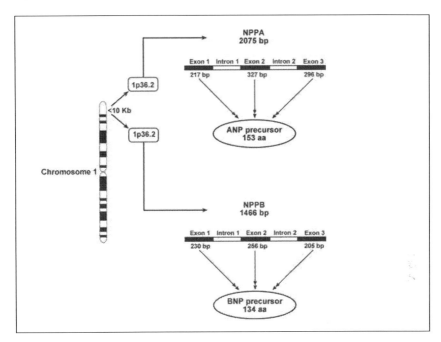

Fig. 3.7. Structure of ANP and BNP genes

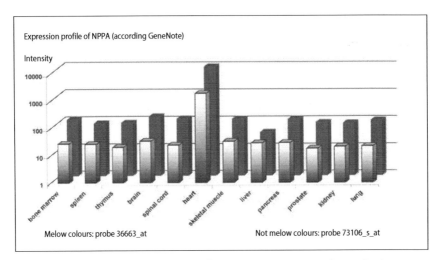

Fig. 3.8. Expression of ANP gene (NPPA) in different human tissues according to the data reported by GeneNote (<*http://genecards.weizmann.ac.il/cgi-bin/genenote/home_page.pl*>*http://genecards.weizmann.ac.il/cgi-bin/genenote/home_page.pl*)

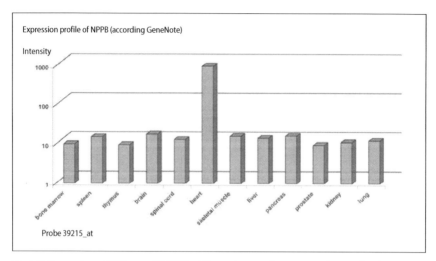

Expression profile of NPPB (according GeneNote)

Probe 39215_at

Fig. 3.9. Expression of BNP gene (NPPB) in different human tissues according to the data reported by GeneNote (*<http://genecards.weizmann.ac.il/cgi-bin/genenote/home_page.pl>http://genecards.weizmann.ac.il/cgi-bin/genenote/home_page.pl*)

On the basis of PCR-analyzed microsatellite length polymorphisms among recombinant inbred strains of mice, Ogawa et al. [10] found that the CNP gene is located on mouse chromosome 1 (Fig. 3.10). Using somatic hybrid cell methodology, the human CNP gene was assigned to chromosome 2 [10]. Extrapolating from studies of homology of synteny, they suggested that the gene endocing CNP may lie in the 2q24-qter region. This gene constitutes 824 bp, organized in two exons separated by an intron, and its mRNA (of 381 bp) gives a C natriuretic peptide precursor of 126 amino acids (Fig. 3.10).

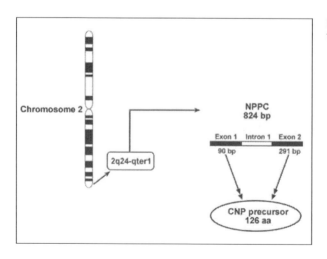

Fig. 3.10. Structure of the human CNP gene

The natriuretic peptide genes encode for the precursor sequences of these hormones, named pre-pro-hormones, which are then split into pro-hormones by proteolytic cleavage of an N-terminal hydrophobic signal peptide. This cleavage occurs cotranslationally during protein synthesis in the rough endoplasmic reticulum, before the synthesis of the C-terminal part of the pro-hormone sequence is completed [11-13].

The pro-hormone of ANP is stored as a 126-amino acid peptide, $proANP_{1-126}$ (also called γANP), which is produced by cleavage of the signal peptide (Fig. 3.11). When appropriate signals for hormone release are given, $proANP_{1-126}$ is further split into an NH_2-terminal fragment, $proANP_{1-98}$ (actually called NT-proANP) and the COOH-terminal peptide ANP_{99-126} (ANP), which is generally considered to be the biologically active hormone [11-13].

The human BNP gene encodes for a preproBNP molecule of 134 amino acid residues with a signal peptide of 26 amino acids (Fig. 3.12). BNP is produced from a pro-hormone molecule of 108 amino acids, the $proBNP_{1-108}$, usually indicated as proBNP. Before secretion, proBNP is split by proteolytic enzymes into two peptides: the $proBNP_{1-76}$ (NH_2-terminal peptide fragment, usually indicated as NT-proBNP), which is biologically inactive, and the $proBNP_{77-108}$ (COOH-terminal peptide fragment), which is the active hormone (BNP) [14].

It is important to note that the preproBNP precursor is not detectable, and its existence is only a theoretical concept, deduced from the BNP cDNA sequence of the human (or other mammalian) gene [14]. On the other hand, intact proBNP, NT-proBNP, and BNP can be identified in plasma by chromatography and immunoassay [14-17]. Moreover, ANP and BNP can be produced and co-stored in the same granule in different stages of peptide maturation [11-13].

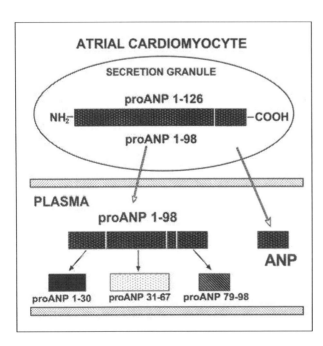

Fig. 3.11. Production and secretion of ANP from atrial cardiomyocytes

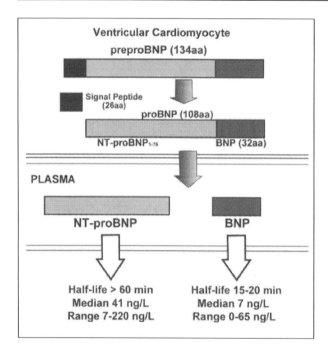

Fig. 3.12. Production and secretion of BNP from ventricular cardiomyocytes

3.3 Regulation of Production/Secretion of ANP and BNP in Cardiac Tissue

Atrial natriuretic peptide and BNP are synthesized and secreted mainly by cardiomyocytes. However, it is generally thought that ANP is preferentially produced in the atria, while BNP is produced in the ventricles, particularly in patients with chronic cardiac diseases. Synthesis and secretion of the two different peptides may be differently regulated in atrial and ventricular myocytes, and, probably, even at different stages of life (neonatal or adult life) [12-14, 18-23]. Furthermore, there could be some differences in regulation of expression of CNH genes among mammalian species; for example, between rat and human in *cis*-acting regulatory elements responsible for BNP promoters [22]. These findings suggest some caution in the use of study results performed in experimental animals to interpret specific pathophysiological conditions in humans. Unfortunately, our present knowledge on regulation of CNH gene expression derives in great part from experimental studies in rodents [18-23].

Some recent data suggest that not only cardiomyocytes, but also fibroblasts may produce CNH in human heart [24]; however, the clinical relevance of this finding has not been ascertained. According to studies performed in experimental animals, it has also been proposed that the endocrine response of the heart to pressure or volume load varies depending on whether the stimulus is acute, subacute, or chronic [12, 13, 18, 22].

Atrial cardiomyocytes store pro-hormones (proANP and proBNP) in secretory granules, and split them into ANP and BNP before secretion. ANP and BNP are produced and stored in different stages of peptide maturation even though they are co-stored in the same granule. It was suggested that the prevalent peptide form in the atrial granules is unprocessed proANP, whereas BNP is mainly stored in atrial granules as the processed and mature form of the active peptide hormone [12, 13, 18].

Peptide hormones are secreted via several pathways including regulated secretion, constitutive secretion and constitutive-like secretion. Regulated secretion occurs upon stimulation by agonists whereby the hormone packaged is released from the storage granules, thus allowing endocrine cells to secrete hormones at a rate that exceeds its biosynthesis [13]. The constitutive-like pathway is independent from both regulated and constitutive secretion and is insensitive to cycloheximide treatment [13]. The constitutive pathway involves the passive diffusion of hormone in the absence of stimuli. The presence of clathrin-coated vesicles in the atrial cardiocytes is indicative of the existence of this constitutive pathway [13].

CNH (especially ANP) should be predominantly secreted throughout a regulated pathway [12, 13, 18]. There is also the possibility that a small amount of CNH is released via a constitutive pathway involving passive diffusion of secretory products [12, 13, 18]. Indeed, protein synthesis inhibition by cycloheximide significantly, though partially, decreases ANP secretion; this suggests that basal ANP secretion is to a degree, dependent on newly synthesized hormone [13]. However, a component of basal secretion appears to depend upon stored hormone. Some studies have demonstrated that 60% of the newly synthesized ANP is intended for storage, whereas the remaining 40% is secreted under unstimulated conditions [13].

It is likely that circulating CNH (especially ANP) mostly derives from atria in healthy subjects [12-14, 18]. An acute atrial stretch may result in an immediate, sharp increase in the release rate of ANP at the expense of a rapidly depleting pool of newly synthesized hormone. The BNP pool that is utilized in response to stretch remains to be determined but in terms of peptide release, the ratio of ANP/BNP released is roughly the same as found in tissue storage, i.e., the response is in keeping with the lesser proportion of BNP present in mature atrial granules [18]. The response of the CNH system to stretch may not be strictly reflected *in vivo* by an increase in plasma levels of ANP and BNP, probably because the amount of peptide released is masked by dilutional effects and different clearance rates of the two peptide hormones.

The BNP gene is expressed in both atrial and ventricular myocytes of normal and diseased heart [12-14, 18]. Ventricular myocytes in the normal heart of adult mammals do not usually show any evident secretory granules on electron microscopy [13, 14]. However, some authors have identified secretory granules, similar to the atrial ones, in samples of ventricular myocardium collected during surgery or in endocardial biopsies studied by electron microscopy and immunohistocytochemistry in patients with cardiac disease [14, 25, 26]. These studies suggest that normal ventricular myocardium may produce only a limited amount of BNP in response to an acute and appropriate stimulation, probably via a constitutive secretory pathway, while the amount of hormone produced and secreted after chronic stimulation could be greatly increased via an upregulated secretory pathway. However, further studies are necessary in order to confirm the presence of secretory granules in human ventricular cardiomyocytes and in particular to evaluate their peptide content and pathophysiological relevance.

BNP mRNA levels increase predominantly by upregulated gene transcription and to a lesser degree, by post-transcriptional mechanisms [22]. BNP transcription can increase with the activation of numerous positive *cis*-acting regulating elements or the inhibition of negative *cis*-acting elements on the 5'-flanking region on the BNP promoter, as recently reviewed in detail [18, 22]. The type of the element depends on whether the stimulus is a mechanical or a neuro-humoral agonist [22, 23]. Due to their ability to cooperate with a diverse group of transcription factors and to react to a variety of different stimuli, some proteins of the GATA family (especially GATA-4 and GATA-6) emerge as crucial factors in regulating basal expression and inducible ANP and BNP promoter activity [18, 23]. The transcription factors of the GATA family (from GATA-1 to GATA-6) are zinc-finger proteins that bind to the consensus sequence (A/T)GATA(A/G) via a DNA-binding domain containing two zinc fingers to activate target genes. GATA proteins play important roles in cell differentiation and homeostasis in all eukaryotes [23]. It has been suggested that endothelin-1, angiotensin II and adrenergic agonists increase the expression of BNP mRNA in cultured isolated cardiomyocytes by activating the proximal GATA elements [22]. The muscle-CATTCCT (M-CAT) consensus element, the shear stress responsive element (SSRE), and the thyroid hormone response element (TRE) could be other additional *cis*-acting factors regulating inducible BNP expression [18, 22]. Like GATA proteins, these elements can also be selectively activated by specific stimuli, especially by some neuro-hormones (such as b-adrenergic agonist and thyroid hormones) and cytokines (such as interleukin-1β [IL-1β] and tumor necrosis factor-α [TNF-α]) [22].

From a clinical point of view, it is important to note that chronic stimulation produces a greater amount of BNP than ANP, probably because the former is produced mainly by ventricular myocardium, which has a relatively greater mass than atria. However, ventricular BNP gene expression can be selectively upregulated during the evolution of diseases affecting the ventricles, as demonstrated in an experimental model of heart failure (HF), i.e., the rapid ventricular pacing-induced congestive HF in dog [27]. In fact, on average, the molar ratio of circulating BNP over ANP increases progressively with the severity of HF from a value of about 0.5 in healthy subjects up to about 3 in patients with NYHA functional class IV (Table 3.1, Fig. 3.13) [28].

Table 3.1. ANP and BNP values (mean and median, ng/L) in healthy subjects (age: 43.9, SD 13.6, range 16-85 years) and patients with heart failure grouped according to NYHA functional class (age: mean 64.4, SD 12.7, range 20-89 years). For the healthy subjects the 97.5th percentile of distribution values was also reported for both hormones. Plasma ANP and BNP concentrations were measured with IRMA methods. Molar ratio was calculated as the ratio between the respective mean values of BNP and ANP (BNP mean/ANP mean, expressed as pmol/L). The number (n) of subjects/patients studied for each group are reported within brackets

	ANP			BNP			
	Mean (SD)	Median	97.5th perc.	Mean (SD)	Median	97.5th perc.	Molar ratio
Healthy subjects (n = 292)	17.9 (10.7)	15.8	48	10.4 (8.9)	8.0	39	0.52
NYHA I (n = 33)	52.3 (43.9)	36.9		62.2 (92.7)	29.9		1.06
NYHA II (n = 132)	100.9 (95.6)	68.6		195.5 (251.4)	130.2		1.72
NYHA III (n = 80)	175.7 (124.5)	155.4		445.9 (377.5)	353.5		2.26
NYHA IV (n = 31)	205.5 (156.5)	259.3		621.8 (592.2)	390.0		2.70

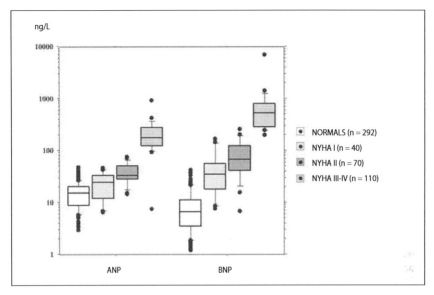

ng/L

Fig. 3.13. Circulating levels of ANP and BNP measured in healthy subjects and in patients with heart failure (HF), divided according to severity of disease (mild HF: patients in NYHA class I and II; severe HF: patients in NYHA class III-IV). The number of subjects included in each group is indicated in brackets. The results are expressed as boxes with five horizontal lines, displaying the 10th, 25th, 50th (median), 75th, and 90th percentiles of the variable. All values above the 90th percentile and below the 10th percentile (outliers) are plotted separately (as circles). Log scale in y-axis

These data explain why the BNP assay usually shows a better diagnostic accuracy in patients with cardiac disease than the ANP assay [28].

ANP and BNP are secreted from the heart into the circulation, thus providing for a baseline level of the hormones in blood [13]. The response of the heart to pressure or volume load varies in relation to whether the challenge is acute, subacute or chronic [12, 13].

Wall stretch is the most important stimulus for synthesis and secretion of ANP at the atrial level [12, 13, 21-23]. The increased secretion of ANP following acute mechanical atrial stretch is based on a phenomenon referred to as "stretch-secretion coupling". This effect is dependent upon a depletable ANP pool and is characterized by a phasic, short-term (i.e. minutes) burst of CNH secretion with no apparent effect on synthesis [13]. The precise mechanism by which force is translated into biochemical stimulus has not been completely elucidated. However, several studies have documented the importance of outside-in signaling by extracellular matrix proteins (especially integrin) in translating mechanical stress to changes in gene expression and the induction of ANP and BNP in hypertrophic myocardium [22].

Any physiological condition associated with an acute increase in venous return (preload), such as physical exercise, rapid change from standing to supine position, or head-out water immersion, causes a more rapid augmentation in ANP than in BNP plasma concentration. For instance, changes in ANP and BNP secretion have been well characterized during and after the tachyarrhythmia induced in pigs by rapid atrial pacing

(225 beats per minute). In this model, ANP plasma concentration shows a sharp initial peak followed by a decline, but remains significantly increased throughout a 24-hour post-pacing period, while BNP increases significantly after an 8-hour pacing, and even more after a 24-hour pacing [29]. Even acute changes in the effective plasma circulating volume, such as during a dialysis session in patients with chronic renal failure, cause greater variations in circulating levels of ANP than BNP [30].

Whereas chronic stimulated CNH secretion results in increased synthesis and secretion in both atria and ventricles, there is an intermediate level stimulation of the endocrine heart whereby increased synthesis and secretion of CNH is evident only in the atria [12, 13]. This can be observed during the "mineralocorticoid escape", a pathophysiological condition characterized by a transient period of positive sodium balance resulting from chronic exposure to mineralocorticoid excess, such as aldosterone or deoxycorticosterone acetate followed by a vigorous natriuresis leading to a new steady state of sodium balance [12, 13]. The rise in intravascular volume and central venous pressure leads to increased CNH production by the atria.

Wall distension is generally considered the main mechanical stimulus for CNH (especially BNP) production by ventricular tissue. This occurs in long-standing conditions characterized by electrolyte and fluid retention, and therefore expansion of effective plasma volume, such as primary [31] and secondary hyperaldosteronism, including cardiac, renal and liver failure [12, 13, 18, 30]. The changes in the pattern of gene expression are observed not only in the long-term hypertrophic process of ventricular myocardium, but also at the onset of hemodynamic overload. Moreover, expression of the BNP gene takes place with many characteristics of an immediate-early gene. Indeed, hemodynamic overload in the left ventricle has been shown to result in an increase in the BNP gene expression within 1 h, associated with the expression of oncogenes c-*fos* and c-*jun* [32]. A recent study suggested that the stretch-induced activation of BNP gene expression by increased left ventricular wall stress in an isolated perfused rat heart preparation is independent of transcriptional mechanisms and dependent on protein synthesis [32]; other studies are necessary to confirm and clarify these findings.

The presence of ventricular hypertrophy and fibrosis can stimulate hormone production [12, 13, 18-21, 30, 33-36]. However, recent studies have suggested that myocardial fibrosis rather than hypertrophy is associated with increased production of BNP [24, 35, 36].

More recently, several studies indicated that myocardial ischemia and hypoxia per se could also induce the synthesis/secretion of CNH by cardiomyocytes [37-44]. The studies indicating that ANP gene is responsive to hypoxia have been reviewed recently in detail [37]. Several data indicated that hypoxia directly stimulates ANP gene expression and its release in cardiac myocytes *in vitro* [37]. The effect of hypoxia on BNP production/secretion was also studied, demonstrating that surgical reduction of blood in an area of the anterior ventricular wall in pigs increased BNP mRNA by 3.5-fold in hypoxic compared with normoxic ventricular myocardium [44]. Moreover, proBNP peptide accumulated in the medium of freshly harvested ventricular myocyte cultures, but was undetectable in ventricular myocardium, indicating rapid release of the newly synthesized proBNP peptide [44]. The direct stimulating effect of hypoxia on CNH gene expression is probably due to the activation of promoter activity; however, other potential mechanisms could modulate peptide hormone release from cardiomyocytes, including the influx of extracellular Na^+ and Na^+/Ca^{++} exchange (due to the hypoxia-dependent intracellular acidosis) as well as the activation of protein kinase C [37]. Moreover, clinical studies reported that plasma levels of CNH (especially BNP and its related peptides) were found to be closely related to aerobic exercise capacity in patients with HF [45-47]. In particular, plasma NT-proBNP correlates better than indices of left ventricular systolic function, such as ejection fraction, with peak oxygen consumption and exercise duration [47]. These results may explain the elevated levels of BNP found even in patients with acute coronary syndrome (ACS), in the absence of a significant dilatation of the ventricular chambers [40]. This suggests a neuro-hormonal activation secondary to both reversible myocardial ischemia and necrosis [41].

There is increasing evidence from *in vivo* and ex vivo studies supporting the hypothesis that the production/secretion of CNH is regulated by complex interactions with the neuro-hormonal and immune systems, especially in ventricular myocardium [12, 13, 18]. Neuro-hormones, cytokines, and growth factors that can affect the production/secretion of CNH are summarized in Table 3.2.

Table 3.2. Summary list of some neuro-hormones, mediators of inflammation, and growth factors affecting the production/secretion of CNH

Angiotensin II
Endothelin-1
Adrenergic agents
Cytokines and other mediators of inflammation (including IL-1, IL-6, TNF, and lipopolysaccharide)
Growth and coagulation factors
Insulin
Growth hormone
Thyroid hormones
Corticosteroids
Estrogens

Endothelin and angiotensin II are considered the most powerful stimulators of production/secretion of CNH [12, 13, 18, 22]; similarly, glucocorticoids, sex steroid hormones, thyroid hormones, some growth factors and mediators of inflammation (such as some cytokines, especially TNF-α, interleukin-1, interleukin-6, and lipopolyliposaccharide, LPS) share stimulating effects on the CNH system [12, 13, 18, 22, 36, 48-57] (Table 3.2). The interesting finding that CNH production is stimulated by cytokines and growth factors suggests a link between cardiac endocrine activity and remodelling or inflammatory processes in myocardial and smooth muscle cells. A large number of studies have recently contributed to support this hypothesis [33-36, 50-53, 56-62].

More complex, and still in part unknown, is the effect of adrenergic stimulation on CNH production. The α_1-adrenergic agonist phenylephrine enhances the expression of some transcription factors, such as *Egr-1* and *c-myc*, regulating (usually increasing) the natriuretic peptide gene expression in cultured neonatal rat cardiomyocytes [12, 13, 18, 63-66]. Conflicting results were obtained with β-agonists. In one study, the β-agonist isoproterenol reduced the expression of BNP mRNA, but not that of ANP, an effect prevented by the β_1-antagonist CGP20712A in isolated adult mouse cardiomyocytes [67]. In another study, isoproterenol stimulated the BNP mRNA expression in rat ventricular myocyte-enriched cultures [68]. However, it was suggested that the stimulatory effects of both α- and β-adrenergic agonists on BNP gene inducible transcription are principally mediated by GATA elements [22, 23].

Clinical studies performed in hypertensive patients have shown that monotherapy with a β-blocker, either $β_1$-selective or not, is associated with an increase in the plasma concentration of ANP and/or BNP and their related peptides [69-71]. In contrast, CNH response can be heterogeneous during β-blocker therapy in congestive HF [28, 72], probably due to the various additive effects of other co-administered drugs. However, sustained treatment with β-blockers with improvement in cardiac function and exercise capacity and reduction in filling pressure and cardiac volumes is usually associated with a fall in CNH levels in patients with HF [28, 73, 74].

As far as hormones more specifically acting on intermediate metabolism are concerned, insulin (but not hyperglycemia) increased protein synthesis and ANP secretion and gene expression in cultured rat cardiac myocytes [75]. Moreover, in a model of genetic murine dilated cardiomyopathy, short-term RhGH treatment improved left ventricular function and significantly reduced elevated mRNA expression of ANP and BNP gene expression in left ventricular tissue [76].

In conclusion, a huge number of experimental and clinical studies demonstrated that production and secretion of CNH (especially BNP) are not only related to hemodynamic variations, but also subtly regulated by neuro-hormonal and immunological factors. Therefore, the variation of CNH circulating levels can be considered as a sensitive index of the perturbation of the homeostatic systems.

3.4 Biological Action of CNH

It is important to note that specific receptors for CNH have been found in all mammalian tissues, although at different concentrations, thus suggesting that CNH play an important biological role in several tissues. Most of these biological effects of CNH may be due to an autocrine/paracrine, rather than hormonal, action. In this section, we will discuss in detail only the best-known effects of CNH, and in particular those more strictly related to the endocrine function of the heart.

Cardiac natriuretic hormones have powerful physiological effects on the cardiovascular system, body fluid, and electrolyte homeostasis [13, 28, 30, 77, 78]. CNH share a direct diuretic, natriuretic and vasodilator effect and an inhibitory action on ventricular myocyte contraction [79] as well as remodeling and inflammatory processes of myocardium and smooth muscle cells [80-83] (Fig. 3.14). Thus, CNH exert a protective effect on endothelial function by decreasing shear stress, modulating coagulation and fibrinolysis pathways, and inhibiting platelet activation (Fig. 3.15). They can also inhibit vascular remodeling process as well as coronary restenosis post-angioplasty [56, 84-89].

Furthermore, CNH share an inhibitory action on neuro-hormonal and immunological systems, and on some growth factors [13, 28, 30, 77, 78, 90-99]. In particular, the pivotal role of CNH (especially ANP) in modulating the immune response has been reviewed recently [98]. The first evidence for a role of CNH in the immune system was given by the fact that peptide hormones and their receptors are expressed in various immune organs. Furthermore, several studies indicated that the CNH system in immune cells underlies specific regulatory mechanisms by affecting the innate as well as the adaptive immune response [99]. In particular, ANP supports the first line of defense by increasing phagocytotic activity and production of reactive oxygen species of phagocytes. ANP affects the induced innate immune response by regulating the activation of macrophages at various stages. It also reduces production of pro-inflammatory mediators by inhibition of iNOS and COX-2 as well as TNF-α synthesis. ANP also affects TNF-α action, i.e. it interferes with the inflammatory effects of TNF-α on the endothelium. The peptide hormone counteracts TNF-α-induced endothelial permeability and adhesion and attraction of inflammatory cells. Finally, it affects thymopoesis and T-cell maturation by acting on dendritic cells and regulates the balance between TH1 and TH2 responses [99].

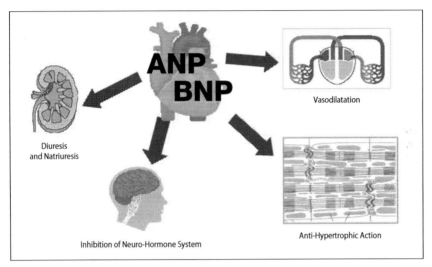

Fig. 3.14. Main effects of CNH on the cardiovascular system

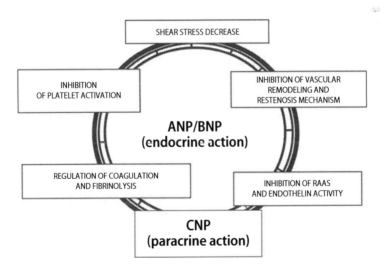

Fig. 3.15. Protective actions of CNH on endothelial function

The cited effects on the cardiovascular system and body fluid and electrolyte homeostasis can be explained at least in part by the inhibition of control systems, including the sympathetic nervous system, the renin-angiotensin-aldosterone system (RAAS), the vasopressin/antidiuretic hormone system, the endothelin system, cytokines and growth factors [90-99]. The endocrine action, shared by plasma ANP and BNP, can be enhanced by natriuretic peptides produced locally in target tissues (paracrine action). Indeed, endothelial cells synthesize CNP, which in turn exerts a paracrine action on vessels [57, 84-88]. Moreover, renal tubular cells produce urodilatin, another member of the peptide natriuretic family, which has powerful diuretic and natriuretic properties [100]. Genes for natriuretic peptides (including ANP, BNP and CNP) are also expressed in the central nervous system, where they likely act as neurotransmitters and/or neuromodulators [91-93, 100-102]. In particular, it was demonstrated that intranasal ANP acts as central nervous inhibitor of the hypothalamus-pituitary-adrenal stress system in humans [103]. Finally, co-expression of CNH and of their receptors was observed in rat thymus cells and macrophages [104,105], suggesting that CNH may have immunomodulatory and anti-inflammatory functions in mammals [106].

A recent detailed review [107] has highlighted a possible major role for CNH in the development of certain systems, in particular skeleton, brain, and vessels. This review cites recent studies showing severe skeletal defects and impaired recovery after vascular and renal injury in CNH transgenic and knockout (KO) mice [108]. In addition, CNH may have a role in the regulation of proliferation, survival, and neurite outgrowth of cultured neuronal and/or glial cells [108].

Changes in plasma ANP are also correlated with alcohol-associated psychological variables [108]. Acute administration of alcohol stimulates the release of ANP independently of volume-loading effects. Patients whose ANP levels fell markedly during abstinence also reported more intense and frequent craving as well as more anxiety [108].

Several reports have shown that CNH stimulate the synthesis and release of testosterone in a dose-dependent manner in isolated and purified normal Leydig cells [109-112]. It has been suggested that this effect on normal Leydig cell steroidogenesis does not involve classical mechanisms of cAMP-mediated regulation of steroidogenic activity by gonadotropins [112]. The stimulated levels of testosterone production by ANP, BNP, and gonadotropins were comparable, whereas CNP has been found to be a weak stimulator of testosterone production in Leydig cells [112]. Moreover, testicular cells contain immunoreactive ANP-like materials and a high density of natriuretic peptide receptor-A (NRP-A) [112]. These findings suggest that CNH play paracrine and/or autocrine roles in testis and testicular cells. Furthermore, the presence of ANP and its receptors has been reported in ovarian cells, too. Increasing evidence strongly support that CNH are present and probably locally synthesized in ovarian cells of different mammalian species and also play an important physiological role in stimulating estradiol synthesis and secretion in the female gonad [112-115]. However, further studies are necessary in order to clarify completely the role played by CNH in the regulation of gonadal function and also to assess the inter-relationship between heart endocrine function and gonadal function in humans.

The huge amount of data reported above strongly supports the hypothesis that CNH are active components of the body integrative network that includes nervous, endocrine and immune systems. According to this hypothesis, the heart can no longer be seen as a passive automaton driven by nervous, endocrine or hemodynamic inputs, but as a leading actor on the stage. Thus, CNH, together with other neuro-hormonal factors, regulate cardiovascular hemodynamics and body fluid and electrolyte homeostasis, and probably modulate inflammatory response in some districts, including the cardiovascular one. This hypothesis implies that there are two counteracting systems in the body: one has sodium-retaining, vasoconstrictive, thrombophylic, pro-inflammatory and hypertrophic actions, while the second one promotes natriuresis and vasodilatation, and inhibits thrombosis, inflammation and hypertrophy. CNH are the main effectors of the latter system, and work in concert with NO, some prostaglandins, and other vasodilator peptides (such as bradykinin) [116-120]. Under physiological conditions, the effects of these two systems are well balanced via feedback mechanisms, and result in a beat-to-beat regulation of cardiac output and blood pressure in response to endogenous and exogenous stimuli. In patients with HF, the action of the first system is predominant, as a compensatory mechanism, initially, that progressively leads to detrimental effects.

The knowledge so far accumulated regarding CNH suggests that a continuous and intense information exchange flows from the endocrine heart system to nervous and immunological systems and to other organs (including kidney, endocrine glands, liver, adipose tissue, immuno-competent cells) and vice versa (Fig. 3.16). From a pathophysiological point of view, the close link between the CNH system and counter-regulatory systems could explain the increase in circulating levels of CNH in some non-cardiac-related clinical conditions. Increased or decreased BNP levels were frequently reported in acute and chronic respiratory diseases [121-129], some endocrine and metabolic diseases [130-141], liver cirrhosis [142-144], renal failure [100, 144], septic shock, chronic inflammatory diseases [145-149], subarachnoid hemorrhage [150-153], and some paraneoplastic syndromes [154-156]. In addition, any myocardial damage leading to the release of sarcoplasma constituents (including CNH) in extracellular fluid, for instance that due to cardiotoxic agents [157-161], cardiac trauma or ischemic necrosis [162, 163], also causes an increase in plasma concentration of CNH.

Furthermore, the inter-relationships between the CNH system and pro-inflammatory cytokines suggest that cardiac hormones play an important role in mechanisms respon-

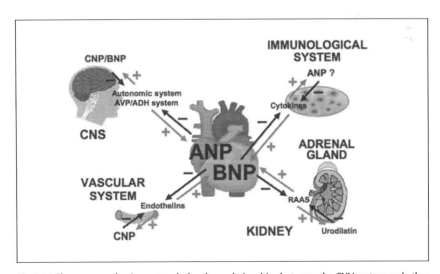

Fig. 3.16. The neuro-endocrine network: the close relationships between the CNH system and other organs and regulatory systems

sible for cardiac and vascular adaptation, maladaptation and remodeling in response to various physiological and pathological stimuli [32, 35, 62, 162].

Elevated BNP levels in extra-cardiac diseases reveal an endocrine heart response to a "cardiovascular stress" (Fig. 3.17). Indeed, recent studies reported that plasma BNP concentration is an independent risk factor for mortality (cardiac and/or total) in pulmonary embolism [121, 123, 124] and hypertension [127], renal failure [28, 100, 144], septic shock [145], amyloidosis [149], and diabetes mellitus [141] (see Chapter 6 for more details). According to this hypothesis, a BNP assay should be considered as a marker of cardiac stress (Fig. 3.17).

In conclusion, CNH share a powerful action on the cardiovascular system, including diuretic, natriuretic and vasodilator effects and an inhibitory action on ventricular myocyte contraction, as well as on remodeling and inflammatory processes of myocardium and smooth muscle cells. Furthermore, CNH exert a protective effect on endothelial function by decreasing shear stress, modulating coagulation and fibrinolysis pathways, and inhibiting platelet activation. They can also inhibit the vascular remodeling process as well as coronary restenosis post-angioplasty. These effects can be explained, at least in part, by the inhibition of control systems, including the sympathetic nervous system, the RAAS, the vasopressin/antidiuretic hormone system, the endothelin system, cytokines and growth factors. Finally, the endocrine action of ANP and BNP is potentiated at the periphery (target tissues) by the paracrine action of other members of the peptide natriuretic family, such as CNP (in the vascular tissue) and urodilatin (in renal tissue).

Finally, some experimental studies performed in KO mice suggest a distinct pathophysiological role for BNP in respect to ANP [18]. While BNP KO mice are no different

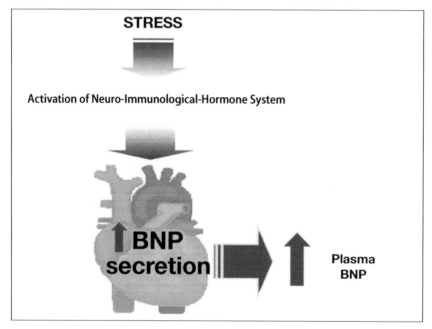

Fig. 3.17. Elevated BNP levels in the absence of cardiac diseases reveal an endocrine heart response to "stress", not necessarily involving the cardiovascular system

from control mice with regard to blood pressure, urine volume, and urinary electrolyte excretion, they have more extensive ventricular fibrosis, accompanied by increased transforming growth factor-b3 (TGF-b3) and collagen mRNA [18]. These data suggest that BNP may function more as an autocrine/paracrine inhibitor of cell growth in the heart; while ANP may be considered as a traditional circulating hormone with pronounced diuretic, natriuretic, and antihypertensive effects.

3.5 Natriuretic Peptide Receptors and Intracellular Second Messenger Signaling

Cardiac natriuretic hormones share their biological action by means of specific receptors (NPR), which are present within the cell membranes of target tissues. Three different subtypes of NPRs have so far been identified in mammalian tissues [112, 164, 165].

3.5.1 Genes Encoding for NPRs

NPR1 is the gene coding the NPR-A receptor (natriuretic peptide receptor A/guanylate cyclase A) and it is located on 1q21-q22 spanning 15,534 bp with 22 exons. The relative mRNA of 3,805 bp leads to a protein of 1,061 amino acids.

The NPR-B receptor (natriuretic peptide receptor B/guanylate cyclase B) is codified by the gene NPR2. This gene of 17,303 bp is on chromosome 9 (9p21-p12) and it is organized in 22 exons, which can give two types of mRNA. NPR2 Ia is an mRNA of 3,482 bp that has a 71 nucleotide insertion relative to isoform b, which results in a different, and shorter (995 aa), carboxy-terminus that may disrupt the guanylyl cyclase activity. NPR2 Ib (3,411 bp, 1,047 aa) does not include the alternate exon found in isoform a, and thus isoform b contains a longer carboxy-terminus. The natriuretic peptide receptor C gene, also named NPR3, is on 5p14-p13 and spans 74,698 bp (8 exons), giving an mRNA of 1,753 bp that is translated into a protein of 540 amino acids.

3.5.2 Biological Function of NPRs

NPR-A and NPR-B are generally considered to mediate all known biological actions throughout the guanylate cyclase (GC) intracellular domain, while the third member of the natriuretic peptide receptor family, the NPR-C receptor, does not have a GC domain (Figs. 3.18, 3.19 and 3.20).

The GC receptors for ANP/BNP (NPR-GC-A) and CNP (NPR-GC-B) belong to a family of seven isoforms of transmembrane enzymes (from GC-A to GC-G), which all convert guanosine triphosphate into the second messenger cyclic 3',5'-guanosine monophosphate (cGMP) [164].

Although partly homologous to soluble GC, the receptor for NO, the membrane GCs share a different and unique topology. The single transmembrane span domain divides the protein structure into an extracellular ligand binding domain and an intracellular region consisting of a protein kinase-homology domain, an amphipathic helical or hing region, and a cyclase-homology domain [165] (Figs. 3.18, 3.19 and 3.20). The cyclase-homology domain represents the catalytic cGMP synthesizing domain. The function of the intracellular region consisting of a protein kinase-homology domain is incompletely understood. Although it probably binds ATP and contains many residues conserved in the catalytic domain of protein kinases, kinase activity has not been detected [165]. It represses the enzyme activity of the catalytic cGMP-synthesizing domain and at the same time is necessary for its ligand-dependent activation [154]. The coiled-coil hing region is involved in receptor dimerization, which is also essential for the activation of the catalytic domain [165].

The cGMP produced modulates the activity of specific downstream regulatory proteins, such as cGMP-regulated phosphodiesterases, ion channels and cGMP-dependent

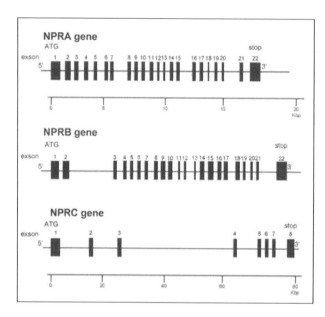

Fig. 3.18. Schematic structure of the natriuretic peptide receptor genes

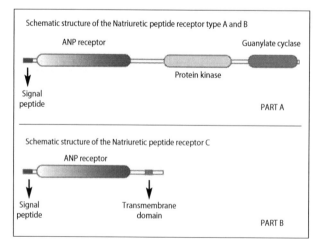

Fig. 3.19. Schematic structure of the natriuretic peptide receptors. *Part A* Domain structure of NPR-A and NPR-B. *Part B* Domain structure of NPR-C

protein kinases type I (PKG I) and type II (PKG II) (Fig. 3.20). These proteins should be considered to be third messengers, which are differentially expressed in different cell types, ultimately modifying cellular functions [166, 167]. This specific action of CNH on target tissues depends essentially on two different mechanisms.

The physiological expression of NPR-A and NPR-B differs quite significantly in human tissues (Fig. 3.21). NPR-A is found in abundance in larger, conduit blood vessels, whereas the NPR-B is found predominantly in the central nervous system [168]. Both receptors have been localized in adrenal glands and kidney [168]. On the other hand, several studies indicate that phosphorylation of the kinase homology domain is a critical event in the regulation of NPRs [169-171].

The affinity for ANP, BNP and CNP also varies greatly among the different NPRs. ANP shows a greater affinity for NPR-A and NPR-C, and CNP for NPR-B, while BNP shows a lower affinity for all NPRs compared to the other two peptides (Fig. 3.21).

Activation of the GC-linked NPRs is incompletely understood [172]. NPR-A and NPR-B are homo-oligomers in the absence and presence of their respective ligands, indicating that receptor activation does not simply result from ligand-dependent dimerization [173]. However, ANP binding does cause a conformational change of each monomer closer together [172-176]. The stoichiometry of the ligand-receptor complex is 1:2 [177].

Initial *in vitro* data suggested that direct phosphorylation of NPR-A by protein kinase C mediated its "desensitization" (i.e., the process by which an activated receptor is turned off) [178]. However, subsequent studies conducted in live cells indicated that desensitization in response to prolonged natriuretic peptide exposure or activators of protein kinase C results in a net loss of phosphate from NPR-A and NPR-B [171, 179-182].

Although ligand-dependent internalization and degradation of NPR-A has been intensely studied by several groups for many years, a consensus understanding of the importance of this process in the regulation of NPRs has not emerged [182]. Early studies conducted

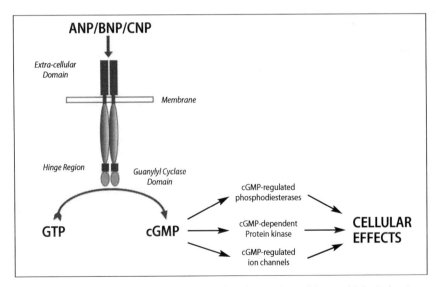

Fig. 3.20. NPR-A and NPR-B are generally considered to mediate all known biological actions, while NPR-C is independent of guanylate cyclase (GC)

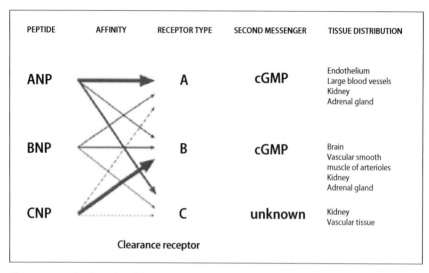

Fig. 3.21. Main biological and functional characteristics of natriuretic peptide receptors

on PC-12 pheochromocytoma cells suggested that both NPR-A and NPR-C internalize ANP and that both receptors are recycled back to the cell surface [184]. Other studies, using Leydig, Cos, and 293 cell lines, have reported that ANP binding to NPR-A stimulates its internalization, which results in the majority of the receptors being degraded with a smaller portion being recycled to the plasma membrane [184-187]. In contrast, other studies performed in cultured glomerular mesangial and renomedullary interstitial cells from the rat or Chinese hamster ovary cells reported that NPR-A is a constitutively membrane-resident protein that neither undergoes endocytosis nor mediates lysosomal hydrolysis of ANP [188, 189]. A more recent study using 293T cells suggested that NPR-A and NPR-B are neither internalized nor degraded in response to receptor occupation [173]. Furthermore, this study did not support the hypothesis that down-regulation is responsible for NPR desensitization observed in response to various physiological or pathological stimuli [182]. Further studies are necessary to clarify whether or not ANP binding to NPR-A stimulates its internalization, and whether this process is tissue- and/or species-specific.

It is generally thought that the NPR-C is not linked to GC and so serves as a clearance receptor [28, 77, 78]. NPR-C is present in higher concentration than NPR-A or NPR-B in several tissues (especially vascular tissue), and it is known constitutively to internalize CNH [172] (Fig. 3.22). However, recent studies have found that CNH interact with NPR-C to suppress the cAMP concentration by inhibition of adenylyl cyclase [190, 191]. Specific binding to NPR-C increases inositol triphosphate and diacylglycerol concentrations by activating phospholipase C activity or inhibits DNA synthesis stimulated by endothelin, platelet-derived growth factor and phorbol ester by inhibiting MAPK activity, as recently reviewed [190]. The NPR-C-mediated inhibition of adenylyl cyclase is mediated through Gi (inhibitory guanine nucleotide regulatory) proteins. According to this hypothesis, NPR-C, which is present in large amounts, especially on the endothelial cell wall, may mediate some paracrine effects of CNP on vascular tissue [168, 190]. However, further studies are necessary to elucidate the possible role of NPR-C receptors as modulators of CNH action and/or degradation in peripheral tissues.

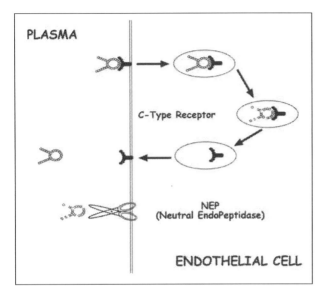

Fig. 3.22. Degradation pathways of CNH. CNH are degraded via two different metabolic pathways: (1) internalization and intracellular degradation after binding with the specific receptor NPR-C; (2) degradation by several plasma and tissue proteases, especially a membrane-bound endopeptidase (NEP 24.11)

3.6 Metabolic Pathways and Circulating Levels of CNH

Atrial natriuretic peptide and BNP are secreted directly from the heart. In the circulation, CNHs are metabolized via two principal mechanisms: degradation by a membrane-bound endopeptidase (NEP 24.11) and receptor-mediated cellular uptake via NPR-C [14] (Fig. 3.22). Some biological characteristics of ANP, BNP and CNP (as well as of their precursors) are summarized in Table 3.3.

Table 3.3. A comparison of respective biological characteristics of ANP, BNP and CNP

Precursors	proANP		proBNP		proCNP	
Main synthesis site	Heart		Heart		Endothelial vessels	
Molecules in blood	ANP	NT-proANP	BNP	NT-proBNP	CNP	NT-proCNP
Amino acids	28	98	32	76	CNP-22 (CNP_{82-103}) CNP-53 (CNP_{51-103})	50
Weight (Daltons)	3,078	10,615	3,462	8,457	2,199 5,802	~5,000
Biological activity	Yes	Probably yes	Yes	Not yet found	Yes Yes	Not yet found
Half-life in plasma (min)	2–4	40–50	15–25	60–120	1–3	Unknown

3.6.1 ANP Metabolism

Atrial natriuretic peptides are a family of peptides derived from a common precursor, called preproANP, which in humans contains 151 amino acids and has a signal peptide sequence at its amino-terminal end (Fig. 3.11). The pro-hormone is stored in secretion granules of cardiomyocytes as a 126-amino-acid peptide, $proANP_{1-126}$, which is produced by cleavage of the signal peptide. When appropriate signals for hormone release are given, $proANP_{1-126}$ is further split by some proteases (especially the serine protease corin) [192] into N-terminal fragment NT-proANP and the COOH-terminal peptide ANP, which is generally considered to be the biologically active hormone, because it contains the cysteine ring (Figs. 3.1 and 3.11).

Studies from the group of Vesely et al. suggested that the NT-proANP can be metabolized *in vivo* in three peptide hormones with blood pressure-lowering, natriuretic, diuretic and/or kaliuretic properties [100]. These peptide hormones, numbered by their amino acid sequences, beginning at the N-terminal end of the proANP pro-hormone, include: 1) the peptide $proANP_{1-30}$, also called long-acting natriuretic peptide (LANP); 2) the peptide $proANP_{31-67}$ with vessel dilator properties; 3) the peptide $proANP_{79-98}$ with kaliuretic properties [98]. However, these three peptides do not bind to the same NPRs of CNHs, because they do not have the cysteine ring. Further studies are necessary to confirm and elucidate the biological action of these putative peptide hormones, as well as their *in vivo* metabolism.

There is some evidence that ANP is secreted according to a pulsatile pattern in humans [193-197]. Upon secretion, ANP is rapidly distributed and degraded (the metabolic clearance rate of ANP is on average about 2,000 ml/min in healthy subjects) with a plasma half-life of about 4-6 minutes in healthy adult subjects. In humans, about 50% of the ANP secreted into the right atrium is extracted by the peripheral tissues during the first pass throughout the body [198-201]. Furthermore, circulating ANP represents only a small fraction of the total body pool (no more than 1/15) in normal subjects and plasma ANP concentration shows rapid and wide fluctuations in healthy subjects, even at rest in the recumbent position [198-201]. The turnover data suggest that circulating levels of ANP may not represent a close estimate of their disposal, and therefore of the activity of the CNH system, as implicitly accepted in physiological or clinical studies in which only the plasma concentration of the hormone is measured, without an estimation of turnover rate. However, it was demonstrated that ANP clearance mechanisms are constant in the presence of rapid and large changes in endogenous ANP plasma levels induced by atrial and/or ventricular pacing, thus indicating that, at least for studies lasting only a few hours, changes in ANP circulating levels may provide a reliable estimate of production rate variations [201].

3.6.2 BNP Metabolism

The biological action, metabolic pathways, and turnover parameters of BNP are not as well known as those of ANP [14]. However, it is commonly believed that the BNP turnover is less rapid than that of ANP with a plasma half-life of about 13-20 minutes; indeed, circulating levels of BNP are more stable than those of ANP in adult healthy subjects (Fig. 3.23). Bentzen et al. [197] analyzed the secretion pattern of ANP and BNP in 12 patients with chronic HF and in 12 healthy adult subjects. ANP

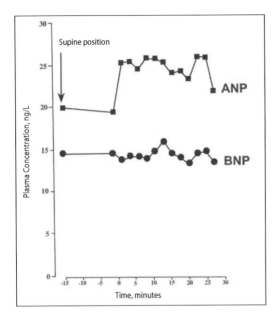

Fig. 3.23. Variations of plasma ANP and BNP, both measured by immunoradiometric assay, in a normal subject (woman, aged 23 years) throughout 45 min at rest in the recumbent position. Supine position at rest was attained at -15 min; starting from time 0, blood samples (5 ml) were drawn every 2.5 min for the following 30 min. A saline infusion was used to flush the catheter and to replace the same volume of fluid withdrawn

and BNP in plasma were determined by radioimmunoassay (RIA) at 2 min intervals during a 2-h period and were subsequently analyzed for pulsatile behavior using the method of Fourier transformation. All patients and healthy subjects had significant rhythmic oscillations in plasma ANP levels, and 11 patients with HF and 10 healthy subjects had significant rhythmic oscillations in plasma BNP levels [197]. The amplitude of the main frequency was considerably higher in patients than in healthy subjects, but the main frequency did not differ significantly between patients and healthy subjects for either ANP or BNP. Patients with HF demonstrated pulsatile secretion of ANP and BNP with a much higher absolute amplitude, but with the same main frequency as healthy subjects [197]. Finally, rhythmic oscillations in plasma ANP levels of healthy subjects showed significantly higher mean amplitude, but not frequency, than those of BNP [197].

A very small amount of immunoreactive BNP has been found in urine [202, 203], but the precise mechanism of renal excretion has not yet been fully clarified. In contrast to BNP, the biologically active peptide, other proBNP-derived inactive fragments also circulate in plasma. These fragments are commonly referred to as "N-terminal proBNP" (NT-proBNP), but the molecular heterogeneity also includes the intact precursor, particularly in patients with HF [14, 204]. Cardiac secretion of proBNP and its N-terminal fragments has been demonstrated by blood sampling from the coronary sinus [205]. Some data suggest that the major part of proBNP produced in myocardiocytes is apparently processed prior to release [14]; however, intact proBNP peptide was also found in plasma of patients with HF as well as healthy adult subjects [14, 205, 206].

A recent study, employing a new method for the total and equimolar assay of all proBNP-related peptides (i.e., intact proBNP precursor plus NT-proBNP concentrations), found comparable peripheral concentrations of BNP (measured by immunoradiometric assay) and proBNP-related peptides in patients with HF [206]. Moreover, the BNP concentration (median 125 pmol/l) was higher than that of total proBNP (103 pmol/l) in the coronary sinus, suggesting that the cardiac secretion of these two peptides could be different [206]. Alternatively, this finding could also reflect some difference in peripheral elimination of peptides because total proBNP concentration is significantly higher in the pulmonary artery than the aortic root in patients with right ventricular failure [207].

While NEP enzymes are mainly involved in natriuretic peptide inactivation *in vivo*, the degradation of BNP seen *in vitro* is most likely due to other enzymes, such as peptyl arginine aldehyde proteases, kallikrein, and serine proteases [15]. However, the role of these enzymes in the degradation of BNP *in vivo* is unclear.

A recent study reported that both the BNP and total proBNP concentrations were increased more than 2-fold in the coronary sinus compared to the inferior caval vein (BNP-32: median 125 pmol/l, range 21-993 vs median 52 pmol/l, range 7-705; proBNP: median 103 pmol/l, range 16-691 vs 47 pmol/l, 8-500) [206]. These findings are in accordance with previous studies suggesting that the cardiac gradient for BNP secretion (as estimated by the difference between BNP concentration in coronary sinus and inferior caval vein) ranges from 1.6-fold to 2.9-fold [204,208-210]. Taking these studies as a whole, ANP and BNP share a similar peripheral extraction value (of about 30-50%). Further studies are necessary to elucidate the metabolism of BNP and in particular the predominant form of the circulating BNP-related peptides.

3.7 CNH System in Fetal Heart and Circulation

In human fetal ventricles, ANP mRNA is considerably higher than in adult ventricles and tends to decrease with gestational age [211, 212]. Peptide levels of ANP and BNP in fetal ventricles have also been reported to be greater than in the adult ventricle, although there are some differences among mammals [212]. No CNP expression has been detected in developing hearts of human embryos [213].

In general, these studies indicate that the relative contribution of ventricular ANP is significantly greater in the embryo than in the adult, and in some species the ventricle is the predominant site of ANP and BNP expression during fetal development [212]. During the molecular processes underlying "physiological" hypertrophy (such as physical training and pregnancy) or myocardial remodeling in patients with arterial hypertension or myocardial infarction, numerous genes normally expressed during development are reactivated, including ventricular ANP and BNP [19-23, 214, 215].

In mice, the peaks of ANP and BNP mRNA coincide with a landmark in the development of the embryonic heart, including the start of regular beating of the primitive heart (day 9 of gestation), septal formation (day 12), and alteration of heart axis (day 15) [212].

CNH are secreted in response to similar physiological stimuli during development as in the adult animals [211], including volume loading [216, 217], hyperosmolarity [216], hypoxia [218], and the stimulatory action of angiotensin II, phenylephrine, vasopressin, and endothelin [219-221]. These data suggest that CNH may play an important role in regulating blood pressure and salt and water balance in the developing embryo in mammals [221].

Expression of BNP and CNP has been demonstrated within the decidua of the mouse placenta [222], while the expression of ANP has been demonstrated in the human placenta, particularly in the cytotrophoblast tissue [223, 224]. Furthermore, ANP or BNP administered into the fetal placental circulation have been shown to inhibit the effects of vasoconstrictor agents [225-227]. These studies suggest that CNH act as a vasodilator in the fetal-placental vasculature and may help regulate the blood supply to the fetus [221].

CNH modulate cell growth and proliferation, including inhibition of proliferation of vascular smooth muscle cells [228], inhibition of hypertrophy [229], and induction of apoptosis in cultured cardiac myocytes [230]. Furthermore, CNH suppress cardiac fibroblast growth [231]. These data suggest that natriuretic peptides may play a role in cardiac organogenesis of the embryonal heart and cardiovascular system.

Further support for a role of CNH in regulating cardiac growth is provided by some studies in KO mice. The phenotype of the NPR-A KO (*Npr1-/-*) mouse lacks the receptor that mediates the biological actions of both ANP and BNP and has elevated CNH levels and blood pressure, with marked cardiac hypertrophy and fibrosis [232-234]. Furthermore, the *Npr1-/-* mice show enlarged hearts at birth, with *Npr1-/-* neonates having heart-weight to body-weight ratios 140% greater than wild-type littermates [233], confirming that the ANP/BNP system is an important regulator of myocyte growth during development [221]. On the other hand, KO mice for the ANP [234] or BNP [236] gene show no such changes in size or structure in the hearts of neonates, thus suggesting that the presence of only one peptide hormone can compensate for the absence of the other.

It should be noted that BNP-overexpressing mice [237] and natriuretic peptide clearance receptor (NPR-C)-KO mice [238] show skeletal overgrowth, whereas CNP-KO mice show dwarfism and bone malformation [239]. Fetal bone growth is regulated by CNP, via stimulation of chondrocyte proliferation and cartilage matrix production [240]. Thus, the natriuretic peptides have effects on the development of other tissues besides the heart [107]. However, further research will be needed before we fully understand all the roles of the natriuretic peptides during embryogenesis.

It is well known that CNH increase progressively during pregnancy in the mother's circulation [241, 242]. Several mechanisms may play a role in activating the CNH system during pregnancy; the most important (and well known) may be the progressive increase in plasma volume, the direct and progressive stimulating effect of female steroid hormones on CNH production [48, 49] and the activation of counter-regulatory systems (especially the hypophysis-adrenal axis and the RAAS) [243, 244].

Moreover, plasma CNH levels are frequently increased in women with hypertensive pregnancy and eclampsia compared to normal pregnancy [245-250]. The higher levels of CNH (especially BNP or NT-proBNP) in pre-eclamptic women may be an indicator of high left-ventricular filling pressure, and indicate left-ventricular diastolic dysfunction [248, 250].

These data confirm that the CNH system plays a relevant role in the regulation of fluid and electrolyte homeostasis, as well as in cardiovascular hemodynamics, even during pregnancy.

3.8 CNH Genes and Cardiovascular Diseases

Since CNH have a potent diuretic antihypertensive action, and the impaired action of the peptides may cause hypertension, their genes may be candidates for cardiovascular disease, especially arterial hypertension. Furthermore, transgenic animals (especially mice), overexpressing CNH or knockout for ANP/BNP genes or their specific receptors, have been used to evaluate the pathophysiological role of the CNH system in cardiovascular diseases [251].

In transgenic mice with overexpression of ANP and BNP in liver, plasma ANP and BNP levels are from 10- to 100-fold higher than in control mice, with a blood pressure of 20-25 mmHg lower. These mice also have lighter hearts, but with the same cardiac output and rate, than controls [251, 253-255]. The BNP-overexpressing mice show the same hemodynamic changes; on the other hand, ANP KO mice develop NaCl-sensitive hypertension [251]. Transgenic mice overexpressing the NPRA gene have also been created; these animals have a lower blood pressure than wild-type mice [251]. The corresponding KO mice show an increase in blood pressure compared with controls (on average 10 mmHg in heterozygous and 30 mmHg in homozygous animals), which is not affected by NaCl intake [254, 255]. These data suggest a different pathophysiological mechanism for hypertension between KO mice for the ANP gene and its specific receptor; this difference does not yet have an explanation [251]. NPRC heterozygous KO mice do not show blood pressure variation, whereas homozygous mice show on average a decrease in blood pressure of about 8 mmHg [251].

The function of natriuretic peptides was also studied after induction of myocardial infarction in KO mice lacking the natriuretic peptide receptor guanylyl cyclase-A, the receptor for ANP and BNP [89]. KO and wild-type mice were subjected to left coronary artery ligation and then followed-up for 4 weeks. KO mice showed significantly higher mortality because of a higher incidence of acute HF, which was associated with diminished water and sodium excretion and with higher cardiac levels of mRNAs encoding ANP, BNP, TGF-b1, and type I collagen. By 4 weeks after infarction, left ventricular remodeling, including myocardial hypertrophy and fibrosis, and impairment of left ventricular systolic function were significantly more severe in KO than wild-type mice [89]. These data confirm that the CNH system has powerful anti-remodeling properties on ventricular cardiomyocytes.

In recent years, molecular genetic techniques have been introduced in etiological studies of polygenetic diseases, in linkage studies, in sib-pair linkage studies of various candidate genes, and in related studies [251, 252]. The association between some abnormalities in genes, coding for the CNH and their receptors, and some cardiovascular (in particular hypertension) and metabolic (such as diabetes mellitus) diseases has been tested in a large number of clinical studies (see also Chapter 6 for more details). To date, the results obtained are conflicting and seem to depend strictly on the ethnic population of the study.

The restriction fragment length polymorphism for the enzyme HpaII, located in intron 2 of NPPA (polymorphism also called Sma I), was reported to be more common in hypertensive African-Americans than in normotensive black controls [257]; these data were then confirmed in two [258, 259], but not a third [260], Caucasian populations. Furthermore, another study found that the HpaII polymorphism was not associated with hypertension in the Chinese population of Hong Kong [261].

Regarding other NPPA polymorphisms, Japanese studies reported that both G1837A and T2238C polymorphisms are associated with essential hypertension [262], while only a marginally significant association was found with an ANP polymorphism located in the 5'-untranslated region (C664G) [263].

The possible association between mutations of the ANP gene and some complications of diabetes mellitus and obesity will be discussed in detail in Chap. 6 (Cardiac Natriuretic Peptides as Possible Markers of Extra-cardiac Diseases: Clinical Considerations and Applications).

Several allelic variants have also been described for genes coding for CNH receptors (see the recent revew by Nakayama [251] for a more detailed discussion of this topic). The clearance receptor for natriuretic peptides (NPR-C) is highly expressed in adipose tissue, and its bi-allelic (A/C) polymorphism was detected at position -55 in the conserved promoter element named P1. This variant of the NPR-C P1 promoter is associated with lower ANP levels and higher systolic blood pressure and mean blood pressure in obese hypertensives: the C(-55) variant, in the presence of increased adiposity, might reduce plasma ANP through increased NPR-C-mediated ANP clearance, contributing to higher blood pressure [264].

In the Japanese population an insertion/deletion (GCTGAGCC) polymorphism has been identified in the 5'-flanking region of the NPRA gene that is associated with essential hypertension and left ventricular hypertrophy [265]. Another insertion/deletion polymorphism is on the 3'-untranslated region of the NPRA gene, on exon 22, and it seems to be associated with familial hypertension [266]. However, these data should be confirmed in larger studies, including other ethnic populations.

3.9 An Integrated Neuro-Hormonal System Regulates Vascular Function

Endothelial cells release an array of vasoactive mediators that alter the tone and growth of the underlying smooth muscle and regulate the reactivity of circulating white blood cells, erythrocytes and platelets. These endogenous factors are usually called endothelium-derived vasorelaxant mediators [267]. Moreover, it appears that alterations in the capacity of the endothelium to release some mediators in response to pathophysiological stimuli (the so-called endothelium dysfunction) are a major precipitating factor in many cardiovascular diseases. Perhaps the most important of these paracrine mediators are prostacyclin (PGI$_2$) and nitric oxide (NO). More recently, a third endothelium-derived vasorelaxant mediator has been described [267]. This is termed endothelium-derived hyperpolarizing factor (EDHF) because it elicits a characteristic smooth-muscle hyperpolarization and relaxation. Much attention has focused on identifying EDHF(s), with diverse candidates, including cytochrome P450 metabolites, KC ions, anandamide and hydrogen peroxide [267]. However, the role of each of these as EDHF remains unsubstantiated.

There is now compelling evidence that CNH (and especially CNP) act as EDHFs in some vascular beds [267-271]. Indeed, numerous studies have demonstrated that ANP, BNP and CNP bind to NPR-A and NPR-B receptors on vascular smooth muscle cells (either freshly isolated or in culture), stimulate cGMP accumulation, and cause a dose-dependent vasodilation [268-271]. This increase in cGMP causes vasodilatation by reducing intracellular calcium levels, as occur when cGMP accumulation is stimulated by NO and its analogs [268].

It is theoretically conceivable that ANP and BNP act like hormones in vascular tissue by reaching the smooth muscle cells from the circulation after secretion by the heart, while CNP shows a paracrine action, being secreted by endothelial cells [57, 84, 87, 88] (Fig. 3.15). However, Casco et al. [272] demonstrated the existence of a complete CNH system (including the production and secretion of ANP, BNP and CNP) in atherosclerotic human coronary vessels by means of *in situ* hybridization and immunocytochemistry methods. In particular, the expression of mRNAs of ANP, BNP and CNP, measured by RT PCR, tended to be increased in macroscopically diseased arteries compared to normal vessels, although only the values for BNP expression were significantly different [272]. This study suggests that the CNH system is involved in the pathobiology of intimal plaque formation as well as in vascular remodeling in humans.

Some studies indicated that there are complex interactions even among CNH themselves. Nazario et al. [273] reported that ANP and BNP can stimulate CNP production through a guanylate cyclase receptor on endothelial cells. As a result, vasodilatory, and anti-mitogenic effects of ANP and BNP in the vasculature could occur in part through CNP production and subsequent action if these interactions occur *in vivo*. In other words, ANP/BNP and CNP paracrine system should share a synergic action on vascular tissues.

Several studies have demonstrated complex interactions betwen CNH and the other endothelium-derived vasorelaxant mediators [267]. Indeed, evidence from cellular, animal, and human studies suggests that all CNH are able to stimulate NO production by endothelial NO synthase (eNOS); this effect is probably mediated by clearance receptor NPR-C [270]. Stimulation of this NPR-C receptor results in decreased cAMP levels by adenyl cyclase inhibition through an inhibitory guanine nucleotide-regulating protein [270]. Furthermore, ANP treatment increases renal and cardiac NO synthesis in rats [274]. On the other hand, NO, released from endothelial cells, negatively modulates ANP secretion from atrial myocytes, induced by mechanical stretch in perfused rat heart preparation [275]. Furthermore, ANP expression is markedly upregulated in eNOS$^{-/-}$ mice, and exogenous ANP restores ventricular relaxation in wild-type mice treated with NOS inhibitors [276]. These data suggest that the CNH and NO systems are linked by a negative feedback mechanism. Finally, CNH (and especially CNP) mimic many of the anti-atherogenic actions of PGI$_2$ and NO [267]. This gives rise to the possibility that CNP might compensate for the loss of these mediators in cardiovascular pathologies to restore the vasodilator capacity of the endothelium, in addition to its anti-adhesive and anti-aggregatory influences.

CNH also strongly interact with the effectors of counter-regulatory systems at the vascular tissue level [13, 28, 30, 77, 78, 90-99]. In particular, interactions between CNH and ET-1 also appear to be important physiologically; indeed, the vascular effects of CNH are directly opposite to those of ET-1 [267, 269]; in particular, ET-1-induced vasoconstriction and myocyte hypertrophy is inhibited by CNH. While CNP has little natriuretic and diuretic action compared to ANP or BNP, it is capable of modulating the vascular effects of the local RAAS by opposing potent vasoconstriction to angiotensin II [269]. CNP not only functionally antagonizes ET-1 and angiotensin II, but it also directly modulates ET-1 [277] and angiotensin II [278] synthesis. On the other hand, ET-1 induces an increase in the number of endothelial cells that secrete CNP [279]. Therefore, the parallel production and activity of vasodilator CNP and vasoconstrictors such as ET-1 and angiotensin II allows for tight local regulation of these vasoactive peptides and thus blood flow [267, 269, 279].

Furthermore, the inter-relationships between the CNH system and pro-inflammatory cytokines suggest that cardiac hormones play an important role in mechanisms responsible for cardiac and vascular adaptation, maladaptation and remodeling in response to various physiological and pathological stimuli [32, 35, 62, 162]. The identification of CNP as an EDHF, combined with its expression in endothelial cells, indicates that CNP is suited to modulate the activity of circulating cells, particularly leukocytes and platelets. Moreover, inflammatory stimuli such as IL-1b, TNF and lipopolysaccharide [280] stimulate the release of CNP from isolated endothelial cells. As a result, modulation of the biological activity of CNP is likely to have a profound influence on the development of an inflammatory response. Certainly, an anti-atherogenic activity of CNP fits with the cytoprotective, anti-inflammatory actions of NO and PGI$_2$, the other major endothelium-derived vasorelaxants [267, 269-271, 280].

From a clinical point of view, it is important to note that exogenous application of CNP in situations where endothelial NO production is compromised might be therapeutic in disorders that are associated with endothelial dysfunction. For example, overexpression of CNP by adenoviral-gene delivery in veins dramatically reduces the luminal narrowing (neointimal hyperplasia) that develops when it is grafted to the carotid artery, thereby retaining patency of the graft [281]. CNH, including CNP, also suppress the production of pro-inflammatory cyclooxygenase 2 metabolites in isolated cells [106, 282]. Other studies demonstrated a direct effect of CNP on immune-cell recruitment *in vivo* [267, 271]. Therefore, like NO, endothelial CNP (like ANP and BNP) exerts a protective anti-inflammatory effect [104-106, 267, 271, 283]. This inhibitory effect of CNH on leukocytes indicates that these peptides modulate the expression of adhesion molecules on either the endothelium or leukocytes.

Several data support the thesis that CNH (and especially CNP) are important, endogenous, anti-atherogenic mediators. CNP is a potent inhibitor of vascular smooth muscle migration and proliferation that is stimulated by oxidized LDL [277]. CNP also inhibits the proliferation of vascular smooth muscle [284], and enhances endothelial cell regeneration *in vitro* and *in vivo* [281]. The observation that CNP alters leukocyte-endothelial interactions indicates that it might also affect platelet function. In accordance with this, thrombus formation is suppressed significantly in the presence of CNP [280], which indicates that inhibition of coagulation might contribute to the vasoprotective properties of this peptide. Observations that CNP blocks platelet aggregation, induced by thrombin, confirm that endothelium-derived CNP also exerts an anti-thrombotic effect [267].

All the above-mentioned studies demonstrate that CNH (and especially CNP) exert a protective effect on endothelial function by decreasing shear stress, modulating coagulation and fibrinolysis pathways, and inhibiting platelet activation (Fig. 3.15). They can also inhibit the vascular remodeling process as well as coronary restenosis post-angioplasty [56, 84-89, 267, 281, 283]. These vasoprotective actions should be considered as a result of complex inter-relationships between the CNH system and both the synergic (including NO, PGI_2, and other endothelium-derived vasoactive mediators) and the counter-regulatory systems (including endothelins, RAAS, cytokines, and growth factors).

3.10 Summary and Conclusion

Natriuretic peptides (including ANP, BNP, CNP, DNP and urodilatin) constitute a family of peptide hormones and neurotransmitters, sharing a similar peptide chain, characterized by a cysteine bridge (Fig. 3.1). The physiological relevance of these peptides is well demonstrated by their presence since the first dawning of life, from unicellular to pluricellular organisms, including plants and all animals. Furthermore, their genes have been repeatedly doubled during evolution, starting from an ancestral gene, thus suggesting that these peptides are indispensable for life (Fig. 3.6).

CNH have powerful physiological effects on the cardiovascular system, body fluid, and electrolyte homeostasis. These effects can be explained at least in part by the inhibition of counter-regulatory systems, including the sympathetic nervous system, RAAS, the vasopressin/antidiuretic hormone system, the endothelin system, cytokines and growth factors.

The endocrine action shared by plasma ANP and BNP can be enhanced by natriuretic peptides produced locally in target tissues (paracrine action). Indeed, endothelial cells synthesize CNP, which exerts a paracrine action on vessels. Moreover, renal tubular cells produce urodilatin, another member of the peptide natriuretic family, which shows powerful diuretic and natriuretic properties. Genes for natriuretic peptides (including ANP, BNP and CNP) are also expressed in the central nervous system, where they likely act as neurotransmitters and/or neuromodulators. Finally, co-expression of CNH and their receptors was observed in immunocompetent cells, suggesting that CNH may have immunomodulatory and anti-inflammatory functions in mammals. Furthermore, CNH are expressed in almost all the body tissues as well as their specific receptors, including organs and tissues not discussed in this chapter, such as gut [285], skeletal [106] and ocular [286] tissues. In all tissues, CNH could also act as a local mediator or paracrine effector of tissue-specific functions.

These data, taken as a whole, strongly suggest that natriuretic peptides constitute a family sharing endocrine, paracrine and autocrine actions and neurotransmitter and immunomodulator functions. Therefore, it can be hypothesized that the CNH system is closely related to the other regulatory systems (nervous, endocrine and immunological) in a biological hierarchical network (Fig. 3.16) [287, 288].

References

1. Takei Y (2001) Does the natriuretic peptide system exist throughout the animal and plant kingdom? Comp Biochem Physiol Part B 129:559-573
2. Vesely DL, Giordano AT (1991) Atrial natriuretic peptide hormonal system in plants. Biochem Biophys Res Commun 179:695-700
3. Billington T, Pharmawati M, Gehring CA (1997) Isolation and immunoaffinity purification of biologically active plant natriuretic peptide. Biochem Biophys Res Commun 235:722-725
4. Loretz CA, Pollina C (2000) Natriuretic peptides in fish physiology. Comp Biochem Physiol Part A 125:169-187
5. Kawakoshi A, Hyodo S, Yasuda A, Takei Y (2003) A single and novel natriuretic peptide is expressed in the heart and brain of the most primitive vertebrate, the hagfish (*Eptatretus burgeri*). J Mol Endocrinol 31:209-220
6. Kawakoshi A, Hyodo S, Inoue K et al (2004) Four natriuretic peptides (ANP, BNP, VNP and CNP) coexist in the sturgeon: identification of BNP in fish lineage. J Mol Endocrinol 32:547-555
7. Arden KC, Viars CS, Weiss S et al (1995) Localization of the human B-type natriuretic peptide precursor (NPPB) gene to chromosome 1p36. Genomics 26: 385-389
8. Yang-Feng TL, Floyd-Smith G, Nemer M et al (1985) The pronatriodilatin gene is located on the distal short arm of human chromosome 1 and on mouse chromosome 4. Am J Hum Genet 37:1117-1128
9. Steinhelper ME (1993) Structure, expression, and genomic mapping of the mouse natriuretic peptide type-B gene. Circ Res 72:984-992
10. Ogawa Y, Itoh H, Yoshitake Y et al (1994) Molecular cloning and chromosomal assignment of the mouse C-type natriuretic peptide (CNP) gene (Nppc): comparison with the human CNP gene (NPPC). Genomics 24:383-387
11. De Bold AJ, Borenstein HB, Veress AT, Sonnenberg H (1981) A rapid and important natriuretic response to intravenous injection of atrial myocardial extracts in rats. Life Sci 28:89-94
12. De Bold AJ, Bruneau BG, Kuroski de Bold ML (1996) Mechanical and neuroendocrine regulation of the endocrine heart. Cardiovasc Res 31:7-18
13. McGrath MF, de Bold AJ (2005) Determinants of natriuretic peptide gene expression. Peptides 26:933-943
14. Goetze JP (2004) Biochemistry of pro-B-type natriuretic peptide-derived peptides: the endocrine heart revisited. Clin Chem 9:1503-1510
15. Belenky A, Smith A, Zhang B et al (2004) The effect of class-specific protease inhibitors on the stabilization of B-type natriuretic peptide in human plasma. Clin Chim Acta 340:163-172
16. Shimizu H, Masuta K, Aono K et al (2002) Molecular forms of human brain natriuretic peptide in plasma. Clin Chim Acta 316:129-135
17. Shimizu H, Masuta K, Asada H et al (2003) Characterization of molecular forms of probrain natriuretic peptide in human plasma. Clin Chim Acta 334:233-239
18. LaPointe MC (2005) Molecular regulation of the brain natriuretic gene. Peptides 26:944-956
19. Sumida H, Yasue H, Yoshimura M et al (1995) Comparison of secretion pattern between A-

type and B-type natriuretic peptides in patients with old myocardial infarction. J Am Col Cardiol 25:1105-1110

20. Nakagawa O, Ogawa Y, Itoh H et al (1995) Rapid transcriptional activation and early mRNA turnover of brain natriuretic peptide in cardiocyte hypertrophy. J Clin Invest 96:1280-1287

21. Vanderheyden M, Bartunek J, Goethals M (2004) Brain and other natriuretic peptides: molecular aspects. Eur J Heart Fail 6:261-268

22. Ma KK, Banas K, de Bold AJ (2005) Determinants of inducible brain natriuretic peptide promoter activity. Regul Pept 128:169-176

23. Temsah R, Nemer M (2005) GATA factors and transcriptional regulation of cardiac natriuretic peptide genes. Regul Pept 128:177-185

24. Tsuruda T, Boerrigter G, Huntley BK et al (2002) Brain natriuretic peptide is produced in cardiac fibroblasts and induces matrix metalloproteinases. Circ Res 91:1127-1134

25. Nicolau N, Butur G, Laky D (1997) Electronmicroscopic observations regarding the presence of natriuretic granules in the ventricle of patients with cardiopathies. Rom J Morphol Embryol 43:119-137

26. Hasegawa K, Fujiwara H, Doyama K et al (1993) Ventricular expression of atrial and brain natriuretic peptides in dilated cardiomyopathy. An immunohistocytochemical study of the endomyocardial biopsy specimens using specific monoclonal antibodies. Am J Pathol 142:107-116

27. Luchner A, Stevens TL, Borgeson DD et al (1998) Differential atrial and ventricular expression of myocardial BNP during evolution of heart failure. Am J Physiol 274:H1684-1689

28. Clerico A, Emdin M (2004) Diagnostic accuracy and prognostic relevance of the measurement of the cardiac natriuretic peptides: a review. Clin Chem 50:33-50

29. Qi W, Kjekshus J, Hall C (2000) Differential responses of plasma atrial and brain natriuretic peptides to acute alteration in atrial pressure in pigs. Scand J Clin Lab Invest 60:55-63

30. Clerico A (2002) Pathophysiological and clinical relevance of circulating levels of cardiac natriuretic hormones: is their assay merely a marker of cardiac disease? Clin Chem Lab Med 40:752-760

31. Kato J, Etoh T, Kitamura K, Eto T (2005) Atrial and brain natriuretic peptides as markers of cardiac load and volume retention in primary aldosteronism. Am J Hypertens 18:354-357

32. Tenhunen O, Szokodi I, Ruskoaho H (2005) Posttranscriptional activation of BNP gene expression in response to increased left ventricular wall stress: role of calcineurin and PKC. Regul Pept 128:187-196

33. Sakata Y, Yamamoto K, Masuyama T et al (2001) Ventricular production of natriuretic peptides and ventricular structural remodelling in hypertensive heart failure. J Hypertens 19:1905-1909

34. Takahashi N, Saito Y, Kuwahara K et al (2003) Angiotensin II-induced ventricular hypertrophy and extracellular signal-regulated kinase activation are suppressed in mice overexpressing brain natriuretic peptide in circulation. Hypertens Res 26:847-853

35. Walther T, Klostermann K, Hering-Walther S et al (2003) Fibrosis rather than blood pressure determines cardiac BNP expression in mice. Regul Pept 116:95-100

36. Fredj S, Bescond J, Louault C, Potreau D (2004) Interactions between cardiac cells enhance cardiomyocyte hypertrophy and increase fibroblast proliferation. J Cell Physiol (published online, September 7, 2004)

37. Chen YF (2005) Atrial natriuretic peptide in hypoxia. Peptides 26:1068-1077

38. Hama N, Itoh H, Shirakami G et al (1995) Rapid ventricular induction of brain natriuretic peptide gene expression in experimental acute myocardial infarction. Circulation 92:1158-1164

39. Toth M, Vuorinen KH, Vuolteenaho O et al (1994) Hypoxia stimulates release of ANP and BNP from perfused rat ventricular myocardium. Am J Physiol 266(4 Pt2):H1572-580

40. Baxter GF (2004) Natriuretic peptides and myocardial ischaemia. Basic Res Cardiol 99:90-93

41. Jernberg T, James S, Lindahl B et al (2004) Natriuretic peptides in unstable coronary artery disease. Eur Heart J 25:1486-1493

42. Foote RS, Pearlman JD, Siegel AH, Yeo KT (2004) Detection of exercise-induced ischemia by changes in B-type natriuretic peptides. J Am Coll Cardiol 44:1980-1987

43. Sabatine MS, Morrow DA, de Lemos JA et al (2004) TIMI Study Group. Acute changes in circulating natriuretic peptide levels in relation to myocardial ischemia. J Am Coll Cardiol 44:1988-1995

44. Goetze JP, Gore A, Moller CH et al (2004) Acute myocardial hypoxia increases BNP gene expression. FASEB J 18:1928-1930
45. Wu X, Seino Y, Ogura H et al (2001) Plasma natriuretic peptide levels and daily physical activity in patients with pacemaker implantation. Jpn Heart J 42:471-482
46. Kinugawa T, Kato M, Ogino K et al (2003) Neurohormonal determinants of peak oxygen uptake in patients with chronic heart failure. Jpn Heart J 44:725-734
47. Williams SG, Ng LL, O'Brien RJ et al (2004) Comparison of plasma N-brain natriuretic peptide, peak oxygen consumption, and left ventricular ejection fraction for severity of chronic heart failure. Am J Cardiol 93:1560-1561
48. Kuroski de Bold ML (1999) Estrogen, natriuretic peptides and the renin-angiotensin system. Cardiovasc Res 41:524-531
49. Maffei S, Del Ry S, Prontera C, Clerico A (2001) Increase in circulating levels of cardiac natriuretic peptides after hormone replacement therapy in postmenopausal women. Clin Sci 101:447-453
50. Tanaka T, Kanda T, Takahashi T et al (2004) Interleukin-6-induced reciprocal expression of SERCA and natriuretic peptides mRNA in cultured rat ventricular myocytes. J Int Med Res 32:57-61
51. Witthaut R, Busch C, Fraunberger P et al (2003) Plasma atrial natriuretic peptide and brain natriuretic peptide are increased in septic shock: impact of interleukin-6 and sepsis-associated left ventricular dysfunction. Intensive Care Med 29:1696-1702
52. Hiraoka E, Kawashima S, Takahashi T et al (2003) PI 3-kinase-Akt-p70 S6 kinase in hypertrophic responses to leukemia inhibitory factor in cardiac myocytes. Kobe J Med Sci 49:25-37
53. Deten A, Volz HC, Briest W, Zimmer HG (2002) Cardiac cytokine expression is upregulated in the acute phase after myocardial infarction. Experimental studies in rats. Cardiovasc Res 55:329-340
54. Hamanaka I, Saito Y, Nishikimi T et al (2000) Effects of cardiotrophin-1 on hemodynamics and endocrine function of the heart. Am J Physiol Heart Circ Physiol 279:H388-396
55. Takahashi N, Saito Y, Kuwahara K et al (2003) Angiotensin II-induced ventricular hypertrophy and extracellular signal-regulated kinase acivation are suppressed in mice overexpressing brain natriuretic peptide in circulation. Hypertens Res 26:847-853
56. Ma KK, Ogawa T, de Bold AJ (2004) Selective upregulation of cardiac brain natriuretic peptide at the transcriptional and translational levels by pro-inflammatory cytokines and by conditioned medium derived from mixed lymphocyte reactions via p38 MAP kinase. J Mol Cell Cardiol 36:505-513
57. Woodard GE, Rosado JA, Brown J (2002) Expression and control of C-type natriuretic peptide in rat vascular smooth muscle cells. Am J Physiol Reg Int Comp Physiol 282:R156-165
58. Harada E, Hakagawa O, Yoshimura M et al (1999) Effect of interleukin-1β on cardiac hypertrophy and production of natriuretic peptides in rat cardiocyte culture. J Mol Cell Cardiol 31:1997-2006
59. He Q, LaPointe MC (1999) Interleukin-1b regulation of the human brain natriuretic peptide promoter involves Ras-, Rac-, and p38 kinase-dependent pathways in cardiac myocytes. Hypertension 33(part II):283-289
60. Kinugawa T, Kato M, Ogino K et al (2003) Interleukin-6 and tumor necrosis factor-α levels increase in response to maximal exercise in patients with chronic heart failure. Int J Cardiol 87:83-90
61. Witthaut R, Busch C, Fraunberger P et al (2003) Plasma atrial natriuretic peptide and brain natriuretic peptide are increased in septic shock: impact of interleukin-6 and sepsis-associated left ventricular dysfunction. Intensive Care Med 29:1696-1702
62. Glembotski CC, Irons CE, Krown KA et al (1993) Myocardial a-thrombin receptor activation induces hypertrophy and increases atrial natriuretic factor gene expression. J Biol Chem 268:20646-20652
63. Knowlton KU, Baraccini E, Ross RS et al (1991) Co-regulation of the atrial natriuretic factor and cardiac myosin light chain-2 genes during α-adrenergic stimulation of neonatal rat ventricular cells. J Biol Chem 266:7759-7768

64. Sprenkle AB, Murray SF, Glemboski CC (1995) Involvement of multiple *cis* elements in basal- and α-adrenergic agonist-inducible atrial natriuretic factor transcription. Circul Res 77:1060-1069
65. Thuerauf DJ, Arnold ND, Zechner D et al (1998) p38 Mitogen-activated protein kinase mediates the transcriptional induction of the atrial natriuretic factor gene through a serum response element. A potential role for the transcription factor ATF6. J Biol Chem 273:20636-20643
66. King KL, Winer J, Phillips DM et al (1998) Phenylephrine, endothelin, prostaglandin F2 alpha and leukemia inhibitory factor induce different cardiac hypertrophy phenotypes *in vitro*. Endocrine 9:45-55
67. Ander AN, Duggirala SK, Drumm JD, Roth DM (2004) Natriuretic peptide gene expression after beta-adrenergic stimulation in adult mouse cardiac myocytes. DNA Cell Biol 23:586-591
68. He Q, Wu G, LaPointe MC (2000) Isoproterenol and cAMP regulation of the human brain natriuretic peptide gene involves Src and Rac. Am J Physiol Endocrinol Metab 278:E1115-1123
69. Nakaoka H, Kitahara Y, Amano M et al (1987) Effect of beta-adrenergic receptor blockade on atrial natriuretic peptide in essential hypertension. Hypertension 10:221-225
70. Hama J, Nagata S, Takenaka T et al (1995) Atrial natriuretic peptide and antihypertensive action due to beta-blockade in essential hypertensive patients. Angiology 46:511-516
71. van den Meiracker AH, Lameris TW, van de Ven LL, Boomsma F (2003) Increased plasma concentration of natriuretic peptides by selective beta1-blocker bisoprolol. J Cardiovasc Pharmacol 42:462-468
72. Yoshizawa A, Yoshikawa T, Nakamura I et al (2004) Brain natriuretic peptide response is heterogeneous during beta-blocker therapy for congestive heart failure. J Card Fail 10:310-315
73. Richards AM, Lainchbury JG, Nicholls MG et al (2002) BNP in hormone-guided treatment of heart failure. Trends Endocrinol Metab 13:151-155
74. Takeda Y, Fukutomi T, Suzuki S et al (2004) Effects of carvedilol on plasma B-type natriuretic peptide concentration and symptoms in patients with heart failure and preserved ejection fraction. Am J Cardiol 94:448-453
75. Tokudome T, Horio T, Yoshihara F et al (2004) Direct effects of high glucose and insulin on protein synthesis in cultured cardiac myocytes and DNA and collagen synthesis in cardiac fibroblasts. Metabolism 53:710-715
76. Hongo M, Ryoke T, Schoenfeld J et al (2000) Effects of growth hormone on cardiac dysfunction and gene expression in genetic murine dilated cardiomyopathy. Basic Res Cardiol 95:431-441
77. de Lemos JA, McGuire DK, Drazner MH (2003) B-type natriuretic peptide in cardiovascular disease. Lancet 362:316-322
78. Ruskoaho H (2003) Cardiac hormones as diagnostic tools in heart failure. Endocr Rev 24:341-356
79. Zhang Q, Moalem J, Tse J et al (2005) Effects of natriuretic peptides on ventricular myocyte contraction and role of cyclic GMP signaling. Eur J Pharmacol 510:209-215
80. Nagaya N, Nishikimi T, Goto Y et al (1998) Plasma brain natriuretic peptide is a biochemical marker for the prediction of progressive ventricular remodeling after acute myocardial infarction. Am Heart J 135:21-28
81. Hayashi M, Tsutamoto T, Wada A et al (2001) Intravenous atrial natriuretic peptide prevents left ventricular remodeling in patients with first anterior acute myocardial infarction. J Am Coll Cardiol 37:1820-1826
82. Magga J, Puhakka M, Hietakorpi S et al (2004) Atrial natriuretic peptide, B-type natriuretic peptide, and serum collagen markers after acute myocardial infarction. J Appl Physiol 96:1306-1311
83. Hardt SE, Sadoshima J (2004) Negative regulators of cardiac hypertrophy. Cardiovasc Res 63:500-509
84. Chen HH, Burnett JC Jr (1998) C-type natriuretic peptide: the endothelial component of the natriuretic peptide system. J Cardiovasc Pharmacol 32(Suppl.3):S22-28
85. Morishige K, Shimokawa H, Yamawaki T et al (2000) Local adenovirus-mediated transfer of C-type natriuretic peptide suppresses vascular remodeling in porcine coronary arteries *in vivo*. J Am Coll Cardiol 35:1040-1047
86. Takeuchi H, Ohmori K, Kondo I et al (2003) Potentiation of C-type natriuretic peptide with ultrasound and microbubbles to prevent neointimal formation after vascular injury in rats. Cardiovasc Res 58:231-238

87. Yasuda S, Kanna M, Sakuragi S et al (2002) Local delivery of single low-dose of C-type natriuretic peptide, an endogenous vascular modulator, inhibits neointimal hyperplasia in a balloon-injured rabbit iliac artery model. J Cardiovasc Pharmacol 39:784-788

88. Qian JY, Haruno A, Asada Y et al (2002) Local expression of C-type natriuretic peptide suppresses inflammation, eliminates shear stress-induced thrombosis, and prevents neointima formation through enhanced nitric oxide production in rabbit injured carotid arteries. Circ Res 91:1063-1069

89. Nakanishi M, Saito Y, Kishimoto I et al (2005) Role of natriuretic peptide receptor guanylyl cyclase-A in myocardial infarction evaluated using genetically engineered mice. Hypertension 46:1-7

90. Ventura RR, Gomes DA, Reis WL et al (2002) Nitrergic modulation of vasopressin, oxytocin and atrial natriuretic peptide secretion in response to sodium intake and hypertonic blood volume expansion. Braz J Med Biol Res 35:1101-1109

91. Vatta MS, Presas M, Bianciotti LG et al (1996) B and C types natriuretic peptides modulate norepinephrine uptake and release in the rat hypothalamus. Regul Pept 16:175-184

92. Vatta MS, Presas M, Bianciotti LG et al (1997) B and C types natriuretic peptides modify norepinephrine uptake and release in the rat adrenal medulla. Peptides 18:1483-1489

93. Fermepin M, Vatta MS, Presas M et al (2000) B-type and C-type natriuretic peptides modify norepinephrine uptake in discrete encephalic nuclei of the rat. Cell Mol Neurobiol 20:763-771

94. Brunner-La Rocca HP, Kaye DM, Woods RL et al (2001) Effects of intravenous brain natriuretic peptide on regional sympathetic activity in patients with chronic heart failure as compared with healthy control subjects. J Am Coll Cardiol 37:1221-1227

95. Tsukagoshi H, Shimizu Y, Kawata T et al (2001) Atrial natriuretic peptide inhibits tumor necrosis factor-alpha production by interferon-gamma-activated macrophages via suppression of p38 mitogen-activated protein kinase and nuclear factor-kappa B activation. Reg Pept 99:21-29

96. Kiemer AK, Weber NC, Furst R et al (2002) Inhibition of p38 MAPK activation via induction of MKP-1 atrial natriuretic peptide reduces TNF-a-induced actin polymerization and endothelial permeability. Circ Res 90:874-881

97. Weber NC, Blumenthal SB, Hartung T et al (2003) ANP inhibits TNF-alpha-induced endothelial MCP-1 expression - involvement of p38 MAPK and MKP-1. J Leukoc Biol 74:932-941

98. Kapoun AM, Liang F, O'Young G et al (2004) B-type natriuretic peptide exerts broad functional opposition to transforming growth factor-beta in primary human cardiac fibroblasts: fibrosis, myofibroblasts conversion, proliferation, and inflammation. Circ Res 94:453-461

99. Vollmar AM (2005) The role of atrial natriuretic peptide in the immune system. Peptides 26:1086-1094

100. Vesely DL (2003) Natriuretic peptides and acute renal failure. Am J Physiol Renal Physiol 285:F167-177

101. Imura H, Nakao K, Itoh H (1992) The natriuretic peptide system in the brain: implications in the central control of cardiovascular and neuroendocrine functions. Front Neuroendocrinol 13:217-249

102. Langub MC Jr, Watson RE Jr, Herman JP (1995) Distribution of natriuretic peptide precursor mRNAs in the rat brain. J Comp Neurol 356:183-199

103. Perras B, Schultes B, Behn B et al (2004) Intranasal atrial natriuretic peptide acts as central nervous inhibitor of the hypothalamo-pituitary-adrenal stress system in humans. J Clin Endocrinol Metab 89:4642-4648

104. Vollmar AM, Wolf R, Schulz R (1995) Co-expression of the natriuretic peptides (ANP, BNP, CNP) and their receptors in normal and acutely involuted rat thymus. J Neuroimmunol 57:117-127

105. Vollmar AM, Schultz R (1995) Expression and differential regulation of natriuretic peptides in mouse macrophages. J Clin Invest 95:2442-2450

106. Vollmar AM, Kiemer AK (2001) Immunomodulatory and cytoprotective function of atrial natriuretic peptide. Crit Rev Immunol 21:473-485

107. Waschek JA (2004) Developmental actions of natriuretic peptides in the brain and skeleton. Cell Mol Life Sci 61:2332-2342

108. Kiefer F, Wiedemann K (2004) Neuroendocrine pathways of addictive behaviour. Addict Biol 9(205):12
109. Bex F, Corbin A (1985) Atrial natriuretic factor stimulates testosterone production by mouse interstitial cells. Eur J Pharmacol 115:125-126
110. Foresta C, Mioni R, Careto A (1987) Specific binding and steroidogenic effects of atrial natriuretic factor in Leydig cells of rats. Arch Androl 19:253-259
111. El-Gehani F, Tena-Sempere M, Ruskoaho H, Huhtaniemi I (2000) Natriuretic peptides stimulate steroidogenesis in the fetal rat testis. Biol Reprod 65:595-600
112. Pandey KN (2005) Biology of natriuretic peptides and their receptors. Peptides 26:901-932
113. Gutkowska J, Tremblay J, Antakly T et al (1993) The atrial natriuretic peptide system in rat ovaries. Endocrinology 132:693-700
114. Vollmer AM, Mytzka C, Arendt RM, Schulz R (1988) Atrial natriuretic peptide in bovine corpus luteum. Endocrinology 123:762-767
115. Ivanova MD, Gregoraszczuk EL, Augustowska K et al (2003) Localization of atrial natriuretic peptide in pig granulosa cells isolated from ovarian follicles of various size. Reprod Biol 3:173-181
116. Chatterjee PK, Hawksworthy GM, McLay JS (1999) Cytokine-stimulated nitric oxide production in the human renal proximal tubule and its modulation by natriuretic peptides: a novel immunomodulatory mechanism? Exp Nephrol 7:438-448
117. Ruskoaho H, Leskinen H, Magga J et al (1997) Mechanisms of mechanical load-induced atrial natriuretic peptide secretion: role of endothelin, nitric oxide, and angiotensin II. J Mol Med 75:876-885
118. Gyurko R, Kuhlencordt P, Fishman MC, Huang OL (2000) Modulation of mouse cardiac function *in vivo* by eNOS and ANP. Am J Physiol 278:H971-981
119. Tanaka Y, Nagai M, Date T et al (2005) Effects of bradykinin on cardiovascular remodeling in renovascular hypertensive rats. Hypertens Res 27:865-875
120. Booz GW (2005) Putting the brakes on cardiac hypertrophy: exploiting the NO-cGMP counter-regulatory system. Hypertension 45:341-346
121. Kruger S, Graf J, Merx MW et al (2004) Brain natriuretic peptide predicts right heart failure in patients with acute pulmonary embolism. Am Heart J 147:60-65
122. Pruszczyk P, Kostrubiec M, Bochowicz A et al (2003) N-terminal pro-brain natriuretic peptide in patients with acute pulmonary embolism. Eur Respir J 22:649-653
123. Kucher N, Printzen G, Goldhaber SZ (2003) Prognostic role of brain natriuretic peptide in acute pulmonary embolism. Circulation 107:2545-2547
124. ten Wolde M, Tulevski II, Mulder JW et al (2003) Brain natriuretic peptide as a predictor of adverse outcome in patients with pulmonary embolism. Circulation 107:2082-2084
125. Ando T, Ogawa K, Yamaki K et al (1996) Plasma concentrations of atrial, brain, and C-type natriuretic peptides and endothelin-1 in patients with chronic respiratory diseases. Chest 110:462-468
126. Maeder M, Ammann P, Rickli H, Diethelm M (2003) Elevation of B-type natriuretic peptide levels in acute respiratory distress syndrome. Swiss Med Wkly 133:515-518
127. Nagaya N, Nishikimi T, Uematsu M et al (2000) Plasma brain natriuretic peptide as a prognostic indicator in patients with primary pulmonary hypertension. Circulation 102:865-870
128. Leuchte HH, Neurohr C, Baumgartner R et al (2004) Brain natriuretic peptide and exercise capacity in lung fibrosis and pulmonary hypertension. Am J Respir Crit Care Med 170:360-365
129. Leuchte HH, Holzapfel M, Baumgartner RA et al (2004) Clinical significance of brain natriuretic peptide in primary pulmonary hypertension. J Am Coll Cardiol 43:764-770
130. Kohno M, Horio T, Yasunari K et al (1993) Stimulation of brain natriuretic peptide release from heart by thyroid hormone. Metabolism 42:1059-1064
131. Bernstein R, Midtbo K, Urdal P et al (1997) Serum N-terminal pro-atrial natriuretic factor 1-98 before and during thyroxine replacement therapy in severe hypothyroidism. Thyroid 7:415-419
132. Parlapiano C, Campana E, Alessandri N et al (1998) Plasma atrial natriuretic hormone in hyperthyroidism. Endocr Res 24:105-112

133. Schultz M, Faber J, Kistorp C et al (2004) N-terminal-pro-B-type natriuretic peptide (NT-pro-BNP) in different thyroid function states. Clin Endocrinol 60:54-59

134. Jensen KT, Carstens J, Ivarsen P, Pedersen EB (1997) A new, fast and reliable radioiimunoassay of brain natriuretic peptide in human plasma. Reference values in healthy subjects and in patients with different diseases. Scand J Clin Lab Invest 57:529-540

135. Sugawara A, Nakao K, Itoh H et al (1988) Cosecretion of peptides derived from gamma-human atrial natriuretic polypeptide in normal volunteers and patients with essential hypertension and adrenal disorders. J Hypertens 6(Suppl 4):S327-329

136. Fujio N, Ohashi M, Nawata H et al (1989) Cardiovascular, renal and endocrine effects of a-human atrial natriuretic peptide in patients with Cushing's syndrome and primary aldosteronism. J Hypertens 7:653-659

137. Opocher G, Rocco S, Carpene G et al (1990) Atrial natriuretic peptide in Cushing's disease. J Endocrinol Invest 13:133-137

138. Lapinski M, Stepniakowski K, Januszewicz A et al (1991) Plasma atrial natriuretic peptide concentration in patients with primary aldosteronism. J Hypertens 9(Suppl 6):S260-261

139. Cappuccio FP, Markandu ND, Buckley MG et al (1989) Raised plasma levels of atrial natriuretic peptides in Addison's disease. J Endocrinol Invest 12:205-207

140. Straub RH, Hall C, Kramer BK et al (1996) Atrial natriuretic factor and digoxin-like immunoreactive factor in diabetic patients: their interrelation and the influence of the autonomic nervous system. J Clin Endocrinol Metab 81:3385-3389

141. Bhalla MA, Chiang A, Epshteyn VA et al (2004) Prognostic role of B-type natriuretic peptide levels in patients with type 2 diabetes mellitus. J Am Coll Cardiol 44:1047-1052

142. La Villa G, Riccardi D, Lazzeri C et al (1995) Blunted natriuretic response to low-dose brain natriuretic peptide infusion in non azotemic cirrhotic patients with ascites and avid sodium retention. Hepatology 22:1745-1750

143. Salo J, Jimenez W, Kuhn M et al (1996) Urinary excretion of urodilatin in patients with cirrhosis. Hepatology 24:1428-1432

144. Henriksen JH, Gotze JP, Fuglsang S et al (2003) Increased circulating pro-brain natriuretic peptide (proBNP) and brain natriuretic peptide (BNP) in patients with cirrhosis: relation to cardiovascular dysfunction and severity of disease. Gut 52:1511-1517

145. McCullough PA, Kuncheria J, Mathur VS (2004) Diagnostic and therapeutic utility of B-type natriuretic peptide in patients with renal insufficiency and decompensated heart failure. Rev Cardiovasc Med 5:16-25

146. Castillo JR, Zagler A, Carrillo-Jimenez R, Hennekens CH (2004) Brain natriuretic peptide: a potential marker for mortality in septic shock. Int J Infect Dis 8:271-274

147. Witthaut R, Busch C, Fraunberger P et al (2003) Plasma atrial natriuretic peptide and brain natriuretic peptide are increased in septic shock: impact of interleukin-6 and sepsis-associated left ventricular dysfunction. Intensive Care Med 29:1696-1702

148. Takemura G, Takatsu Y, Doyama K et al (1998) Expression of atrial and brain natriuretic peptides and their genes in hearts of patients with cardiac amyloidosis. J Am Coll Cardiol 31:254-265

149. Palladini G, Campana C, Klersy C et al (2003) Serum N-terminal pro-brain natriuretic peptide is a sensitive marker of myocardial dysfunction in AL amyloidosis. Circulation 107:2440-2445

150. McGirt MJ, Blessing R, Nimjee SM et al (2004) Correlation of serum brain natriuretic peptide with hyponatremia and delayed ischemic neurological deficits after subarachnoid hemorrhage. Neurosurgery 54:1369-1373

151. Fukui S, Nawashiro H, Otani N et al (2003) Focal brain edema and natriuretic peptides in patients with subarachnoid hemorrhage. Acta Neurochir Suppl 86:489-491

152. Kurokawa Y, Uede T, Ishiguro M et al (1996) Pathogenesis of hyponatremia following subarachnoid hemorrhage due to ruptured cerebral aneurysm. Surg Neurol 46:500-507

153. Fukui S, Katoh H, Tsuzuki N et al (2004) Focal brain edema and natriuretic peptides in patients with subarachnoid hemorrhage. J Clin Neurosci 11:507-511

154. Mimura Y, Kanauchi H, Ogawa T, Oohara T (1996) Resistance to natriuresis in patients with peritonitis carcinomatosa. Horm Metab Res 28:183-186

155. Marchioli CC, Graziano SL (1997) Paraneoplastic syndromes associated with small cell lung cancer. Chest Surg Clin N Am 7:65-80

156. Johnson BE, Damodaran A, Rushin J et al (1997) Ectopic production and processing of atrial natriuretic peptide in a small cell. Cancer 79:35-44

157. Hayakawa H, Komada Y, Hirayama M et al (2001) Plasma levels of natriuretic peptides in relation to doxorubicin-induced cardiotoxicity and cardiac function in children with cancer. Med Pediatr Oncol 37:4-9

158. Suzuki T, Hayashi D, Yamazaki T et al (1998) Elevated B-type natriuretic peptide levels after anthracycline administration. Am Heart J 136:362-363

159. Nousiainen T, Jantunen E, Vanninen E et al (1998) Acute neurohumoral and cardiovascular effects of idarubicin in leukemia patients. Eur J Haematol 61:347-353

160. Nousiainen T, Jantunen E, Vanninen E et al (1999) Natriuretic peptides as markers of cardiotoxicity during doxorubicin treatment for non-Hodgkin's lymphoma. Eur J Haematol 62:135-141

161. Okumura H, Iuchi K, Yoshida T et al (2000) Brain natriuretic peptide is a predictor of anthracycline-induced cardiotoxicity. Acta Haematol 104:158-163

162. Mukoyama M, Nakao K, Obata K et al (1991) Augmented secretion of brain natriuretic peptide in acute myocardial infarction. Biochem Biophys Res Commun 15: 431-436

163. Morita E, Yasue H, Yoshimura M et al (1993) Increased plasma levels of brain natriuretic peptide in patients with acute myocardial infarction. Circulation 88:82-91

164. Anand-Srivastava MB, Trachte GJ (1993) Atrial natriuretic factor receptors and signal transduction mechanisms. Pharmacol Rev 45:455-497

165. Kuhn M (2004) Molecular physiology of natriuretic peptide signalling. Basic Res Cardiol 99:76-82

166. Lohmann SM, Vaandrager AB, Smolenski A et al (1997) Distinct and specific functions of cGMP-dependent protein kinases. Trend Biochem Sci 22:307-312

167. Pfeifer A, Ruth P, Dostmann W et al (1999) Structure and function of cGMP-dependent protein kinases. Rev Physiol Biochem Pharmacol 135:105-149

168. Ahluwalia A, MacAllister RJ, Hobbs AJ (2004) Vascular actions of natriuretic peptides. Cyclic GMP-dependent and -independent mechanisms. Basic Res Cardiol 99:83-89

169. Potter LR, Hunter T (1998) Identification and characterization of the major phosphorylation sites of the B-type natriuretic peptide receptor. J Biol Chem 273:15533-15539

170. Potter LR, Hunter T (1998) Phosphorylation of the kinase homology domain is essential for activation of the A-type natriuretic peptide receptor. Mol Cell Biol 18:2164-2172

171. Potter LR (1998) Phosphorylation-dependent regulation of the guanylyl cyclase-linked natriuretic peptide receptor B: dephosphorylation is a mechanism of desensitization. Biochemistry 37:2422-2429

172. Fan D, Bryan PM, Antos LK et al (2005) Down-regulation does not mediate natriuretic peptide-dependent desensitization of natriuretic peptide receptor (NPR)-A or NPR-B. Guanylyl cyclase-linked natriuretic peptide receptors do not internalize. Mol Pharmacol 67:1-10

173. Chinkers M, Wilson EM (1992) Ligand-independent oligomerization of natriuretic peptide receptors. Identification of heteromeric receptors and a dominant negative mutant. J Biol Chem 267:18589-18597

174. Huo X, Abe T, Risono KS (1999) Ligand binding-dependent limited proteolysis of the atrial natriuretic peptide receptor juxtamembrane hinge structure essential for transmembrane signal transduction. Biochemistry 38:16941-16951

175. Labrecque J, McNiccol N, Marquis M, De Lean A (1999) A disulfide-bridged mutant of natriuretic peptide receptor-A displays constitutive activity. Role of receptor dimerization in signal transduction. J Biol Chem 274:9752-9759

176. Labrecque J, Deschenes J, McNiccol N, De Lean A (2001) Agonistic induction of a covalent dimer in a mutant of natriuretic peptide receptor-A documents a juxtamembrane interaction that accompanies receptor activation. J Biol Chem 276:8064-8072

177. Ogawa H, Qiu Y, Ogata CM, Risono KS (2004) Crystal structure of hormone-bound atrial natriuretic peptide receptor extracellular domain: rotation mechanism for transmembrane signal transduction. J Biol Chem 279:28625-28631

178. Duda T, Sharma RK (1990) Regulation of guanylate cyclase activity by atrial natriuretic factor and protein kinase C. Mol Cell Biochem 93:179-184
179. Potter LR, Garber DL (1992) Dephosphorylation of the guanyl cyclase-A receptor causes desensitization. J Biol Chem 267:14531-14534
180. Potter LR, Garber DL (1994) Protein kinase C-dependent desensitization of the atrial natriuretic peptide receptor is mediated by dephosphorylation. J Biol Chem 269:14636-14642
181. Foster DC, Garber DL (1998) Dual role for adenine nucleotide in the regulation of the atrial natriuretic factor receptor subtypes by angiotensin II. J Biol Chem 273:16311-16318
182. Joubert S, Labrecque J, De Lean A (2001) Reduced activity of the NPR-A kinase triggers dephosphorylation and homologous desensitization of the receptor. Biochemistry 40:11096-11105
183. Rathinavelu A, Isom GE (1991) Differential internalization and processing of atrial-natriuretic-factor B and C receptor in PC12 cells. Biochem J 276:493-497
184. Pandey KN, Inagami T, Misono KS (1986) Atrial natriuretic factor receptor on cultured Leydig tumor cells: ligand binding and photoaffinity labeling. Biochemistry 25:8467-8472
185. Pandey KN (1993) Stoichiometric analysis of internalization, recycling and redistribution of photoaffinity-labeled guanylate cyclase/atrial natriuretic factor receptors in cultured murine Leydig tumor cells. J Biol Chem 268:4382-4390
186. Pandey KN, Kumar R, Li M, Nguyen H (2000) Functional domains and expression of truncated atrial natriuretic peptide receptor-A: the carboxyl-terminal regions direct the receptor internalization and sequestration in COS-/ cells. Mol Pharmacol 57:259-267
187. Pandey KN (2001) Dynamics of internalization and sequestration of guanylyl cyclase/atrial natriuretic peptide receptor-A. Can J Physiol Pharmacol 79:631-639
188. Koh GY, Nussenzveig DR, Okolicany J et al (1992) Dynamics of atrial natriuretic factor-guanylate cyclase receptor and receptor-ligand complexes in cultured glomerular mesangial and renomedullary interstitial cells. J Biol Chem 267:11987-11994
189. Vieira MA, Gao M, Nikonova LN, Maack T (2001) Molecular and cellular physiology of the dissociation of atrial natriuretic peptide from guanylyl cyclase A receptors. J Biol Chem 276:36438-36445
190. Anand-Srivastava MB (2005) Natriuretic peptide receptor-C signaling and regulation. Peptides 26:1044-1059
191. Drewett JG, Ziegler RJ, Trachte GJ (1992) Neuromodulatory effects of atrial natriuretic peptides correlate with an inhibition of adenylate cyclase but not an activation of guanylate cyclase. J Pharmacol Exp Ther 260:689-696
192. D'Souza SP, Davis M, Baxter GF (2004) Autocrine and paracrine actions of natriuretic peptides in the heart. Pharmacol Ther 101:113-129
193. Haak T, Jungmann E, Schoffling K (1990) 24-hour variation in atrial natriuretic peptide. Lancet 335:167-168
194. Haak T, Jungmann E, Schoffling K, Usadel KH (1992) Evidence for pulsatile secretion of human atrial natriuretic peptide in healthy subjects. Exp Clin Endocrinol 99:108-109
195. Nugent AM, Onuoha GN, McEneaney DJ et al (1994) Variable patterns of atrial natriuretic peptide secretion in man. Eur J Clin Invest 24:267-274
196. Pedersen EB, Pedersen HB, Jensen KT (1999) Pulsatile secretion of atrial natriuretic peptide and brain natriuretic peptide in healthy humans. Clin Sci 97:201-206
197. Bentzen H, Pedersen RS, Pedersen HB et al (2003) Abnormal rhythmic oscillations of atrial natriuretic peptide and brain natriuretic peptide in heart failure. Clin Sci 104:303-312
198. Pilo A, Iervasi G, Clerico A et al (1998) The circulatory model in metabolic studies of rapidly renewed hormones: application to ANP kinetics. Am J Physiol 274:E560-572
199. Iervasi G, Clerico A, Pilo A et al (1998) Atrial natriuretic peptide is not degraded from lungs in humans. J Clin Endocrinol Metab 83:2898-2906
200. Clerico A, Iervasi G (1995) Alterations in metabolic clearance of atrial natriuretic peptides in heart failure: how do they relate to the resistance to atrial natriuretic peptides? J Card Fail 1:323-328
201. Iervasi G, Clerico A, Pilo A et al (1997) Evidence that ANP tissue extraction is not changed by large increases of its plasma levels induced by pacing in humans. J Clin Endocrinol Metab 82:884-888

202. Totsune K, Takahashi K, Satoh F et al (1996) Urinary immunoreactive brain natriuretic peptide in patients with renal disease. Regul Pept 63:141-146
203. Ng LL, Geeranavor S, Jennings SC et al (2004) Diagnosis of heart failure using urinary natriuretic peptides. Clin Sci 106:129-133
204. Shimizu H, Masuta K, Asada H et al (2003) Characterization of molecular forms of probrain natriuretic peptide in human plasma. Clin Chim Acta 334:233-239
205. Hunt PJ, Richards AM, Nicholls MG et al (1997) Immunoreactive amino-terminal pro-brain natriuretic peptide (NT-proBNP): a new marker of cardiac impairment. Clin Endocrinol 47:287-296
206. Goetze JP, Rehfeld JF, Videbaek R et al (2005) B-type natriuretic peptide and its precursor in cardiac venous blood from failing hearts. Eur J Heart Fail 7:69-74
207. Goetze JP, Videbaek R, Boesgaard S et al (2004) Pro-brain natriuretic peptide as marker of cardiovascular or pulmonary causes of dyspnea in patients with terminal parenchymal lung disease. J Heart Lung Transplant 23:80-87
208. Mukoyama M, Nakao K, Hosoda K et al (1991) Brain natriuretic peptide as a novel cardiac hormone in humans. Evidence for an exquisite dual natriuretic peptide system, atrial natriuretic peptide and brain natriuretic peptide. J Clin Invest 87:1402-1412
209. Mizuno Y, Yoshimura M, Yasue H et al (2001) Aldosterone production is activated in failing ventricle in humans. Circulation 103:72-77
210. Kalra PR, Clague JR, Bolger AP et al (2003) Myocardial production of C-type natriuretic peptide in chronic heart failure. Circulation 107:571-573
211. Gardner DG, Hedges BK, Wu J et al (1989) Expression of the atrial natriuretic peptide gene in human fetal heart. J Clin Endocrinol Metab 69:729-737
212. Cameron VA, Ellmers LJ (2003) Minireview: natriuretic peptides during development of the fetal heart and circulation. Endocrinology 144:2191-2194
213. Takahashi T, Allen PD, Izumo S (1992) Expression of A-, B-, and C-type natriuretic peptide genes in failing and developing human ventricles. Correlation with expression of the Ca(2+)-ATPase gene. Circ Res 71:9-17
214. Day ML, Schwartz D, Wiegand RC et al (1987) Ventricular atriopeptin. Unmasking of messenger RNA and peptide synthesis by hypertrophy or dexamethasone. Hypertension 9:485-491
215. Swynghedauw B, Baillard C (2000) Biology of hypertensive cardiopathy. Curr Opin Cardiol 15:247-253
216. Cheung CY (1995) Regulation of atrial natriuretic factor secretion and expression in the ovine fetus. Neurosci Biobehav Rev 19:159-164
217. Deloof S, Chatelain A (1994) Effect of blood volume expansion on basal plasma atrial natriuretic factor and adrenocorticotropic hormone secretions in the fetal rat at term. Biol Neonate 65:390-395
218. Johnson DD, Singh MB, Cheung CY (1997) Effect of three hours of hypoxia on atrial natriuretic factor gene expression in the ovine fetal heart. Am J Obstet Gynecol 176(1 Pt 1):42-48
219. Rosenfeld CR, Samson WK, Roy TA et al (1992) Vasoconstrictor-induced secretion of ANP in fetal sheep. Am J Physiol 263:E526-533
220. Wei YF, Rodi CP, Day ML et al (1987) Developmental changes in the rat atriopeptin hormonal system. J Clin Invest 79:1325-1329
221. Cheung CY (1994) Regulation of atrial natriuretic factor release by endothelin in ovine fetuses. Am J Physiol 267:R380-386
222. Cameron VA, Aitken GD, Ellmers LJ et al (1996) The sites of gene expression of atrial, brain, and C-type natriuretic peptides in mouse fetal development: temporal changes in embryos and placenta. Endocrinology 137:817-824
223. Graham CH, Watson JD, Blumenfeld AJ, Pang SC (1996) Expression of atrial natriuretic peptide by third-trimester placental cytotrophoblasts in women. Biol Reprod 54:834-840
224. Lim AT, Gude NM (1995) Atrial natriuretic factor production by the human placenta. J Clin Endocrinol Metab 80:3091-3093
225. Holcberg G, Kossenjans W, Brewer A et al (1995) The action of two natriuretic peptides (atrial natriuretic peptide and brain natriuretic peptide) in the human placental vasculature. Am J Obstet Gynecol 172:71-77

226. Holcberg G, Kossenjans W, Brewer A et al (1995) Selective vasodilator effects of atrial natriuretic peptide in the human placental vasculature. J Soc Gynecol Investig 2:1-5
227. Stebbing PN, Gude NM, King RG, Brennecke SP (1996) Alpha-atrial natriuretic peptide-induced attenuation of vasoconstriction in the fetal circulation of the human isolated perfused placenta. J Perinat Med 24:253-260
228. Abell TJ, Richards AM, Ikram H et al (1989) Atrial natriuretic factor inhibits proliferation of vascular smooth muscle cells stimulated by platelet-derived growth factor. Biochem Biophys Res Commun 160:1392-1396
229. Horio T, Nishikimi T, Yoshihara F et al (2000) Inhibitory regulation of hypertrophy by endogenous atrial natriuretic peptide in cultured cardiac myocytes. Hypertension 35:19-24
230. Wu C, Bishopric N, Pratt R (1997) Atrial natriuretic peptide induces apoptosis in neonatal rat cardiac myocytes. J Biol Chem 272:14860-14866
231. Cao L, Gardner D (1995) Natriuretic peptides inhibit DNA synthesis in cardiac fibroblasts. Hypertension 25:227-234
232. Oliver P, Fox J, Kim R et al (1997) Hypertension, cardiac hypertrophy and sudden death in mice lacking natriuretic peptide receptor A. Proc Natl Acad Sci USA 94:14730-14735
233. Knowles J, Esposito G, Mao L et al (2001) Pressure independent enhancement of cardiac hypertrophy in natriuretic peptide receptor A deficient mice. J Clin Invest 107:975-984
234. Ellmers L, Knowles J, Kim H-S et al (2002) Ventricular expression of atrial and brain natriuretic peptide in *Npr1* deficient mice with cardiac hypertrophy and fibrosis. Am J Physiol 283:H707-714
235. John SWM, Krege JH, Oliver PM et al (1995) Genetic decreases in atrial natriuretic peptide and salt-sensitive hypertension. Science 267:679-681
236. Tamura N, Ogawa Y, Chusho H et al (2000) Cardiac fibrosis in mice lacking brain natriuretic peptide. Proc Natl Acad Sci USA 97:4239-4244
237. Suda M, Ogawa Y, Tanaka K et al (1998) Skeletal overgrowth in transgenic mice that overexpress brain natriuretic peptide. Proc Natl Acad Sci USA 95:2337-2342
238. Matsukawa N, Grzesik W, Takahashi N et al (1999) The natriuretic peptide clearance receptor locally modulates the physiological effects of the natriuretic peptide system. Proc Natl Acad Sci USA 96:7403-7408
239. Chusho H, Tamura N, Ogawa Y et al (2001) Dwarfism and early death in mice lacking c-type natriuretic peptide. Proc Natl Acad Sci USA 98:4016-4021
240. Mericq V, Uyeda J, Barnes K et al (2000) Regulation of fetal rat bone growth by c-type natriuretic peptide and cGMP. Pediatr Res 47:189-193
241. Irons DW, Bayles PH, Davison JM (1996) Effect of atrial natriuretic peptide on renal hemodynamics and sodium excretion during human pregnancy. Am J Physiol 271:F239-242
242. Rutherford AJ, Anderson JV, Elder MG, Bloom SR (1987) Release of atrial natriuretic peptide during pregnancy and immediate puerperium. Lancet i:928-929
243. Clerico A, Del Chicca MG, Ferdeghini M et al (1980) Progressively elevated levels of biologically active (free) cortisol during pregnancy by a direct radioimmunological assay of diffusible cortisol in an equilibrium dialysis system. J Endocrinol Invest 3:185-187
244. Wilson M, Morganti AA, Zervoudakis I et al (1980) Blood pressure, the renin-aldosterone system and sex steroids throughout normal pregnancy. Am J Med 68:97-104
245. Furuhashi N, Kimura H, Nagae H et al (1994) Brain natriuretic peptide and atrial natriuretic peptide levels in normal pregnancy and preeclampsia. Gynecol Obstet Invest 38:73-77
246. Minegishi T, Nakamura M, Abe K et al (1999) Adrenomedullin and atrial natriuretic peptide concentrations in normal pregnancy and pre-eclampsia. Mol Hum Reprod 5:767-770
247. Okuno S, Hamada H, Yasuoka M et al (1999) Brain natriuretic peptide (BNP) and cyclic guanosine monophosphate (cGMP) levels in normal pregnancy and preeclampsia. J Obstet Gynaecol Res 25:407-410
248. Fleming SM, O'Byrne L, Grimes H et al (2001) Amino-terminal pro-brain natriuretic peptide in normal and hypertensive pregnancy. Hypertens Pregnancy 20:169-175
249. Kale A, Kale E, Yalinkaya A et al (2005) The comparison of amino-terminal probrain natriuretic peptide levels in preeclampsia and normotensive pregnancy. J Perinat Med 33:121-124

250. Resnik JL, Hong C, Resnik R et al (2005) Evaluation of B-type natriuretic peptide (BNP) levels in normal and preeclamptic women. Am J Obstet Gynecol 193:450-454

251. Nakayama T (2005) The genetic contribution of the natriuretic peptide system to cardiovascular diseases. Endocr J 52:11-21

252. Clerico A (2003) Increasing impact of laboratory medicine in clinical cardiology. Clin Chem Lab Med 41:871-883

253. Steinhelper ME, Cochrane KL, Field LJ (1990) Hypotension in transgenic mice expressing atrial natriuretic factor fusion genes. Hypertension 16:301-307

254. Ogawa Y, Itoh H, Tamura N et al (1994) Molecular cloning of the complementary DNA and gene that encode mouse brain natriuretic peptide and generation of transgenic mice that overexpress tha brain natriuretic peptide gene. J Clin Invest 93:1911-1921

255. John SW, Krege JH, Oliver PM et al (1995) Genetic decrease in atrial natriuretic peptide and salt-sensitive hypertension. Science 267:679-681

256. Lopez MJ, Wong SK, Kishimoto I et al (1995) Salt-resistant hypertension in mice lacking the guanylyl cyclase-A receptor for atrial natriuretic peptide. Nature 378:65-68

257. Rutledge DR, Sun Y, Ross EA (1995) Polymorphisms within the atrial natriuretic peptide gene in essential hypertension. J Hypertens 13:953-955

258. Ramasawmy R, Kotea N, Lu C et al (1993) A new polymorphic restriction site at the human atrial natriuretic peptide (hANP) gene locus. Hum Genet 91:509-510

259. Schorr U, Beige J, Ringel J et al (1997) HpaII polymorphism of the atrial natriuretic peptide gene and blood pressure response to salt intake in normotensive men. J Hypertens 15:715-718

260. Widecka K, Ciechanowicz A, Adler G et al (1998) Analysis of polymorphisms Sma (Hpa II) and Sca I gene precursors of atrial natriuretic peptide (ANP) in patients with essential hypertension. Pol Arch Med Wewn 100:27-34

261. Cheung BMY, Leung R, Shiu S et al (1999) HpaII polymorphism in the atrial natriuretic peptide gene and hypertension. Am J Hypertens 12:524-527

262. Rahmutula D, Nakayama T, Soma M et al (2001) Association study between the variants of the human ANP gene and essential hypertension. Hypertens Res 24:291-294

263. Kato N, Sugiyama T, Morita H et al (2000) Genetic analysis of the atrial natriuretic peptide gene in essential hypertension. Clin Sci 98:251-258

264. Sarzani R, Dessi-Fulgheri P, Salvi F et al (1999) A novel promoter variant of the natriuretic peptide clearance receptor gene is associated with lower atrial natriuretic peptide and higher blood pressure in obese hypertensives. J Hypertens 17:1301-1305

265. Nakayama T, Soma M, Takahashi Y et al (2000) Functional deletion mutation of the 5'-flanking region of type A natriuretic peptide receptor gene and its association with essential hypertension and left ventricular hypertrophy in the Japanese. Circ Res 86:841-845

266. Lucarelli K, Iacoviello M, Dessi-Fulgheri P et al (2001) Associazione di una nuova variante genica del recettore A dei peptidi natriuretici con la familiarità per ipertensione arteriosa. Ital Heart J 2(Suppl 6):10

267. Ahluwalia A, Hobbs AJ (2005) Endothelium-derived C-type natriuretic peptide: more than just a hyperpolarized factor. Trends Pharmacol Sci 26:162-167

268. Zeidel ML (2000) Physiological responses to natriuretic hormones. In: Fray JCS, Goodman HM (eds) Handbook of physiology, Section 7, The endocrine system, Volume III: Endocrine regulation of water and electrolyte balance. New York, Oxford University Press, pp 410-435

269. Han B, Hasin Y (2003) Cardiovascular effects of natriuretic peptides and their interrelation with endothelin-1. Cardiovasc Drugs Ther 17:41-52

270. Houben AJ, van der Zander K, de Leeuw PW (2005) Vascular and renal actions of brain natriuretic peptide in man: physiology and pharmacology. Fundam Clin Pharmacol 19:411-419

271. Scotland RS, Ahluwalia A, Hobbs AJ (2005) C-type natriuretic peptide in vascular physiology and disease. Pharmacol Ther 105:85-89

272. Casco VH, Veinot JP, Kuroski de Bold ML et al (2002) Natriuretic peptide system gene expression in human coronary arteries. J Histochem Cytochem 50:799-809

273. Nazario B, Hu RM, Pedram A et al (1995) Atrial and brain natriuretic peptides stimulate the

production and secretion of C-type natriuretic peptide from bovine aortic endothelial cells. J Clin Invest 95:1151-1157

274. De los Angeles Costa M, Elesgaray R, Loria A et al (2004) Atrial natriuretic peptide influence on nitric oxide system in kidney and heart. Regul Pept 118:151-157

275. Ruskoaho H, Leskinen H, Magga J et al (1997) Mechanisms of mechanical load-induced atrial natriuretic peptide secretion: role of endothelin, nitric oxide, and angiotensin II. J Mol Med 75:876-885

276. Gyurko R, Kuhlencordt P, Fishman MC, Huang OL (2000) Modulation of mouse cardiac function *in vivo* by eNOS and ANP. Am J Physiol 278:H971-981

277. Kohno M, Horio T, Yokokawa K (1992) C-type natriuretic peptide inhibits thrombin- and angiotensin II-stimulated endothelin release via cyclic guanosine 3',5'-monophosphate. Hypertension 19:320-325

278. Davidson NC, Barr CS, Struthers AD (1996) C-type natriuretic peptide. An endogenous inhibitor of vascular angiotensin-converting enzyme activity. Circulation 931:155-159

279. Evans JJ, Youssef AH, Yandle TG et al (2002) Effects of endothelin-1 on release of adrenomedullin and C-type natriuretic peptide from individual human vascular endothelial cells. J Endocrinol 175:225-232

280. Suga S, Itoh H, Komatsu Y et al (1993) Cytokine-induced C-type natriuretic peptide (CNP) secretion from vascular endothelial cells - evidence for CNP as a novel autocrine/paracrine regulator from endothelial cells. Endocrinology 133:3038-3041

281. Ohno N, Itoh H, Ikeda T et al (2002) Accelerated reendothelialization with suppressed thrombogenic property and neointimal hyperplasia of rabbit jugular vein grafts by adenovirus-mediated gene transfer of C-type natriuretic peptide. Circulation 105:1623-1626

282. Kiemer AK, Lehner MD, Hartung T, Vollmar AM (2002) Inhibition of cyclooxygenase-2 by natriuretic peptides. Endocrinology 143:846-852

283. Kiemer AK, Furst R, Vollmar AM (2005) Vasoprotective actions of the atrial natriuretic peptide. Curr Med Chem Cardiovasc Hematol Agents 3:11-21

284. Furuya M, Yoshida M, Hayashi Y et al (1991) C-type natriuretic peptide is a growth inhibitor of rat vascular smooth muscle cells. Biochem Biophys Res Commun 177:927-931

285. Gonzalez Bosc LV, Majowicz MP, Vidal NA (2000) Effects of atrial natriuretic peptide in the gut. Peptides 21:875-887

286. Rollin R, Mediero A, Roldan-Pallares M et al (2004) Natriuretic peptide system in the human retina. Mol Vis 10:15-22

287. Barabasi AL, Oltvai ZN (2004) Network biology: understanding the cell's functional organization. Nat Rev Genet 5:101-113

288. Clerico A, Recchia FA, Passino C, Emdin M (2006) Cardiac endocrine function is an essential component of the homeostatic regulation network: physiological and clinical implications. Am J Physiol Heart Circ Physiol 290:H17-29

Cardiac Natriuretic Hormones as Markers of Cardiovascular Disease: Methodological Aspects

Mauro Panteghini · Aldo Clerico

4.1 General Considerations

Cardiac natriuretic hormones (CNH) constitute a complex family of related peptides with similar peptide chains as well as degradation pathways (see Chap. 3 for more details). CNH derive from common precursors, pre-pro-hormones (i.e., preproANP and preproB-NP). Pro-hormone peptides are further split into an inactive longer NT-proANP or NT-proBNP and the biologically active hormones, ANP or BNP, which are secreted in the blood in equimolar amounts. However, ANP and BNP have a shorter plasma half-life and consequently lower plasma concentrations compared to NT-proANP and NT-proBNP (Table 4.1). For these reasons, setting up an immunoassay for N-terminal peptide fragments of proANP and proBNP should be easier than that for ANP and BNP, because the requested analytical sensitivity is not too low [1]. However, immunoassays for NT-proANP and NT-proBNP may be affected by problems related to the different assay specificities: as shown in Table 4.1, different results are produced by different methods

Table 4.1. Characteristics of some commercial competitive (EIA) and non-competitive (IRMA, ELISA, and ECLIA) immunoassays for cardiac natriuretic peptides

Method	Detection limit (pmol/l)	Reference interval (pmol/l)	Mean value of reference distribution (pmol/l)
IRMA ANP	0.7	<0.7–16.6	5.6
IRMA BNP	0.7	<0.7–12.4	2.9
POCT BNP	1.4	<1.4–14.2	2.9
ELISA proANP	76.9	<77–1502	731
IRMA proANP	40.5	63–422	228
EIA proANP$_{1-30}$	9.5	44–1209	708
EIA proANP$_{31-67}$	38.4	193–3339	1422
EIA NT–proBNP$_{8-29}$	13.6	64–488	247
EIA NT-proBNP$_{32-57}$	4.0	<4.0–368	118
ECLIA NT-proBNP	0.6	1.7–21.1	6.1

IRMA ANP (Shionogi & Co., Ltd, Osaka, Japan); IRMA BNP (Shionogi & Co., Ltd); POCT BNP (Biosite Triage, San Diego, USA); ELISA proANP (Biomedica Gruppe, Wien, Austria); IRMA proANP (Shionogi & Co., Ltd); EIA proANP$_{1-30}$ (Biomedica Gruppe); EIA proANP$_{31-67}$ (Biomedica Gruppe); EIA NT-proBNP$_{8-29}$ (Biomedica Gruppe); EIA NT-proBNP$_{32-57}$ (Biomedica Gruppe); ECLIA NT-proBNP (Elecsys System, Roche Diagnostics, Mannheim, Germany)

with a large bias [1-3]. The different analytical performances could have some relevance in the diagnostic accuracy of different assay methods in discriminating between subjects with or without cardiac disease [1-11].

Table 4.2 summarizes the respective advantages of the assay of biologically active peptide hormones (ANP and BNP) compared to those of the assay of NT-proANP and NT-proBNP. The assay of the inactive NT-propeptides better fits the definition of a disease biomarker than that measuring circulating concentrations of ANP or BNP, which, on the other hand, may be considered a more reliable index of the activation (hormonal) status of the CNH system.

Table 4.2. Relative advantages of ANP/BNP and NT-proANP/NT-proBNP measurements

ANP/BNP	NT-proANP/NT-proBNP
Close correlation between hormonal and immunological activities	Higher and more stable circulating concentrations
Better correlation with physiological or clinical conditions after acute hemodynamic changes	Less *in vitro* degradation

Taking into account the biochemical and physiological characteristics of different peptides, it is theoretically conceivable that ANP is a better marker of acute overload and/or rapid cardiovascular hemodynamic changes than BNP and NT-proANP or NT-proBNP. It is well known that the circulating concentrations of ANP are more affected by body position and more decreased by a hemodialysis session in patients with chronic renal failure than those of BNP, while plasma concentrations of NT-proANP or NT-proBNP are not significantly changed [1, 4]. Furthermore, ANP increases more than NT-proANP during rapid ventricular pacing [12].

The first methods commercially available for ANP and BNP determination, set up before 1990, were competitive immunoassays (i.e., radioimmunoassay [RIA] and enzyme immunoassay [EIA] methods). These methods usually required a preliminary chromatographic step because of their poor sensitivity and specificity [1]; this purification step markedly decreased assay precision and practicability. A second generation of immunoassays for ANP- and BNP-related peptides became commercially available during the 1990s; these methods were non-competitive immunoassays, e.g. immunoradiometric assays (IRMAs) [13, 14]. Compared to competitive methods, IRMAs for CNH determination showed better sensitivity, specificity, and did not require a preliminary chromatographic step. However, the long turnaround time did not allow their use in the clinical setting, especially in emergency situations [1-4]. More recently, a new generation of immunoassays for CNH became commercially available, including some point-of-care testing (POCT) methods [15]. These methods are non-competitive sandwich immunoassays, which use non-radioactive materials as labels for the antigen/antibody reaction [3, 4]. The availability of these methods has allowed a wider diffusion of CNH assays (mainly BNP and NT-proBNP assays) in clinical practice, including emergencies.

In summary, several methods for CNH determination have been proposed measuring similar or identical peptides, showing, however, different analytical performance, reference values, clinical results, and, possibly, diagnostic accuracy [3,4]. In addition, there is no general agreement about the CNH terminology used by different researchers and manufacturers; this may increase confusion and cause misleading interpretation. A standardization of terminology and methods is, therefore, required in order to evaluate and compare the diagnostic accuracy of the different CNH assays [4]. In this chapter, the most important analytical characteristics and performances of CNH immunoassays are described.

4.2 Determination of ANP and NT-proANP

4.2.1 Competitive Immunoassay Methods for ANP

Before 2000, tissue or circulating concentrations of ANP were usually measured by competitive immunoassay methods using radiolabeled tracers (RIA), although enzyme immunoassay methods were also set up [16-32]. As ANP determination by competitive immunoassay methods can be affected by many analytical problems, several analytical options were proposed [1, 2, 29, 30]. First, a suitable ANP assay should be targeted only at the biologically active peptide. For this reason, the employed antibodies should be highly specific for the "biologically active" part of the peptide, i.e., the amino acid sequence containing the ring structure formed by the disulfide bridge. As an example, cross-reactivities of four different antisera used in commercial ANP assays are reported in Table 4.3. These data indicate that all assays are more specific for the intact ANP molecule than for the other tested ANP fragments, in which the disulfide bridge is disrupted. However, large differences in specificities of the antisera are also present. The main consequence of this finding is that large differences in ANP values should actually be expected when measured by different assays (Table 4.4) [1, 2, 29, 30].

Theoretically, the major drawback results from the presence of several ANP-related peptides in plasma samples (or tissues; i.e., all the endogenous precursors or metabolites of the hormone and other cardiac or non-cardiac peptide hormones structurally

Table 4.3. Cross-reactivities (in percentages) of four commercial ANP assays against human ANP-related peptide fragments

Peptide	RIA I	RIA II	RIA III	IRMA
$\alpha h_{1-28}ANP$	100	100	100	100
$\alpha h_{1-10}ANP$				<0.001
$\alpha h_{3-28}ANP$	95	90		
$\alpha h_{7-28}ANP$	<0.01		127	118
$\alpha h_{5-28}ANP$	0.16		109	110
$\alpha h_{5-27}ANP$	<0.1			<0.002
$\alpha h_{13-28}ANP$	<0.01	50	<0.2	0.01
$\alpha h_{18-28}ANP$	<0.01		<0.2	<0.001
$\beta h ANP$		94		105
$\gamma r ANP$				13

RIA I RPA 512 kit, Amersham International plc, Bucks, UK; *RIA II* RIK8798 kit (May 1988), Peninsula Laboratories, Inc., Belmont, California, USA; *RIA III* ANP RIA kit (4/92-NIDANP-SS), Nichols Institute Diagnostics, San Juan Capistrano, California; *IRMA* Shionoria ANP, Shionogi & Co., Ltd, Osaka, Japan

Table 4.4. Reference values for plasma ANP concentrations (in ng/l) as measured by RIA and IRMA methods

Author (reference)	Number of subjects (sex)	Mean ± SD (range)
RIA (direct assay)		
Marumo et al. [16]	124 (62 M, 62 F)	31.7 ± 12.0 (10–60)
RIA (with extraction/purification step)		
Yandle et al. [18]	19 (7 M, 12 F)	43.1 ± 13.4 (20–90)*
Ohashi et al. [23]	19 (M)	25.0 ± 21.8 (4–37)
Richards et al. [24]	55 (33 M, 22 F)	23.3 ± 13.3 (5–65)
Rosmalen et al. [25]	25	26.0 ± 15.5
Poiesi et al. [26]	32 (20 M, 12 F)	33.0 ± 22.6 (9–70)
Clerico et al. [29]	33 (20 M, 13 F)	26.8 ± 16.4 (5–55)
Lindberg et al. [31]	19	22.7 ± 17.5*
IRMA (direct assay)		
Lewis et al. [34]	10	20.3 ± 4.7 (8–55)*
Tattersall et al. [35]	11 (6 M, 5 F)	28** (17–57)*
Clerico et al. [37]	59 (25 M, 34 F)	18.0 ± 10.6 (4–63)

* Values originally reported in pmol/l and converted into ng/l (1 pmol/L = 3.078 ng/L);
** Median value

related to ANP), which can interfere with a competitive immunoassay. Moreover, some authors have suggested that platelets can interfere with a direct RIA by producing an enhanced plasma peptide concentration due to the presence of high-affinity receptors for cardiac natriuretic peptides on platelets [24]. As suggested, the "classical" centrifugation (1000 x g for 10 min at 4°C) of blood samples could actually produce platelet-enriched plasma with a platelet count exceeding that in the original whole-blood sample. For these reasons, preliminary extraction and chromatographic purification of plasma (or tissue) samples is suggested with the aim of eliminating these interferences and increasing accuracy (i.e., specificity) [24, 29, 30]. As a matter of fact, RIAs with a preliminary extraction/purification step gave in general more accurate results than the same RIAs without this step [24, 29].

High sensitivity for detection of low ANP concentrations is also required for a plasma ANP assay, due to low circulating concentrations of the hormone in healthy subjects (about 5-50 ng/l, corresponding to about 1.6-16.2 pmol/l) (Table 4.4). Chromatographic extraction of large volumes of plasma (≥3 ml) has therefore been suggested to increase the precision of the measurement in this concentration range [24, 29, 30].

As mentioned above, a preliminary step for the extraction/purification of the peptides from the plasma or tissue samples is generally requested when RIAs for ANP are used. However, this step greatly decreases assay precision and practicability, thus generating conflicting results [30]. The main reasons are: 1) the quantitative recovery of native hormone added to plasma samples after extraction with Sep-Pak C18 cartridges is generally poor for all the most used procedures (~50-70%); 2) the chromatographic pattern of ^{125}I-radiolabeled ANP, generally used for the routine assessment of extraction recovery, may be different from that of native hormone [2, 29, 30], so that the recovery of tracer could not be a suitable estimate of true recovery of native ANP present in plasma samples; 3) the extraction recovery was not verified for all the individual samples assayed, but only a mean run recovery was measured in general. These factors make it difficult to standardize a chromatographic procedure for the preliminary extraction/purification step of ANP present in plasma or tissue [1, 2, 30].

Finally, since a tracer with the highest specific activity must be used to increase the assay sensitivity of the RIA system, the peptide is generally labeled with two atoms of radioiodine (namely ^{125}I) per molecule by adding these isotopes directly to the ring of the last C-terminal amino acid (tyrosine). Unfortunately, this type of di-iodinated tracer is more rapidly degraded *in vitro* than the mono-iodinated tracer [2, 33]. Furthermore, radiolabeled ANP, labeled with one or two ^{125}I atoms in the tyrosine ring, is not stable in aqueous solutions, this representing another important issue for ANP determination by RIA [33].

Because of the different analytical characteristics and performances of RIA methods, it is not surprising that a great variability in ANP measured values was observed in an external quality assessment of five Italian laboratories with long experience in performing ANP assays: between-assay coefficients of variations (CV) >50% were indeed found [30].

4.2.2 Non-Competitive Immunoassay Methods for ANP

Non-competitive IRMA methods for the measurement of plasma ANP have been set up to overcome the problems observed with competitive assays [34-37]. All these methods are "two-site" (sandwich) IRMAs, which use two specific monoclonal antibodies or antisera prepared against two sterically remote epitopes of the ANP molecule. In some methods, using a solid phase as a separation system, one of the two antibodies is radiolabeled with ^{125}I and the other is coated onto wells of a microliter plate [34] or beads [36, 37]. Other IRMAs use a liquid-phase system in which both the specific anti-ANP antibodies (i.e., radiolabeled and non-radiolabeled) are in solution and the bound fraction is separated from the free fraction using a precipitating antiserum with centrifugation [35].

IRMAs have some advantages over RIAs. First, IRMAs do not use radiolabeled ANP as tracer but the more stable radiolabeled antibody; consequently, these methods do not present the tracer instability-related problems that can affect some ANP RIAs. Second, because ANP IRMA methods are in general highly sensitive and not significantly affected by non-specific (so-called "matrix effects") as well as specific interferences, these methods do not generally require preliminary extraction and purification of the plasma sample, which can reduce assay precision and practicability as well as increase the cost. Finally, IRMAs use a lower plasma volume (generally 0.1-0.3 ml) for the assay than RIAs [37].

Figure 4.1 displays the imprecision profiles of three RIAs and an IRMA for ANP measurement [29, 30, 37]. The IRMA method showed better precision than RIAs, especially in the low range concentrations. The detection limit of RIAs ranged between 10 and 20 ng/l (3.2-6.5 pmol/l) [29, 30], while the detection limit of IRMA was ~2 ng/l (0.65 pmol/l) [37]. The working range (arbitrarily defined as the interval of ANP values measured with an imprecision [as CV] <15%) of IRMA was greater (10-2,000 ng/l; 3.2-650 pmol/l) than that of RIA (on average 20-1,000 ng/l; 6.5-325 pmol/l) [30, 37].

It is noteworthy that IRMAs generally have reference intervals superimposable on those obtained with the most accurate RIAs, using a preliminary extraction/purification step (Table 4.4).

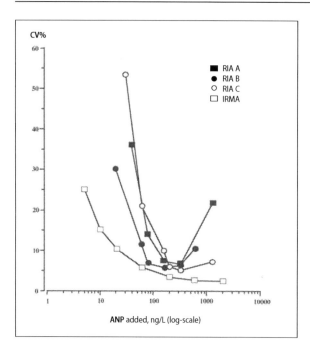

Fig. 4.1. Imprecision profiles of three RIA methods and one IRMA method for ANP

The IRMA system, which uses two monoclonal antibodies, is more specific for the intact ANP than RIAs, as indicated by the results reported in Table 4.3. However, it is theoretically conceivable that the intact peptide proANP$_{1-126}$, containing the biologically active hormone ANP in its C-terminal 99-126 amino acid residues, may also be measured by this IRMA (as well as by all RIAs). This would be a considerable drawback if the assayed concentrations of ANP and intact proANP$_{1-126}$ are similar, which is evidently the case when cardiac tissue extracts are assayed. Under these experimental conditions, if the aim of the study is to measure separately both the biologically active ANP and the intact precursor proANP$_{1-126}$, IRMA methods (as well as all RIAs) require a preliminary extraction/chromatographic step to separate the two molecules accurately before the assay.

On the other hand, an intrinsic problem of the non-competitive "two-site" immunometric methods is the so-called "hook" effect at high concentrations of analyte. Indeed, this effect was found in one IRMA for ANP concentrations >250 pmol/l [35], but not in another IRMA for ANP concentrations of up to 2,000 ng/l (650 pmol/l) [37]. The "hook" effect can probably be avoided by using a monoclonal antibody coated onto the solid phase showing high binding capacity [34].

The only disadvantage of commercially available IRMA compared to RIA is the greater cost. For laboratories that have an opportunity to set up an RIA method without using expensive commercial products (e.g., to prepare specific antibodies and tracers directly), purchasing a commercial IRMA kit may increase the cost by approximately three times. On the other hand, for laboratories in which a commercial RIA kit is already being used, the higher cost of an IRMA kit may be largely counterbalanced by the increase in accuracy, precision, and, especially, practicability.

At the present time, no non-competitive, fully automated immunoassay system for ANP is commercially available.

4.2.3 Determination of NT-proANP

NT-proANP is generally measured by direct RIA methods, i.e., without a preliminary extraction/purification step [1, 2, 20, 38-40]. NT-proANP RIAs are more practicable and cheaper than ANP IRMAs, but they can be affected by some analytical problems. The intact NT-proANP is a long peptide, implying that an anti-NT-proANP antiserum may recognize only a few epitopes of the peptide [1, 2, 39]. Consequently, if low-molecular mass fragments of NT-proANP are present within the circulation, RIA using different antisera or monoclonal antibodies can show significantly different results [1, 2].

In their extensive studies, Vesely and coworkers have suggested that NT-proANP can be degraded *in vivo* with the production of at least three different biologically active peptides (i.e., NT-proANP$_{1-30}$, proANP$_{31-67}$, and proANP$_{79-98}$) [41-46]. These peptides are unable to bind the specific ANP/BNP receptors, but they show peculiar biological effects (such as blood pressure lowering, diuretic, natriuretic, and/or kaliuretic properties) and a considerably longer plasma half-life (hours versus minutes) than that of ANP and BNP. Therefore, these peptides should be considered as distinct peptide hormones too [46]. Further studies are, however, necessary to confirm the physiological relevance of these peptides. Of course, to accurately incasure these NT-proANP related peptides, specific methods for each peptide are necessary [1].

A two-site IRMA for the NT-proANP$_{1-98}$, which uses a first monoclonal antibody against the peptide NT-proANP$_{1-25}$ and a second antibody against the peptide NT-proANP$_{43-66}$, has also been set up [47]. As expected, this IRMA was more sensitive, precise, and specific for the intact NT-proANP than RIA [47].

4.3 Determination of BNP and NT-proBNP

4.3.1 First-Generation (Manual) BNP Assays

The first methods set up for BNP determination were RIAs [48-55]. Because BNP shows circulating values and peptide structure similar to those of ANP, BNP RIAs were also characterized by the same analytical problems (i.e., low degree of precision, sensitivity, accuracy, and practicability). As a consequence, a preliminary extraction/purification step was generally requested and a relatively large volume of plasma sample (3 10 ml) needed for the determination of BNP by RIA [53]. As for ANP, the recovery of BNP after the extraction/purification procedure with Sep-Pack C18 cartridges (generally used in RIA methods) was poor (~70% on average) [50, 53].

To overcome these problems, a two-site, solid-phase (sandwich) IRMA method has been proposed for the determination of the biologically active form of BNP [13, 56, 57]. The IRMA uses two different monoclonal antibodies that recognize the C-terminal region and the intramolecular ring structure of BNP, respectively. One of these antibodies is radiolabeled with ^{125}I and the other is coated on the beads in solid phase. The detection limit of this IRMA was ~2 ng/l (0.6 pmol/l), with a working range (BNP values measured with an imprecision [CV] <15%) of 7-2,000 ng/l (2-578 pmol/l). Only 0.1 ml of plasma was necessary for the assay [13, 57].

4.3.2 Second-Generation (Automated) BNP Assays

In the past few years a new generation of fully automated immunoassays for BNP has become commercially available, including POCT methods. These assays are non-competitive sandwich-type immunoassays that use non-radioactive materials as labels for antigen/antibody reaction and two monoclonal antibodies or a combination of monoclonal and polyclonal antibodies for BNP binding (Fig. 4.2) [7, 8, 15, 58-64]. Usually one antibody binds to the ring structure and the other antibody either to the C- or N-terminal end of BNP, respectively (Table 4.5).

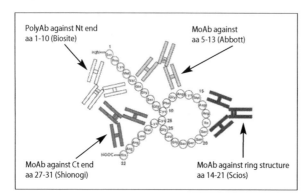

Fig. 4.2. Epitope specificity of antibodies employed in commercially available BNP assays. *PolyAb* polyclonal antibody, *MoAb* monoclonal antibody, *Nt* NH$_2$-terminus of BNP molecule, *Ct* COOH-terminus of BNP molecule, *aa* amino acid

PolyAb against Nt end aa 1-10 (Biosite)

MoAb against aa 5-13 (Abbott)

MoAb against Ct end aa 27-31 (Shionogi)

MoAb against ring structure aa 14-21 (Scios)

Table 4.5. Analytical configuration of commercial fully automated BNP/NT-proBNP assays

Company/platform	Calibrator material	Capture antibody (epitope)	Detection antibody (epitope)
Abbott AxSYM (Abbott Architect)	BNP$_{1-32}$ synthetic peptide (Peptide Institute)	Abbott (amino acids 5–13)	Shionogi (C-terminus)
Bayer Advia Centaur (Bayer ACS:180)	BNP$_{1-32}$ synthetic peptide (Phoenix Pharmaceutical)	Scios (ring)	Shionogi (C-terminus)
Biosite Triage (Beckman Access)	BNP$_{1-32}$ recombinant peptide (Scios)	Scios (ring)	Biosite (N-terminus)
Roche Elecsys (Dade Behring Dimension, Dade Behring Stratus CS, Ortho Clinical Diagnostics Vitros)	NT-proBNP$_{1-76}$ synthetic peptide* (Roche)	Roche (N-terminus)	Roche (amino acids 39–50)

* C-terminus is amidated to improve resistance to proteolysis; methionine at position 67 is replaced by the equivalent amino acid norleucine to reduce susceptibility to oxidation

4.3.3 Determination of NT-proBNP

The first assay for the measurement of NT-proBNP was reported by Hunt et al. [65,66]. Later on, other groups have developed "in-house" methods [67,68]. All these methods were direct (i.e., without extraction) competitive assays. Commercial EIA kits for NT-proBNP related peptides are also available and their analytical performances have been evaluated [5,11,69].

A two-site sandwich immunoassay for NT-proBNP using detection by electro-chemiluminescence (electrochemiluminescence immunoassay [ECLIA]) and fully auto-mated instrumentation has recently been developed and its analytical performance extensively evaluated [69-75]. Two polyclonal antibodies directed against amino acid residues 1-21 and 39-50 of the NT-proBNP molecule are used (Table 4.5). The peptide concentration is measured on the Elecsys systems (Roche Diagnostics). Quite recently, methods using the same antibody combination and calibrator material have been developed by Dade Behring and Ortho Clinical Diagnostics for their automatic platforms. Several others are under development.

As discussed below, the heterogeneity of the NT-proBNP fragments in blood has a major influence on antibody detection and assay specificity (Fig. 4.3) [1,4,76]. Therefore, it is not surprising that different NT-proBNP assays may produce different results (Table 4.6) [3].

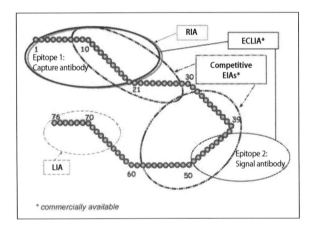

Fig. 4.3. Epitope specificity of antibodies employed in NT-proBNP assays. *RIA* radioimmunoassay, *LIA* immunoluminometric assay, *ECLIA* electrochemilumi-nescence immunoassay, *EIA* enzyme immunoassay

Table 4.6. Reference values for plasma NT-proBNP concentrations (in pmol/l) reported in the literature

Author (reference)	Assay	Median (range)
Hughes et al. [67]	LIA	159 (120–245)
Schulz et al. [68]	RIA	29 (13–75)
Mueller et al. [69]	EIA	78 (38–145)
Prontera et al. [71]	ECLIA	6.1 (4.1)*

* Mean (SD); values originally reported in ng/l and converted into pmol/l (1 pmol/L = 8.457 ng/L) *LIA* immunoluminometric assay, *RIA* radioimmunoassay, *EIA* enzyme immunoassay, *ECLIA* electrochemiluminescence immunoassay

4.3.4 Specificity of BNP/NT-proBNP Assays

It is known that BNP derives from the preproBNP, which contains a signal peptide sequence at the N-terminal end. After the signal peptide is cleaved, proBNP is further split proteolytically into NT-proBNP and the biologically active peptide hormone, BNP. However, the site at which proteolytic cleavage of proBNP takes place is still being debated. Most of it occurs within or on the surface of cardiomyocytes before the secretion in blood, but small amounts of the intact proBNP are also found in the circulation, indicating that some proteolysis may occur in the circulation. Thus, with the exception of preproBNP, all the metabolically BNP-related molecules are likely to be present in plasma, which is the biological sample generally used for measurements (Fig. 4.4) [76-79]. This fact was shown most clearly in the study of Hunt et al. [79], which compared the amounts of proBNP-derived molecular forms found in cardiac tissue and in plasma. Qualitatively, the same peaks were seen after HPLC fractionation of an atrial extract as were seen in plasma from a patient with heart failure, documenting the presence of proBNP, NT-proBNP, and BNP in both samples. The presence of intact proBNP in human plasma, in addition to BNP and NT-proBNP fragments, is important because of the potential that it may create problems regarding analytical specificity in the measurement of these peptides in plasma.

The N-terminal region of proBNP contains a leucine zipper-like sequence motif that may induce peptide oligomerization in plasma under physiological conditions, producing either a trimer or tetramer of proBNP [80]. These oligomerized molecules may expose or obscure epitopes recognized by the antibodies used in commercial assays. However, a more recent study indicated that human synthetic NT-proBNP exists as a monomer with an unordered random coil in neutral pH physiological salt solution [81].

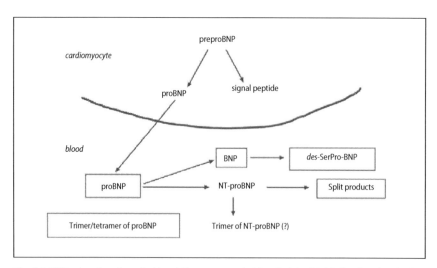

Fig. 4.4. BNP-related analytes in blood. The presence in blood of the highlighted molecules has been demonstrated in experimental studies. Splitting of proBNP into BNP and NT-proBNP peptides occurring in the cardiomyocyte is not shown

Experimental data also support the cleavage of BNP by plasma proteases. Proteolysis of the C-terminal structure by kallikrein occurs after activation of the coagulation contact activation system by a negatively charged surface. This can occur *in vivo* on the intraluminal surface of a damaged vessel and/or *in vitro* on the glass wall of blood collection tubes [82, 83]. Proteolytic cleavage of the two N-terminal amino acid residues, serine and proline, may occur immediately after blood collection or still within the circulation, making the N-terminal residue of BNP very sensitive to degradation [78]. It may be critical to take these enzymatic cleavages, particularly the one at the N-terminus, into account when choosing epitopes for antibody production and immunoassay design. The disulfide-bond-mediated ring structure appears to be stable in blood samples. However, this does not mean that degradation can never occur even in this site [83].

Finally, a recent study has shown that circulating NT-proBNP is heterogeneous and that most immunoreactive NT-proBNP is significantly smaller in size than NT-proBNP$_{1-76}$ because of truncation at both termini [84]. This fragmentation is more pronounced in serum than in plasma.

In the light of all these data, the complexity of the measurement of BNP and related peptides is clear. Assays with critical epitope requirements may differ in their reactivity with circulating peptides, so that commercial assays, nominally measuring the same analyte, may be differently affected by cross-reactivity problems (Table 4.7). Plasma BNP may be overestimated if the sandwich against BNP is formed by an antibody directed against the ring structure of the molecule and the second antibody is directed to the C-terminal end. In this case, plasma intact proBNP is also detected by the assay [78]. On the other hand, the combination of an antibody directed against the ring structure with an antibody against the N-terminal part of the molecule appears to be specific for the BNP, being, however, more prone to the peptide degradation by plasma proteases which can affect the N-terminus position [63, 77, 78]. This may result in a significant instability of the sample [70].

As regards NT-proBNP measurement, the recognized antibody epitopes are also crucial for immunoassay specificity. It is likely, although frequently not reported, that the antibodies used in many so-called "NT-proBNP" assays may also detect many of the circulating NT-proBNP split products, in addition to measuring proBNP. Further, several clinical studies reported in the literature have been performed by home-made non-commercial methods, which are not available to other research groups. To obviate the NT-proBNP heterogeneity in plasma, Goetze et al. developed a processing-independent analysis (PIA) for quantification of total proBNP, i.e. intact proBNP and its fragments in plasma

Table 4.7. Recovery of BNP-related peptides by commercially available BNP assays. Modified from [63]

Peptide	Beckman Access (Biosite)	Bayer Advia	Abbott AxSYM
BNP$_{1-32}$	100%	100%	100%
BNP$_{3-32}$	84%	100%	111%
BNP$_{10-32}$*	<1%	139%	<1%
BNP$_{1-31}$	106%	<1%	<1%

* Not found in plasma

[85]. Calibrators were prepared from synthetic tyrosine-extended proBNP$_{1-10}$ and an antibody directed against amino acid sequence 1-10 of human proBNP was used. Before measurement, plasma was treated with a proteinase (trypsin) that cleaved all proBNP peptides present in plasma to the 1-21 fragment. In this way, intact proBNP and all biologically derived fragments in the sample are cleaved into the same analyte and assayed together as equimolar amounts by RIA. The clinical utility of this approach remains to be determined, but it would overcome the issue of differential detection of circulating proBNP-derived fragments by different assays.

Different assays, theoretically measuring the same analyte, may thus produce significantly different results, not only in terms of proportional bias, but also displaying significant intercept values, meaning different analytical specificities [7, 8, 62, 69]. Generally speaking, it would be correct to assert that there are currently two types of commercially available assays. The former group, which uses a sandwich with an antibody against the ring portion and a second antibody against the N-terminal part of BNP peptide, is specific for the measurement of biologically active hormone, BNP. The latter, which is more heterogeneous, comprises methods that measure proBNP and all (or some) of its metabolic products, including BNP and NT-proBNP, with variable specificity. Nevertheless, when using these cardiac natriuretic peptides as biomarkers of cardiac dysfunction (and not for the evaluation of a biologically active hormone and its possible alterations), both analytical approaches can be acceptable, once their clinical usefulness has been proven. No two assays are, however, analytically equivalent at present. The BNP/NT-proBNP values are significantly dependent on the type of assay used, as a result of the specificity of the employed antibodies and of different calibration materials. As results are heavily method-dependent, it should clearly be stated that reference intervals and decision limits derived from clinical studies are only valid for the particular assay used and must not be extrapolated to other assays (Table 4.8).

Therefore, there is a need for assay standardization that, through the selection of appropriate reference materials and an adequate reference measurement procedure useful for their certification, and especially through the definition of the analyte to be measured, allows the same results to be obtained even when the measurements are performed with different methods [86]. In the meantime, in order to employ correctly the measurement of these markers in clinical practice, it is mandatory to use method-dependent reference limits and cut-off values without extrapolations from one method to another [87].

Table 4.8. Reference values (in ng/l) for BNP obtained with different commercial assays [4, 6, 62, 64]

Company/platform	Mean ± SD	Median value	Range	Upper reference limit (97.5th percentile)
Shionogi/IRMA (manual)	10.7 ± 9.9	7.1	<2.0–66.1	40
Abbott/AxSYM	22.2 ± 29.7	13.4	<5–221	105
Bayer/Advia Centaur	13.5 ± 11.9	9.4	<3–65.9	45
Biosite/Triage	10.4 ± 7.2	7.6	<8–62.5	40
Beckman/Access	12.4 ± 10.1	8.9	0.5–51.9	35

4.3.5 Quality Specifications for BNP/NT-proBNP Assays

With the clinical meaning of these markers of cardiac function being firmly documented, it now seems important to focus more on the biology of these peptides and related analytical issues. Only after appropriate analytical quality specifications are addressed, will the many issues pertaining to methodological differences that lead to non-harmonized concentration values and clinical interpretation of natriuretic peptide concentrations be reconciled. The responsibility of defining and implementing these issues should be shared among laboratories, industry, clinicians, and regulatory agencies on an international front.

A report was recently published by the Committee on Standardization of Markers of Cardiac Damage of the International Federation of Clinical Chemistry and Laboratory Medicine (IFCC), concerning quality specifications for BNP assays [88]. The recommendations proposed in this report are mainly intended for use by manufacturers of commercial assays and regulatory agencies. However, several points are also relevant for clinical trial groups and research investigators, as well as for clinical laboratories interested in measuring BNP or NT-proBNP. Both analytical and pre-analytical factors were addressed, as shown in Table 4.9.

Table 4.9. Quality specifications for BNP and NT-proBNP assays

Analytical factors to be considered:
- Calibration characterization (e.g. type of antigen used for calibration)
- Assay specificity (including identification of epitopes recognized by the employed antibodies and cross-reactivity characteristics to structurally related molecules present in blood, e.g. intact proBNP1–108)
- Assay imprecision
- Interferences (e.g. by endogenous constituents, such as hemoglobin, bilirubin, triglycerides, or by heterophilic antibodies)

Pre-analytical factors to be considered:
- Sample type (including type of biological sample – serum, plasma, whole blood – and type of specimen collection tubes)
- Sample stability at different temperatures of storage

First, definitive information about the synthesis and catabolism of BNP-related peptides is needed to determine the characteristics of the calibrator materials to be used in standardizing clinical assays. Their composition should closely resemble that of the molecule showing the greatest utility in a given clinical situation. For this type of definition, an evidence-based international agreement is required.

Second, assay specifications including antibody specificity and cross-reactivity characteristics to structurally related (e.g., metabolized and degraded) molecules need to be clearly delineated.

Third, assay imprecision and interferences have to be entirely described. Because of a consistently high biological variation for both BNP and NT-proBNP, very low assay imprecision may be unnecessary (see Chapter 5, section 5.1.5, for a more detailed discussion of this point). A desirable total imprecision (as CV) of <15% at BNP/NT-proB-NP concentrations within the reference interval has been recommended [88]. Acceptable imprecision was observed with different commercial automated assays, the Abbott AxSYM method having the largest CV range (Fig. 4.5). In general, no problems have been reported with the most important endogenous interferents (hemolysis, hyperbilirubinemia, hypertriglyceridemia) (Table 4.10) [8, 70, 89-92]. Grossly hemolyzed samples might, however, be a problem in the Beckman Access BNP assay [90].

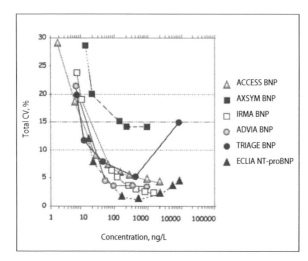

Fig. 4.5. Imprecision profiles of some commercial BNP and NT-proBNP assays. *MEIA* microparticle enzyme immunoassay (Abbott AxSYM), *IRMA* immunoradiometric assay (Shionogi), *POCT* point-of-care testing (Biosite Triage), *ECLIA* electrochemiluminescence immunoassay (Roche Elecsys)

Table 4.10. Relevant endogenous interferents and corresponding tested concentrations for some automated BNP and NT-proBNP assays

Company/ platform	Hemoglobin	Recovery	Bilirubin	Recovery	Triglycerides	Recovery	Author (reference)
Abbott/ AxSYM	1.00 g/dl	91%	20 mg/dl	101%	3000 mg/dl	103%	Daghfal et al. [89]
Bayer/Advia Centaur	1.00 g/dl	99%	25 mg/dl	93%	800 mg/dl	96%	Wu et al. [8]
Beckman/ Access	1.25 g/dl	80%	20 mg/dl	>90%	3000 mg/dl	>90%	Beyne et al. [90], Oswall et al. [91]
Dade Behring/ Dimension	0.50 g/dl	>90%	60 mg/dl	>90%	3000 mg/dl	>90%	Wei et al. [92]
Roche/ Elecsys	2.00 g/dl	95%	60 mg/dl	94%	2,100 mg/dl	103%	Yeo et al. [70]

Table 4.11. Sample stability at different storage temperatures for some commercial BNP/NT-proBNP assays

Company/platform	Sample type	Stability	Author (reference)
Abbott/AxSYM	EDTA plasma	4 h at RT 24 h at 2–8°C <1 day at –20°C	Daghfal et al. [95] Mueller et al. [96]
Bayer/Advia Centaur	EDTA plasma	<1 day at RT <1 day at 2–8°C	Smith & Wu [93]
Biosite/Triage	EDTA plasma	<4 h at RT <1 day at 2–8°C <3 days at –20°C	Yeo et al. [70]
Beckman/Access	EDTA plasma	4 h at RT <1 day at –4°C	Prontera et al. [64]
Roche/Elecsys	Serum, heparinized plasma	2 days at RT 6 days at 2–8°C 3 months at –20°C 1 year at –80°C	Yeo et al. [70] Mueller T et al. [96] Nowatzke & Cole [97]

RT room temperature

Finally, there are important issues related to the type of sample to be used for BNP/NT-proBNP measurements and the *in vitro* stability of these analytes. For BNP assays, the EDTA plasma is the only suitable specimen [93]. Conversely, it appears that for measuring NT-proBNP by the ECLIA method, serum is the sample of choice [72]. With this assay, EDTA plasma gave a consistent negative bias (8% on average) compared with matched serum samples, although studies did not indicate the variability among samples.

Blood samples should not be collected in glass tubes when using an immunoassay employing in the sandwich an antibody against the C-terminus for BNP measurement. It has been demonstrated that the above antibody is highly susceptible to the effect of kallikrein, a plasma protease activated by contact with the wall of the glass tube, that degrades the C-terminal portion of BNP (and proBNP), making impossible the identification of the molecule by the immunoassay using the above-reported antibody in the sandwich [82, 83, 94]. The stability of the blood sample can therefore be obtained by the use of plastic collection tubes. The *in vitro* stability is not a problem for NT-proBNP, while BNP is more unstable as proteolytic phenomena deprive it of the two N-terminal amino acids (Table 4.11). In general, BNP should be measured within 4 hours of collection if the sample is stored at room temperature. If the testing cannot be performed within 4 hours, the plasma should be separated, a kallikrein- or serine-specific protease inhibitor added, and the specimen stored refrigerated at 2-8°C for up to 24 hours or frozen at -70°C if stored for longer periods.

4.4 Determination of Other Natriuretic Peptides (CNP, DNP, and Urodilatin)

The methods set up for determination of CNP [98], DNP [99], and urodilatin [100, 101] were all RIAs. Because these peptides show circulating values and peptide structure similar to those of ANP and BNP, these RIAs were also characterized by the same analytical problems (i.e., low degree of precision, sensitivity, accuracy, and practicability). As a consequence, a preliminary extraction/purification step was generally requested and a relatively large volume of plasma sample (i.e., 1-2 ml for CNP assay) needed for the determination [95]. The assay recovery after the extraction/purification procedure with Sep-Pack C18 cartridges is usually not complete; for example, it is only about 80-85% for the CNP assay [98]. As expected for manual methods with a preliminary extraction step, assay precision is relatively poor. Indeed, the total between-assay variability of the CNP assay is 25.2% [98].

Due to their poor experimental practicability and long TAT, these immunoassay methods are usually used only in clinical or pathophysiological studies rather than in routine clinical practice. It is important to point out that the lack of suitable immunoassays could be an explanation for the relatively small amount of clinical data available for CNP, DNP and urodilatin compared with ANP and BNP.

Some specific points should be taken into account about the measurement of CNP, DNP an urodilatin, respectively.

DNP was first identified in venom of the green mamba snake [103], and then in mammal plasma and tissues, but its origin, biochemical and pathophysiological characteristics, and so the clinical relevance of its assay, are still unclear [102, 104].

Urodilatin is identical in structure to the circulating 28 amino acid human ANP (99-126), with addition of four amino acids (Thr-Ala-Pro-Arg) at the NH_2-terminus (Fig. 4.6). Urodilatin is synthesized by the same gene that synthesizes ANP, but in the kidney, as opposed to all other tissues that have been investigated, the ANP pro-hormone is processed differently, resulting in urodilatin rather than ANP being formed [100-102]. Urodilatin seems to be produced only in renal tissue and is not present in plasma (or at very low concentration), but only in urine [100-102]; consequently, only urine or renal tissue samples must be used for urodilatin assay. The clinical relevance of urodilatin assay should be limited only to renal diseases [102]. From a theoretical point of view, the set-up of a suitable urodilatin immunoassay presents some difficulties due to the very close structural similarity between ANP and urodilatin (Fig. 4.6). In order to distinguish better between these two peptides, an antibody against the first N-terminus four amino acids of urodilatin should be used [100]. However, immunoreactivity and biological activity may be

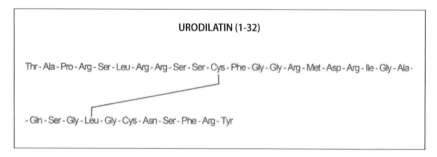

Fig. 4.6. Peptide chain structure of urodilatin (1–32). Urodilatin is identical in structure to the circulating 28 amino acid human atrial natriuretic peptide (ANP) (99–126), with addition of four amino acids (Thr-Ala-Pro-Arg) at the NH_2-terminus

poorly correlated if a competitive immunoassay based on this antibody is used. Indeed, the biological acivity of CNH depends on the integrity of the cysteine bridge, so that only the use of a non-competitive immunoassay using two antibodies (one against the N-terminus and the other against the part of the peptide including the cysteine bridge) should allow a better correlation between immunoreactivity and biological activity.

More information is available about the biochemical and pathophysiological characteristics of CNP, as well as the clinical relevance of its assay in plasma or tissue samples.

CNP is a peptide that was initially identified in the central nervous system [105]. CNP is expressed predominantly in the endothelium, but the central nervous system, myocardium, and gastrointestinal and genitourinary tracts can also express the peptide [106, 107]. CNP has both structural and physiological similarities to other known natriuretic peptides, and a shorter circulatory half-life, and is the most highly conserved form of the natriuretic peptides between species [106-110]. Studies in fish, based on nucleotide and amino acid sequence similarity, suggest that the natriuretic peptide family of iso-hormones may have evolved from a neuromodulatory CNP-like brain peptide (Fig. 3.6) [109, 110].

Two mature forms of the peptide exist, being derived from a 126 amino acid pre-pro-hormone. Both contain the 17 amino acid ring common to all members of the natriuretic peptide family (Fig. 4.7). The peptide with higher molecular weight, CNP-53, predominates in tissues, whereas CNP-22 is found mainly in plasma and in cerebrospinal fluid. It has been suggested that CNP-53 may function, at least in part, as a storage form of the peptide, while CNP-22 circulates in the plasma [106, 108, 111-113].

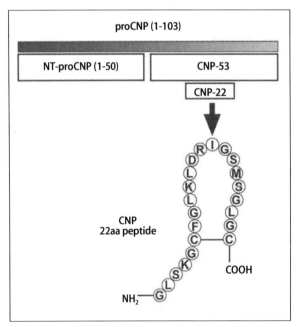

Fig. 4.7. Molecular forms of CNP and its related peptides

Most data on the biological effects of the peptide relate to the 22 amino acid form and its biological effects are currently being investigated at different sites in various species. Moreover, the endothelial site of production of CNP peptide and the proximal location of its receptor in vascular smooth muscle suggest that this vascular natriuretic peptide system may play a role in concert with other local systems (nitric oxide, prostaglandins) in the control of vascular tone, counteracting the vasoconstrictor systems (endothelin, angiotensin II; see Chap. 3 for more details) [107, 114, 115]. Several studies demonstrated that CNP exerts a protective effect on endothelial function by decreasing shear stress, modulating coagulation and fibrinolysis pathways, and inhibiting platelet activation (Fig. 3.15) [114, 115]. CNP can also inhibit the vascular remodeling process as well as coronary restenosis post-angioplasty and the adverse effects of ischemia/reperfusion injury [107, 113-120].

These studies suggest that the assay of CNP and the N-terminus fragment of pro-peptide (NT-proCNP) should have some clinical relevance in all pathophysiological conditions characterized by endothelium dysfunction. Indeed, increased plasma levels of CNP/NT-proCNP have already been identified in a number of pathological conditions (such as hypoxia, sepsis, chronic liver, renal or heart failure) likely characterized by endothelial dysfunction [106, 114, 121-129]. However, clinical interpretation of results of CNP assays may be difficult because this peptide has paracrine rather than hormonal action [112-115]; as a result, variations of circulating levels of CNP may be poorly (or even not at all) correlated to biological effects actually performed by the peptide in vascular tissue. Furthermore, blood collection, pre-analytical purification step and analytical assay performance may strongly affect the results of CNP/NT-proCNP assay [98].

4.5 Summary and Perspectives

The important role of CNH (especially BNP and NT-proBNP) assay in screening for heart disease, detection of left ventricular systolic and/or diastolic dysfunction, and differential diagnosis of dyspnea, prognostic stratification of patients with congestive heart failure has been confirmed even more recently [4, 87, 88, 130, 131]. In particular, the BNP/NT-proBNP assay was included in the first step of the algorithm for the diagnosis of acute heart failure along with the electrocardiogram and chest X-ray examination, as recently confirmed by the Task Force of the European Society of Cardiology for the diagnosis and treatment of chronic heart failure [132]. According to these recommendations, in order to introduce the routine measurement of BNP or NT-proBNP in clinical practice, reliable immunoassay methods should be commercially available.

CNH can be measured with competitive or non-competitive immunoassays. Non-competitive immunoassays generally share better degree of sensitivity, precision and specificity than the respective competitive immunoassays. In the last years a new generation of fully automated immunoassays, for BNP and NT-proBNP, including some POCT methods, became commercially available. These assays are non-competitive sandwich-type immunoassays which uses non-radioactive materials as labels for antigen/antibody reaction and two monoclonal antibodies or a combination of monoclonal and polyclonal antibodies for peptide binding [1, 7, 8, 15, 58-64]. In particular, for BNP assay, usually one antibody binds to the ring structure and the other antibody either to the Cor N-terminal end, respectively (Tables 4, 5). Although these fully automated commercial assays produce results in a short time and with excellent analytical imprecision, the BNP/NT-proBNP values continue to significantly depend on the type of assay used, as a result of the specificity of the employed antibodies and of different analytical standardization deriving from the different calibration materials [86-88]. The mentioned discrepancies among the concentrations obtained with different methods are directly reflected over reference and decisional limits, which often change according to the method used [62, 87, 88] (Tables 4 - 8). Therefore, there is a need for standardization that, through the selection of appropriate reference materials and adequate reference measurement procedures useful for their certification, and especially through the definition of the analyte to be measured, would allow to obtain comparable results, even when the measurements are performed with different methods [1, 86-88].

References

1. Clerico A, Del Ry S, Giannessi D (2000) Measurement of natriuretic cardiac hormones (ANP, BNP, and related peptides) in clinical practice: the need for a new generation of immunoassay methods. Clin Chem 46:1529-1534
2. Clerico A, Del Ry S, Giannessi D et al (2001) Evaluation and comparison of commercial immunoassay methods for the determination of N-terminal proANP in plasma and atrial tissue. J Clin Ligand Assay 24:112-118
3. Panteghini M, Clerico A (2004) Understanding the clinical biochemistry of N-terminal pro-B-type natriuretic peptide: the prerequisite for its optimal clinical use. Clin Lab 50:325-331
4. Clerico A, Emdin M (2004) Diagnostic accuracy and prognostic relevance of the measurement of the cardiac natriuretic peptides: a review. Clin Chem 50:33-50
5. Hammerer-Lercher A, Neubauer E, Muller S (2001) Head-to-head comparison of N-terminal pro-brain natriuretic peptide, brain natriuretic peptide and N-terminal pro-atrial natriuretic peptide in diagnosing left ventricular dysfunction. Clin Chim Acta 310:193-197
6. Prontera C, Emdin M, Zucchelli GC et al (2003) Fully-automated NT-proBNP and IRMA methods for BNP and ANP in heart failure and healthy subjects. Clin Chem 49:1552-1554
7. Storti S, Prontera C, Emdin M et al (2004) Analytical performance and clinical results of a fully automated MEIA system for BNP assay: comparison with a POCT method. Clin Chem Lab Med 42:1178-1185
8. Wu AH, Packer M, Smith A et al (2004) Analytical and clinical evaluation of the Bayer ADVIA Centaur automated B-type natriuretic peptide assay in patients with heart failure: a multisite study. Clin Chem 50:867-873
9. Mueller T, Gegenhuber A, Poelz W, Haltmayer M (2004) Head-to-head comparison of the diagnostic utility of BNP and NT-proBNP in symptomatic and asymptomatic structural heart disease. Clin Chim Acta 341:41-48
10. Mueller T, Gegenhuber A, Poelz W, Haltmayer M (2004) Biochemical diagnosis of impaired left ventricular ejection fraction - comparison of the diagnostic accuracy of brain natriuretic peptide (BNP) and amino terminal proBNP (NT-proBNP). Clin Chem Lab Med 42:159-163
11. Hammerer-Lercher A, Ludwig W, Falkensammer G et al (2004) Natriuretic peptides as markers of mild forms of left ventricular dysfunction: effects of assays on diagnostic performance of markers. Clin Chem 50:1174-1183
12. Ylitalo K, Uusimaa P, Vuolteenaho O et al (1999) Vasoactive peptide release in relation to hemodynamic and metabolic changes during rapid ventricular pacing. Pacing Clin Electrophysiol 22:1064-1070
13. Clerico A, Iervasi G, Del Chicca MG et al (1998) Circulating levels of cardiac natriuretic peptides (ANP and BNP) measured by highly sensitive and specific immunoradiometric assays

in normal subjects and in patients with different degrees of heart failure. J Endocrinol Invest 21:170-178

14. Numata Y, Dohi K, Furukawa A et al (1998) Immunoradiometric assay for the N-terminal fragment of proatrial natriuretic peptide in human plasma. Clin Chem 44:1008-1013

15. Del Ry S, Giannessi D, Clerico A (2001) Plasma brain natriuretic peptide measured by fully-automated immunoassay and by immunoradiometric assay compared. Clin Chem Lab Med 39:446-450

16. Marumo F, Sakamoto H, Ando K et al (1986) highly sensitive radioimmunoassay of atrial natriuretic peptide (ANP) in human plasma and urine. Biochem Biophys Res Commun 137:231-236

17. Gutkowska J, Genst J, Thibault G et al (1987) Circulating forms and radioimmunoassay of atrial natriuretic factor. Endocrinol Metab Clinics North Am 16:183-198

18. Yandle TG, Espiner EA, Nicholls MG, Duff H (1986) Radioimmunoassay and characterization of atrial natriuretic peptide in human plasma. J Clin Endocrinol Metab 63:72-79

19. Kato J, Kida O, Kita T et al (1988) Free and bound forms of atrial natriuretic peptide (ANP) in rat plasma: preferential increase of free ANP in spontaneously hypertensive rats (SHR) and stroke-prone SHR (SHRSP). Biochem Biophys Res Commun 153:1084-1089

20. Itoh H, Nakao K, Sugawara A et al (1988) Gamma-atrial natriuretic polypeptide (gamma-ANP)-derived peptides in human plasma: cosecretion of N-terminal gamma-ANP fragment and alpha-ANP. J Clin Endocrinol Metab 67:429-437

21. Gutkowska J, Bourassa M, Roy D et al (1985) Immunoreactive atrial natriuretic factor (IR-ANF) in human plasma. Biochem Biophys Res Commun 128:1350-1357

22. Hartter E, Woloszczuk W, Stummvoll HK (1986) Radioimmunoassay of atrial natriuretic peptide in human plasma. Clin Chem 32:441-445

23. Ohashi M, Fujio N, Nawata H et al (1987) High plasma concentrations of human atrial natriuretic polypeptide in aged men. J Clin Endocrinol Metab 64:81-85

24. Richards AM, Tonolo G, McIntyre GD et al (1987) Radio-immunoassay for plasma alpha human atrial natriuretic peptide; a comparison of direct and preextracted methods. J Hypertension 5:227-236

25. Rosmalen FMA, Tan ACITL, Tan HS, Benraad TJ (1987) A sensitive radioimmunoassay of atrial natriuretic peptide in human plasma, using a tracer with an immobilized glycouril agent. Clin Chim Acta 165:331-340

26. Poiesi C, Rodella A, Mantero G et al (1989) Improved radioimmunoassay of atrial natriuretic peptide in plasma. Clin Chem 35:1431-1434

27. Capper SJ, Smith SW, Spensley CA, Whateley JG (1990) Specificities compared for a radioreceptor assay and a radioimmunoasay of atrial natriuretic peptide. Clin Chem 36:656-658

28. Rasmussen PH, Nielsen MD, Giese J (1990) Solid-phase double-antibody radio-immunoassay for atrial natriuretic factor. Scand J Clin Lab Invest 50:319-324

29. Clerico A, Del Chicca MG, Giganti M et al (1990) Evaluation and comparison of the analytical performances of two RIA kits for the assay of atrial natriuretic peptides (ANP). J Nucl Med All Sci 34:81-87

30. Clerico A, Giuseppe O, Pelizzola D et al (1991) Evaluation of the analytical performance of RIA methods for measurement of ANP. J Clin Immunoassay 14:251-256

31. Lindberg BF, Nilsson LG, Bergquist S, Andersson KE (1992) Radio-immunoassay of atrial natriuretic peptide (ANP) and characterization of ANP immunoreactivity in human plasma and atrial tissue. Scand J Clin Lab Invest 52:447-456

32. McLaughlin LL, Wei Y, Stockmann PT et al (1987) Development, validation and application of an enzyme immunoassay (EIA) of atriopeptin. Biochem Biophys Res Commun 144:469-476

33. Clerico A, Iervasi G, Manfredi C et al (1995) Preparation of mono-radio-iodinated tracers for studying the in vivo metabolism of atrial natriuretic peptide in humans. Eur J Nucl Med 22:997-1004

34. Lewis HM, Ratcliffe WA, Stott RAW et al (1989) Development and validation of a two-site immunoradiometric assay for human atrial natriuretic factor in unextracted plasma. Clin Chem 35:953-957

35. Tattersal JE, Dawnay A, McLean C, Cattel WR (1990) Immunoradiometric assay of atrial natriuretic peptide in unextracted plasma. Clin Chem 36:855-859

36. Tsuji T, Masuda H, Imagawa K et al (1994) Stability of human atrial natriuretic peptide in blood samples. Clin Chim Acta 225:171-177

37. Clerico A, Iervasi G, Del Chicca MG et al (1996) Analytical performance and clinical usefulness of a commercially available IRMA kit for the measurement of atrial natriuretic peptide in patients with heart failure. Clin Chem 42:1627-1633

38. Sundsfiord JA, Thibault G, Larochelle P, Cantin M (1988) Identification and plasma concentration of the N-terminal fragment of atrial natriuretic factor in man. J Clin Endocrinol Metab 66:605-610

39. Buckley MG, Markandu ND, Sagnella GA, MacGregor GA (1994) N-terminal atrial natriuretic peptide and atrial natriuretic peptide in human plasma: investigation of plasma levels and molecular circulating form(s) using radioimmunoassay for pro-atrial natriuretic peptide (31-67), pro-atrial natriuretic peptide (1-30) and atrial natriuretic peptide (99-126). Clin Sci 87:311-317

40. Mathisen P, Hall C, Simonsen S (1993) Comparative study of atrial peptides ANF(1-98) and ANF(99-126) as diagnostic markers of atrial distension in patients with cardiac disease. Scand J Clin Lab Invest 53:41-49

41. Winters CJ, Sallman AL, Baker BJ et al (1989) The N-terminus and a 4,000-MW peptide from the midportion of the N-terminus of the atrial natriuretic factor prohormone each circulate in humans and increase in congestive heart failure. Circulation 80:438-449

42. Gower WR Jr, Chiou S, Skolnick KA, Vesely DL (1994) Molecular forms of circulating atrial natriuretic peptides in human plasma and their metabolites. Peptides 15:861-867

43. Vesely DL, Douglass MA, Dietz JR et al (1994) Three peptides from the atrial natriuretic factor prohormone amino terminus lower blood pressure and produce diuresis, natriuresis, and/or kaliuresis in humans. Circulation 90:1129-1140

44. Overton RM, Vesely DL (1996) Processing of kaliuretic peptide in human plasma and serum. Peptides 17:1041-1046

45. Overton RM, Vesely DL (1996) Processing of long-acting natriuretic peptide and vessel dilator in human plasma and serum. Peptides 17:1155-1162

46. Vesely DL (2003) Natriuretic peptides and acute renal failure. Am J Physiol Renal Physiol 285:F167-177

47. Numata Y, Dohi K, Furukawa A et al (1998) Immunoradiometric assay for the N-terminal fragment of proatrial natriuretic peptide in human plasma. Clin Chem 44:1008-1013

48. Togashi K, Hirata Y, Ando K et al (1989) Brain natriuretic peptide-like immunoreactivity is present in human plasma. FEBS Lett 250:235-237

49. Lang CC, Coutie WJ, Khong TK et al (1991) Dietary sodium loading increases plasma brain natriuretic peptide levels in man. J Hypertens 9:779-782

50. Hasegawa K, Fujiwara H, Doyama K et al (1993) Ventricular expression of brain natriuretic peptide in hypertrophic cardiomyopathy. Circulation 88:372-380

51. Motwani JG, McAlpine H, Kennedy N, Struthers AD (1993) Plasma brain natriuretic peptide as an indicator for angiotensin-converting-enzyme inhibitor after myocardial infarction. Lancet 341:1109-1113

52. Morita E, Yasue H, Ypshimura M et al (1993) Increased plasma levels of brain natriuretic peptide in patients with acute myocardial infarction. Circulation 88:82-91

53. Yandle TG, Richards AM, Gilbert A et al (1993) Assay of brain natriuretic petide (BNP) in human plasma: evidence for high molecular weight BNP as a major plasma component in heart failure. J Clin Endocrinol Metab 76:832-838

54. Tharaux PL, Dussaule JC, Hubert-Brierre J et al (1994) Plasma atrial and brain natriuretic peptides in mitral stenosis treated by valvulotomy. Clin Sci 87:67-77

55. Davidson NC, Naas AA, Hanson JK et al (1996) Comparison of atrial natriuretic peptide, B-type natriuretic peptide, and n-terminal proatrial natriuretic peptide as indicators of left ventricular systolic dysfunction. Am J Cardiol 77:828-831

56. Kono M, Yamauchi A, Tsuji T et al (1993) An immunoradiometric assay for brain natriuretic peptide in human plasma. Kaku Igaku 13:2-7

57. Del Ry S, Clerico A, Giannessi D et al (2000) Measurement of brain natriuretic peptide in plasma samples and cardiac tissue extracts by means of an IRMA method. Scand J Clin Lab Invest 60:81-90
58. Fisher Y, Filzmaier K, Stiegler H et al (2001) Evaluation of a new, rapid bedside test for quantitative determination of B-type natriuretic peptide. Clin Chem 47:591-594
59. Vogeser M, Jacob C (2001) B-type natriuretic peptide (BNP) - validation of an immediate response assay. Clin Lab 47:29-33
60. Mueller T, Gegenhuber A, Poelz W, Haltmayer M (2004) Preliminary evaluation of the AxSYM B-type natriuretic peptide (BNP) assay and comparison with the ADVIA Centaur BNP assay. Clin Chem 50:1104-1106
61. Wians FH Jr, Wilson BA, Grant A et al (2005) Evaluation of the analytical performance characteristics of the Bayer ACS: 180 B-type natriuretic peptide (BNP) assay. Chim Clin Acta 353:147-155
62. Clerico A, Prontera C, Emdin M et al (2005) Analytical performance and diagnostic accuracy of immunometric assays for the measurement of plasma B-type natriuretic peptide (BNP) and N-terminal proBNP. Clin Chem 51:445-447
63. Rawlins ML, Owen WE, Roberts WL (2005) Performance characteristics of four automated natriuretic peptide assays. Am J Clin Pathol 123:439-445
64. Prontera C, Storti S, Emdin M et al (2005) Comparison of a fully automated immunoassay with a point-of-care testing method for B-type natriuretic peptide. Clin Chem 51:1274-1276
65. Hunt PJ, Yandle TG, Nicholls MG et al (1995) The amino-terminal portion of pro-brain natriuretic peptide (Pro-BNP) circulates in human plasma. Biochem Biophys Res Commun 214:1175-1183
66. Hunt PJ, Richards AM, Nicholls MG et al (1997) Immunoreactive amino-terminal pro-brain natriuretic peptide (NT-PROBNP): a new marker of cardiac impairment. Clin Endocrinol 47:287-296
67. Hughes D, Talwar S, Squire IB et al (1999) An immunoluminometric assay for N-terminal pro-brain natriuretic peptide: development of a test for left ventricular dysfunction. Clin Sci 96:373-380
68. Schulz H, Langvik TA, Lund Sagen E et al (2001) Radioimmunoassay for N-terminal probrain natriuretic peptide in human plasma. Scand J Clin Lab Invest 61:33-42
69. Mueller T, Gegenhuber A, Poelz W, Haltmayer M (2003) Comparison of the Biomedica NT-proBNP enzyme immunoassay and the Roche NT-proBNP chemiluminescence immunoassay: implications for the prediction of symptomatic and asymptomatic structural heart disease. Clin Chem 49:976-979
70. Yeo KTJ, Wu AHB, Apple FS et al (2003) Multicenter evaluation of the Roche NT-proBNP assay and comparison to the Biosite Triage BNP assay. Clin Chim Acta 338:107-115
71. Prontera C, Emdin M, Zucchelli GC et al (2003) Natriuretic peptides (NPs): automated electrochemiluminescent immunoassay for N-terminal pro-BNP compared with IRMAs for ANP and BNP in heart failure patients and healthy individuals. Clin Chem 49:1552-1554
72. Collinson PO, Barnes SC, Gaze DC et al (2004) Analytical performance of the N terminal pro B type natriuretic peptide (NT-proBNP) assay on the Elecsys 1010 and 2010 analysers. Eur J Heart Fail 6:365-368
73. Barnes SC, Collinson PO, Galasko G et al (2004) Evaluation of N-terminal pro-B type natriuretic peptide analysis on the Elecsys 1010 and 2010 analysers. Ann Clin Biochem 41:459-463
74. Prontera C, Emdin M, Zucchelli GC et al (2004) Analytical performance and diagnostic accuracy of a fully-automated electrochemiluminescent assay for the N-terminal fragment of the pro-peptide of brain natriuretic peptide in patients with cardiomyopathy: comparison with immunoradiometric assay methods for brain natriuretic peptide and atrial natriuretic peptide. Clin Chem Lab Med 42:37-44
75. Sokoll LJ, Baum H, Collinson PO et al (2004) Multicenter analytical performance evaluation of the Elecsys proBNP assay. Clin Chem Lab Med 42:965-972
76. Goetze JP (2004) Biochemistry of pro-B-type natriuretic peptide-derived peptides: the endocrine heart revisited. Clin Chem 50:1503-1510
77. Shimizu H, Masuta K, Aono K et al (2002) Molecular forms of human brain natriuretic peptide in plasma. Clin Chim Acta 316:129-135

78. Shimizu H, Masuta K, Asada H et al (2003) Characterization of molecular forms of probrain natriuretic peptide in human plasma. Clin Chim Acta 334:233-239

79. Hunt PJ, Espiner EA, Nicholls MG et al (1997) The role of the circulation in processing pro-brain natriuretic peptide (proBNP) to amino-terminal BNP and BNP-32. Peptides 18:1475-1481

80. Seidler T, Pemberton C, Yandle T et al (1999) The amino terminal regions of proBNP and proANP oligomerise through leucine zipper-like coiled-coil motifs. Biochem Biophys Res Commun 255:495-501

81. Crimmins DL (2005) N-terminal proBNP is a monomer. Clin Chem 51:1035-1038

82. Shimizu H, Aono K, Masuta K et al (2001) Degradation of human brain natriuretic peptide (BNP) by contact activation of blood coagulation system. Clin Chim Acta 305:181-186

83. Belenky A, Smith A, Zhang B et al (2004) The effect of class-specific protease inhibitors on the stabilization of B-type natriuretic peptide in human plasma. Clin Chim Acta 340:163-172

84. Ala-Kopsala M, Magga J, Peuhkurinen K et al (2004) Molecular heterogeneity has a major impact on the measurement of circulating N-terminal fragments of A- and B-type natriuretic peptides. Clin Chem 50:1576-1588

85. Goetze JP, Kastrup J, Pedersen F, Rehfeld JF (2002) Quantification of pro-B-type natriuretic peptide and its products in human plasma by use of an analysis independent of precursor processing. Clin Chem 48:1035-1042

86. Panteghini M (2004) Current concepts in standardization of cardiac markers immunoassay. Clin Chem Lab Med 42:3-8

87. Emdin M, Clerico A, Clemenza F et al (2005) Recommendations for the clinical use of cardiac natriuretic peptides. Ital Heart J 6:430-446

88. Apple FS, Panteghini M, Ravkilde J et al (2005) Quality specifications for B-type natriuretic peptide assays. Clin Chem 51:486-493

89. Daghfal DJ, Kelly P, Foreman P et al (2004) Analytical performance evaluation of the Abbott AxSYM assay. Clin Chem 50(suppl):A22

90. Beyne P, Benoit MO, Cambillau M et al (2005) Multicenter analytical performance of Triage Access BNP assay. Clin Chim Acta 355(suppl):S120

91. Oswal H, Inn M, Jarvinen C, Devaraj S (2005) Evaluation of a rapid automated immunoassay for B-type natriuretic peptide (BNP) - comparison with the Biosite Triage BNP assay. Clin Chem 51(suppl):A21

92. Wei T, Tuhy P, Bantum L et al (2004) Development of an automated immunoassay for NT-proBNP on the Dade Behring Dimension clinical chemistry system. Clin Chem 50(suppl):A13

93. Smith AC, Wu AH (2003) Analytical performance evaluation of the Bayer Advia Centaur BNP immunoassay. Clin Chem 49(suppl):A71

94. Shimizu H, Aono K, Masuta K et al (1999) Stability of brain natriuretic peptide (BNP) in human blood samples. Clin Chim Acta 285:169-172

95. Daghfal DJ, Parsons R, Kelly P et al (2004) Stability of BNP in whole blood and plasma. Clin Chem 50(suppl):A3

96. Mueller T, Gegenhuber A, Dieplinger B et al (2004) Long-term stability of endogenous B-type natriuretic peptide (BNP) and amino terminal proBNP (NT-proBNP) in frozen plasma samples. Clin Chem Lab Med 42:942-944

97. Nowatzke WL, Cole TG (2003) Stability of N-terminal pro-brain natriuretic peptide after storage frozen for one year and after multiple freeze thaw cycles. Clin Chem 49:1560-1562

98. Del Ry S, Maltinti M, Emdin M et al (2005) Radioimmunoassay for plasma C-type natriuretic peptide determination: a methodological evaluation. Clin Chem Lab Med 43:641-645

99. Piao FL, Park SH, Han JH et al (2004) Dendroaspis natriuretic peptide and its functions in pig ovarian granulosa cells. Regul Pept 118:193-198

100. Carstens J, Jensen KT, Ivarsen P et al (1997) Development of a urodilatin-specific antibody and radioimmunoassay for urodilatin in human urine. Clin Chem 43:638-643

101. Schulz-Knappe P, Forssmann K, Hock D et al (1988) Isolation and structural analysis of "urodilatin", a new peptide of the cardiodilatin-(ANP)-family, extracted from human urine. Klin Wochenschr 66:752-759

102. Vesely DL (2003) Natriuretic peptides and acute renal failure. Am J Physiol Renal Physiol 285:F167-177
103. Schweitz H, Vigne P, Moinier D et al (1992) A new member of the natriuretic peptide family is present in the venom of the green mamba (Dendroaspis angusticeps). J Biol Chem 267:13928-13932
104. Richards AM, Lainchbury JG, Nicholls MG et al (2002) Dendroaspis natriuretic peptide: endogenous or dubious? Lancet 359:5-6
105. Sudoh T, Minamino N, Kangawa K, Matsuo H (1990) C-Type natriuretic peptide (CNP): a new member of the natriuretic peptide family identified in porcine brain. Biochem Biophys Res Commun 168:863-870
106. Barr CS, Rhodes P, Struthers AD (1996) C-Type natriuretic peptide. Peptides 17:1243-1251
107. Chen HH, Burnett JC Jr (1998) C-type natriuretic peptide: the endothelial component of the natriuretic peptide system. J Cardiovasc Pharmacol 32(suppl 3):S22-28
108. Kalra PR, Anker SD, Struthers AD, Coats AJS (2001) The role of C-type natriuretic peptide in cardiovascular medicine. Eur Heart J 22:997-1007
109. Takei Y (2001) Does the natriuretic peptide system exist throughout the animal and plant kingdom? Comp Biochem Physiol Part B 129:559-573
110. Loretz CA, Pollina C (2000) Natriuretic peptides in fish physiology. Comp Biochem Physiol Part A 125:169-187
111. Prickett TCR, Yandle TG, Nicholls MG et al (2001) Identification of amino-terminal pro-C-type natriuretic peptide in human plasma. Biochem Biophys Res Commun 286:513-517
112. D'Souza SP, Davis M, Baxter GF (2004) Autocrine and paracrine actions of natriuretic peptides in the heart. Pharmacol Ther 101:113-129
113. Baxter GF (2004) The natriuretic peptides. Basic Res Cardiol 99:71-75
114. Ahluwalia A, Hobbs AJ (2005) Endothelium-derived C-type natriuretic peptide: more than just a hyperpolarized factor. Trends Pharmacol Sci 26:162-167
115. Scotland RS, Ahluwalia A, Hobbs AJ (2005) C-type natriuretic peptide in vascular physiology and disease. Pharmacol Ther 105:85-93
116. Furuya M, Yoshida M, Hayashi Y et al (1991) C-type natriuretic peptide is a growth inhibitor of rat vascular smooth muscle cells. Biochem Biophys Res Commun 177:927-931
117. Morishige K, Shimokawa H, Yamawaki T et al (2000) Local adenovirus-mediated transfer of C-type natriuretic peptide suppresses vascular remodeling in porcine coronary arteries *in vivo*. J Am Coll Cardiol 35:1040-1047
118. Ohno N, Itoh H, Ikeda T et al (2002) Accelerated reendothelialization with suppressed thrombogenic property and neointimal hyperplasia of rabbit jugular vein grafts by adenovirus-mediated gene transfer of C-type natriuretic peptide. Circulation 105:1623-1626
119. Qian JY, Haruno A, Asada Y et al (2002) Local expression of C-type natriuretic peptide suppresses inflammation, eliminates shear stress-induced thrombosis, and prevents neointima formation through enhanced nitric oxide production in rabbit injured carotid arteries. Circ Res 91:1063-1069
120. Yasuda S, Kanna M, Sakuragi S et al (2002) Local delivery of single low-dose of C-type natriuretic peptide, an endogenous vascular modulator, inhibits neointimal hyperplasia in a balloon-injured rabbit iliac artery model. J Cardiovasc Pharmacol 39:784-788
121. Takeuchi H, Ohmori K, Kondo I et al (2003) Potentiation of C-type natriuretic peptide with ultrasound and microbubbles to prevent neointimal formation after vascular injury in rats. Cardiovasc Res 58:231-238
122. Wei CM, Heublein DM, Perella MA et al (1993) Natriuretic peptide system in human heart failure. Circulation 88:1004-1009
123. Totsune K, Takahashi K, Murakami O et al (1994) Elevated plasma C-type natriuretic peptide concentrations in patients with chronic renal failure. Clin Sci 87:319-322
124. Cargill RI, Barr CS, Coutie WJ et al (1994) C-Type natriuretic peptide levels in cor pulmonale and in congestive cardiac failure. Thorax 49:1247-1249
125. Kalra PR, Clague JR, Bolger AP et al (2003) Myocardial production of C-type natriuretic peptide in chronic heart failure. Circulation 107:571-573

126. Wright SP, Prickett TC, Doughty RN et al (2004) Amino-terminal pro-C-type natriuretic peptide in heart failure. Hypertension 43:94-100
127. Potter LR (2004) CNP, cardiac natriuretic peptide? Endocrinology 145:2129-2130
128. Gulberg V, Moller S, Henriksen JH, Gerbes AL (2000) Increased renal production of C-type natriuretic peptide (CNP) in patients with cirrhosis and functional renal failure. Gut 47:852-857
129. Del Ry S, Passino C, Maltinti M et al (2005) C-Type natriuretic peptide plasma levels increase in patients with chronic heart failure as a function of clinical severity. Eur J Heart Fail 7:1145-1148

Clinical Considerations and Applications in Cardiac Diseases

Aldo Clerico • Claudio Passino • Michele Emdin

5.1 Circulating Levels of Cardiac Natriuretic Hormones: Physiological Considerations and Clinical Interpretation

CNH are powerful hormones with important physiological effects. Consequently, by considering their assay only as a marker for cardiac disease may result in a misinterpretation or underestimation of their biological action and of their pathophysiological role in cardiovascular as well as other diseases. In the first part of Chapter 5 (from section 5.1.1 to 5.1.5), some physiological conditions in which the interpretations of increased levels of CNH may be difficult or provoke misunderstanding will be discussed in detail. In particular, the influence of age and sex hormones on circulating levels of CNH will be reviewed (section 5.1.1). As far as the clinical interpretation of variations of circulating levels of CNH is concerned, some important points will be stressed: 1) the pathophysiological and clinical consequence of the progressive resistance to biological actions of CNH in patients with heart failure (section 5.1.3); 2) the inter-relationship between hemodynamic mechanisms and activity of neuro-endocrine system in determining the variation of circulating levels of CNH (section 5.1.4); 3) the clinical relevance of variation of CNH levels (section 5.1.5). The discussion of these points will lay the pathophysiological foundations for better understanding of the second part of this Chapter, which concerns the diagnostic and prognostic role of CNH assay in patients with cardiovascular disease (sections from 5.2 to 5.5).

5.1.1 Influence of Age and Gender

The circulating levels of CNH are regulated or modified by several physiological factors (such as circadian variations, age, gender, exercise, body posture, and water immersion), eating habits (especially sodium intake), clinical conditions (Table 5.1), and drugs (including corticosteroids, sex steroid hormones, thyroid hormones, diuretics, angiotensin-converting enzyme [ACE] inhibitors, and adrenergic agonists and antagonists) [1-6].

The wide variations of circulating levels of CNH in adult healthy subjects in relation to aging and gender could have a particular clinical relevance [7-10] (Figs. 5.1 and 5.2, Table 5.2). Indeed, Vasan et al. [9] recently demonstrated that the diagnostic accuracy of CNH assay for community screening is gender-dependent.

In order to explain these variations, the possible influence of sex steroid hormones on the CNH system, as well as the modification of the cardiovascular system with aging, should be taken into account [11-14]. According to these mechanisms, the higher CNH values of women during the fertile adult period could be explained by the physiological stimulation of female sex steroid hormones. In particular, the BNP concentration is on average 36% higher in women than in men aged less than 50 years [7] (Figs. 5.1 and

Table 5.1. Conditions characterized by altered BNP plasma concentration

Clinical condition	BNP concentration
Cardiovascular diseases	
Chronic heart failure	Highly increased
Acute coronary syndromes	Increased
Hypertension with LVH and fibrosis	Slightly increased
Supraventricular tachyarrhythmias	Increased
Respiratory diseases	
Acute dyspnea	Normal or slightly increased
Pulmonary embolism	Increased
Chronic respiratory disorders	Normal or slightly increased
Primitive pulmonary hypertension	Increased
Endocrine-metabolic diseases	
Hyperthyroidism	Slightly increased
Hypothyroidism	Slightly decreased
Cushing's syndrome	Increased
Hyperaldosteronism	Increased
Diabetes	Normal or increased
Hepatic cirrhosis with ascites	Increased
Renal failure (acute or chronic)	Increased
Septic shock	Increased
Chronic inflammatory diseases	
Amiloidosis and sarcoidosis	Normal or increased
Subarachnoid hemorrhage	Normal or increased
Paraneoplastic syndromes	Normal or increased
Anti-neoplastic therapies	Normal or increased

LVH Left ventricular hypertrophy

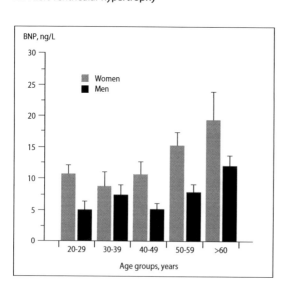

Fig. 5.1. Mean (SEM) BNP values divided according to gender and age groups. Data obtained in the author's laboratory with an IRMA method [7]

5.2, Table 5.2). The increase in CNH with aging may be due to the para-physiological decline in myocardial function and other organs (including kidney), typical of senescence [15]. In this case, the CNH assay may be considered as a biochemical marker of increased risk of cardiac morbidity in old age [16]. Moreover, the increase in CNH with aging may be due to a decrease in their clearance rate. Indeed, an age modulation of maximum binding capacity of clearance (C-type) receptors for CNH was reported in platelets of elderly persons [17].

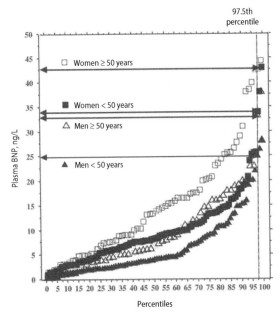

Fig. 5.2. Percentile distribution of plasma BNP divided according to gender and two age groups (≥50 and <50 years). The 97.5th percentile (*dotted line*) and the corresponding BNP values (*arrows*) are indicated. Data obtained in the author's laboratory with an IRMA method [7]

Table 5.2. Mean (± SD) circulating levels of ANP and BNP (ng/l) divided into eight groups according to sex and age. The number of subjects studied for each group is reported within brackets. Data obtained in the author's laboratory with an IRMA method [7]

	Men	Women	*p*-value*
ANP			
Age <50 years	13.8 ± 7.0 (79)	16.1 ± 9.5 (92)	0.0001
Age ≥50 years	21.3 ± 10.3 (56)	22.1 ± 13.2 (67)	0.8529
p-value*	0.0001	0.0013	
BNP			
Age <50 years	6.4 ± 6.2 (95)	10.0 ± 7.5 (104)	<0.0001
Age ≥50 years	9.8 ± 8.0.8 (57)	15.2 ± 11.8 (70)	0.0025
p-value*	0.0001	0.0047	

*Fisher's protected least significant difference test after ANOVA using the logarithmic transformation of original set of data

5.1.2 Comparison between the CNH Assay and that of CNH-Related Pro-Hormone Peptides

All CNH derive from pre-pro-hormones (i.e., preproANP and preproBNP), containing a signal peptide sequence at the amino-terminal end. The pro-hormones (i.e., proANP and proBNP) are produced by cleavage of signal peptide, and then are further split into inactive longer NH_2-terminal fragments (i.e., NT-proANP or NT-proBNP), and a biologically active shorter COOH-terminal peptide (i.e., ANP or BNP), which are secreted in the blood in equimolar amounts (Figs. 3.11 and 3.12). However, ANP and BNP have a shorter plasma half-life and consequently lower plasma concentration, compared to NT-proANP and NT-proBNP (Table 4.1) [1-7, 18].

Studies on structure-activity relationships have shown the importance for the binding to the specific receptors of the central ring structure of CNH, formed by a disulfide bridge between the two cysteine residues. For this reason, only ANP and BNP, which present the disulfide bridge in the peptide chain, share the typical hormonal activity of CNH, while the NT-proANP and NT-proBNP do not [1-7].

Theoretically, setting up an immunoassay for NT-proANP and NT-proBNP should be easier because their plasma concentrations are higher than ANP and BNP [18]. On the other hand, NT-proANP and NT-proBNP immunoassays may be affected by several analytical problems, mainly concerning the different assay specificities; consequently, very different results are produced by different methods with a large bias [2, 5, 6, 18] (Table 4.1). The different analytical performance might affect the diagnostic accuracy of the assays, in discriminating between subjects with or without cardiac disease [2, 5, 6, 18-21] (see Chapter 4 for more details).

The respective advantages of measuring biologically active peptide hormones (ANP and BNP), or inactive peptides (NT-proANP and NT-proBNP) are summarized in Table 4.2. The assay of the inactive propeptides better fits the definition of disease marker than the assay of circulating levels of ANP or BNP, which, on the other hand, may be considered a more reliable index of the activation status of the CNH system.

Considering the biochemical and physiological characteristics of the different peptides, it is conceivable that ANP is a better marker of acute overload and/or rapid cardiovascular hemodynamic changes than BNP and, especially, than NT-proANP or NT-proBNP [2, 5]. For example, circulating levels of ANP are known to be more affected by body position and decreased to a greater extent by a hemodialysis session in patients with chronic renal failure than those of BNP, while plasma NT-proANP is unchanged [22]. Furthermore, ANP increases more than NT-proANP during rapid ventricular pacing [23].

5.1.3 Resistance to the Biological Action of CNH

Deficiencies in the activity of the CNH system could explain altered electrolyte and fluid homeostasis occurring in chronic heart failure (HF) [24-26]. However, the hypothesis proposing HF as a syndrome of CNH deficiency was challenged when the CNH system was more carefully investigated in experimental animals and humans [24-26]. Patients with chronic HF show increased CNH plasma levels compared to normal subjects (Table 3.1, Fig. 3.13). These findings have been recently defined the "endocrine paradox" in HF [6], i.e., extremely high circulating levels of hormones with powerful natriuretic activity in patients with congestive HF, who show physical signs of fluid retention and vasoconstriction due to a relatively poor biological activity of the CNH system.

A blunted natriuretic response after pharmacological doses of ANP and BNP has been observed in experimental models and in patients with chronic HF, suggesting a resistance to the biological effects of CNH, principally natriuresis [24-31]. This resistance syndrome was also demonstrated by *in vivo* turnover studies using radioactive tracers in patients with HF [32, 33].

Resistance to the biological action of CNH could, theoretically, have three different causes (Table 5.3). First, circulating CNH could be, at least in part, inactive. Furthermore, a great fraction of CNH could be inactivated by plasma and tissue proteases before they bind to specific receptors. These two conditions account for all possible mechanisms acting at the pre-receptor level. Second, down-regulation of specific receptors could explain a reduced CNH activity. Finally, some mechanisms can act at post-receptor level, counteracting the biological effects of CNH.

Mechanisms acting at pre-receptor level: Some peptides, derived *in vivo* or *in vitro* from degradation of intact proBNP, are biologically inactive, although they can be measured by immunoassay methods [5, 6, 18]. Since the circulating levels of intact proBNP and of its derived peptides increase progressively with severity of HF, immunoassay methods can greatly overestimate the true biological activity of CNH in patients with severe HF [6]. Unfortunately, at present, it is not possible to estimate the inaccuracy of CNH immunoassays because these methods use different, not standardized antibodies and calibrators, leading to highly different clinical results [5, 6, 18, 34, 35].

A resistance to the biological action of CNH may be theoretically due to an increase in degradation (turnover) of circulating biologically active peptides. CNH are degraded *in vivo* and *in vitro* by several types of proteolytic enzymes, including serin-proteases, peptidyl arginine aldehyde proteases, kallikrein-like proteases, and neutral endopeptidases (NEP) [5, 6, 18, 34-38].

Individual differences in the ability of heart tissue to mature the precursor of CNH pep-

Table 5.3. Classification of mechanisms of resistance to biological effects of CNH

Causes acting at pre-receptor level
    a) Presence of inactive peptides in plasma
    b) Changes in renal filtration
    c) Changes in degradation pathways of active peptides:
        1. Upregulation of NPR-C
        2. Increased activity of proteases

Causes acting at receptor level
    a) Down-regulation of NPR-A and NPR-B in target tissues
    b) Altered CNH receptor binding or desensitization

Causes acting at post-receptor level (activated counter-regulatory mechanisms)
    a) Altered intracellular signalling:
        1. Decreased cGMP cellular accumulation (decreased production or increased degradation)
        2. Altered intracellular pathways beyond cGMP

tides, or of peripheral tissues to degrade them, may help to explain why there are some differences in the clinical presentation among patients with HF with similar clinical severity and ventricular function [6]. However, further studies are necessary to confirm this hypothesis. From a clinical point of view, it is important to note that some drugs sharing an inhibitory action on both NEP and ACE (so called vasopeptidase inhibitors) may have some beneficial effects in patients with arterial hypertension and/or HF because the administration of these durgs can potentiate the biological activity of CNH system by increasing the concentration of biologically active peptides [39-42] (see Chapter 7, sections 7.4 and 7.5, for more details). It is important to note that renal function can affect the biological action of CNH in different ways [5] (see also section 6.3 for more details). CNH are small peptides freely filtrated by renal glomerulus; the kidneys are probably responsible for about 50% of metabolic clerance rate of plasma ANP and BNP and in this way renal diseases can affect the circulating levels of CNH. Indeed, a decreased renal function greatly increases the plasma CNH concentration and consequently more peptide hormones are available for other target tissues (such as brain, vascular tissue, adrenal gland and so on) [5]. However, luminal perfusion with ANP has been shown to reduce sodium efflux from the inner medullar collecting duct, suggesting that this hormone has also luminal sites of action [25]. As a consequence, a reduction in the filtration can potentially induce renal hypo-responsiveness to CNH. To date, however, ANP has been detected only on tubular basolateral membranes [25]. Thus, the mechanisms of CNH luminal action need to be elucidated before conclusions are drawn about the functional significance of reduced natriuretic peptide filtrations in the renal hypo-responsiveness to ANP and other natriuretic peptides. Finally, a resistance to the biological action of CNH may be theoretically also due to an increased renal filtration (clearance) of active peptides; at this moment, however, there are no consistent data to confirm this hypothesis.

Mechanisms acting at receptor level: Some studies suggest that the resistance to biological effects of CNH in HF may be due, in part, to variations in the relative amount of the three different types of natriuretic peptide-specific receptors. In particular, there could be an upregulation of type C receptors (NPR-C) with a parallel down-regulation of type A and B receptors (NPR-A and NPR-B) [43-47]. NPR-A and NPR-B mediate all known hormonal actions of CNH, therefore their down-regulation should induce a deactivation of the CNH system. The upregulation of NPR-C receptors that strongly contribute to the clearance of biologically active peptides could further increase the resistance to CNH in patients with HF [43].

These findings are well in accordance with the results of *in vivo* kinetic studies obtained using radioactive tracers in patients with HF [32, 33]. Moreover, a recent study confirmed that mRNA expression levels of ANP, BNP and the NPR-C receptor were markedly increased in human failing hearts [46]. Reversal of cardiomyocyte hypertrophy during left ventricular assist device support was accompanied by normalization of ANP, BNP and NPR-C mRNA levels and a significant recovery of responsiveness to ANP [47].

However, a very recent study [48] found that neither NPR-A nor NPR-B were internalized or degraded in response to natriuretic peptide binding in 293T cultured cells. Another well-characterized deactivation mechanism is the process by which an activated receptor is turned off, commonly referred to as "desensitization" [48-50]. Phosphorylation of the intracellular kinase homology domain of NRP-A and NPR-B is required for hormone-dependent activation of the receptor, while dephosphorylation at this site causes desensitization. Deactivation of the CNH system via desensitization of NRP-A and NPR-B can occur in response to various pathophysiological stimuli [48-50] (see Chapter 3, section 3.5.2, for more details).

Further studies are necessary to clarify what is the most important mechanism of deactivation of CNH system acting *in vivo* at receptor level in patients with heart failure: the down-regulation (of NPR-A and NPR-B), the upregulation (of NPR-C), or the desensitization (of NPR-A and NPR-B).

A peripheral resistance to the biological effects of CNH may play an important role in other clinical conditions, besides HF. For example, NPR-C is also present on cellular membranes of adipose tissue. It was suggested that the increase in NPR-C receptors observed in obese subjects can in turn increase the peripheral degradation of CNH and consequently blunt the action of the CNH system [51, 52]. Indeed, recent studies have documented decreased circulating levels of CNH (especially BNP) in obese subjects, compared to non-obese subjects matched for age and gender [51, 54]. This reduced activity of the CNH system may increase the risk of developing arterial hypertension and other cardiovascular diseases due to the non-contrasted and therefore prevailing effects of the counter-regulatory system with sodium-retentive and vasoconstrictive properties [52-54] (see Chapter 6, section 6.9, and Chapter 7, section 7.5, for more detailed clinical information).

However, recent studies found that the NPR-C receptor could be coupled to a G-protein that inhibits cyclic AMP synthesis. These receptors, which are present in great amount especially on the endothelial cell wall, may mediate some paracrine effects of CNP on vascular tissue [55-57]. Therefore, further studies will be necessary to elucidate the possible role of NPR-C receptors as modulators of CNH action and/or degradation in peripheral tissues.

Mechanisms acting at post-receptor level: A large number of studies demonstrated that the activation of the neuro-hormonal system accelerates the left ventricular functional impairment in patients with HF [1-6, 58-60]. Drugs that contrast the detrimental effects of the neuro-hormonal system activation play a key role for the current pharmacological treatment of HF. Some of these, such as ACE inhibitors, angiotensin II receptor blockers, β-blockers, and spironolactone decrease the circulating levels of CNH [5, 61-65], "normalize" their kinetics, and increase their biological activity [24, 26]. Furthermore, they enhance the natriuretic effect of ANP or BNP analogs administered to patients. In other words, the treatment with this type of pharmacological agents decreases the systemic resistance to the biological effects of CNH [24, 26].

Patients with HF show a progressive and parallel increase in CNH levels and in some neuro-hormones and cytokines. This increase can be closely related to disease severity, as assessed by functional NYHA class (Table 3.1, Fig. 3.13) [60]. Plasma BNP values, normalized by mean values found in healthy subjects, are significantly higher than other normalized neuro-hormone and cytokine values in HF (Fig. 5.3, Table 5.4) [60]; these data well support the so-called "endocrine paradox" of HF [6]. On average, the response of the CNH system to the increasing challenge of disease severity may not be linear (Fig. 5.4). The curve reported in Figure 5.4 suggests that the CNH system responds with a sharp increase in BNP plasma concentration in the early phase of HF (NYHA class I-II patients), followed, with the clinical progression of the disease, by a blunted increase (NYHA class III), and finally by a plateau (NYHA class IV) (Table 3.1, Fig. 5.4).

These findings are consistent with the results from *in vivo* kinetic studies, indicating that ANP turnover (i.e., metabolic clearance rate and production rate) and natriuresis are both increased in patients in the early phase of HF (NYHA class I), as compared to patients with congestive HF [24, 26]. This suggests that resistance to the biological action of CNH is characteristic only of the congestive stage of HF. During the asymp-

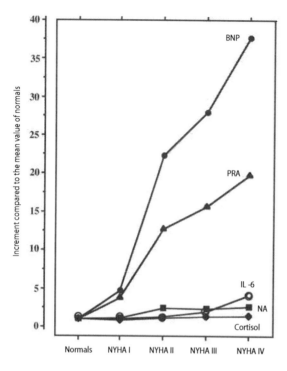

Fig. 5.3. Per cent mean ratio increment of BNP, cortisol, interleukin-6 (IL-6), plasma renin activity (PRA) and noradrenaline (NA) values. The values were calculated by dividing the mean value of the patient's group by the value found in normal subjects (expressed as ratio). These data show a progressively greater increment of BNP compared with those of other biological markers in patients with heart failure. Data obtained in the author's laboratory [7]

Table 5.4. Mean (± SD) levels of CNH, neuro-hormones, thyroid hormones, and cytokines in normal subjects over 50 years of age and patients with heart failure. Data obtained in the author's laboratory

	Normal subjects	Patients	p-value*
ANP (ng/L)	25.4 ± 15.8	184.1 ± 137.8	<0.0001
BNP (ng/L)	14.4 ± 21.0	382.0 ± 364.3	<0.0001
Adrenaline (pg/ml)	52.2 ± 20.4	55.5 ± 66.8	0.7500
NorA (pg/ml)	341.6 ± 133.9	797.9 ± 470.4	<0.0001
TNF-α (pg/ml)	6.9 ± 4.9	9.9 ± 8.4	0.0250
IL-6 (pg/ml)	< 6.0	10.9 ± 18.2	0.0243
PRA (ng/ml/h)	0.5 ± 0.4	7.5 ± 10.2	<0.0001
Aldosterone (pg/ml)	96.2 ± 46.8	204.4 ± 218.7	0.0008
Cortisol (ng/ml)	167.6 ± 46.5	207.5 ± 107.7	0.0127
TSH (µUI/ml)	1.44 ± 0.91	1.78 ± 2.67	0.3875
T4 (µg/100 ml)	6.4 ± 1.6	8.6 ± 2.9	<0.0001
T3 (µg/100 ml)	100.6 ± 17.0	83.5 ± 30.3	0.0007
FT4 (pg/ml)	11.2 ± 2.1	14.2 ± 4.8	<0.0001
FT3 (pg/ml)	2.6 ± 0.4	2.3 ± 0.8	0.0115

NorA noradrenaline, *TNF-α* tumor necrosis factor-a, *IL-6* interleukin-6, *PRA* plasma renin activity, *TSH* thyroid-stimulating hormone, *T4* thyroxine, *T3* tri-iodothyronine, *FT4* free thyroxine, *FT3* free tri-iodothyronine
* Unpaired *t* test after log-transformation of original data

tomatic, early phase of the disease, the CNH system is able to compensate for the over-activity of the counter-regulatory system (Fig. 5.4).

In conclusion, several mechanisms occurring at the pre-receptorial, receptorial and post-receptorial levels may play a role in inducing peripheral resistance to the biological effects of CNH in HF. However, the overwhelming activation of the counter-regulatory system should be considered the predominant pathophysiological mechanism. The data discussed so far also suggest that monitoring the degree of systemic resistance to the biological effects of CNH could be clinically useful in the follow-up of patients with HF.

5.1.4 Diagnostic Accuracy of CNH Assay in Plasma from Patients with Cardiac Diseases

The CNH system activation is modulated not only by hemodynamic factors, but also by the activity of the counter-regulatory neuro-hormonal system. The response of the CNH system to chronic pathophysiological stimuli may be log-like (Figs. 3.13 and 5.4). Consequently, it is likely that very small changes in hemodynamics, not assessable by echocardiographic examination, may produce significant (and measurable) variations in plasma concentrations of CNH. Moreover, recent studies have indicated that very small changes in some neuro-hormones and cytokines can produce wider variations in BNP circulating levels [60] (Fig. 5.3).

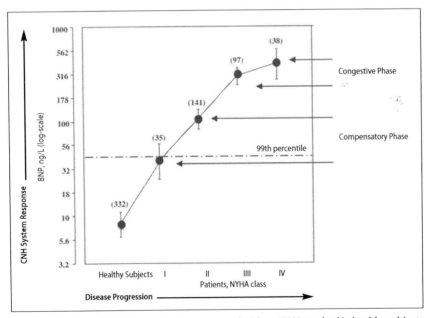

Fig. 5.4. Mean (95% CI) BNP concentration measured with an IRMA method in healthy subjects and patients with heart failure grouped according to the NYHA functional class (the number of subjects/patients enrolled for each group is indicated within brackets). Data obtained in the author's laboratory. The 99th percentile of normal distribution is indicated by a dotted line

It is well known that changes in hemodynamic parameters (such as left ventricular ejection fraction, EF) and plasma CNH levels (expressed in a log scale) are closely related in patients with cardiovascular diseases (Fig. 5.5) [2-5, 19, 58-65]. However, correlations between plasma CNH levels and echocardiographically measured parameters, such as left ventricular EF, myocardial mass and chamber volumes, are usually less close in the general population (large community-based sample, including healthy subjects with or without individuals with asymptomatic myocardial dysfunction) [8, 9, 66, 67], as well shown dy data reported in Figure 5.6.

It should be emphasized that the recognition of HF syndrome is not equivalent to the clinical diagnosis of cardiomyopathy or to the assessment of left ventricular dysfunction, these latter terms describing possible structural reasons for the development of HF [68-70]. Instead, HF is a clinical syndrome that is characterized by specific symptoms (namely dyspnea and fatigue) and signs (namely fluid retention) [68]. There is no diagnostic test for HF, because it is largely a clinical diagnosis based on a careful history and physical examination [68]. Therefore, there are no objective criteria for the identification and/or clinical stratification of patients with suspected HF; several "reference (gold) standards" [71], based on clinical, laboratory and instrumental examinations, can be used to evaluate the diagnostic accuracy of the CNH assay [5]. For this evaluation, some studies took into consideration only echocardiographic assessment of ventricular dysfunction, while in others either results of echocardiography or all clinical data have been used for the diagnosis of HF [5, 72].

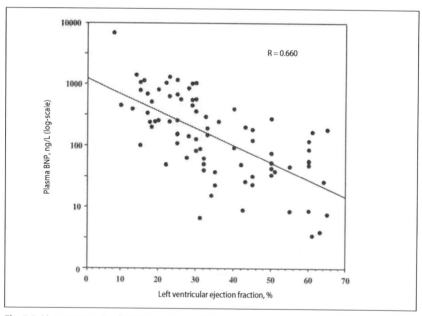

Fig. 5.5. Linear regression between plasma BNP values (measured with an IRMA method) and left ventricular ejection fraction (%), assessed by nuclear medicine imaging, in 84 patients with primary or secondary cardiomyopathy. Data obtained in the author's laboratory

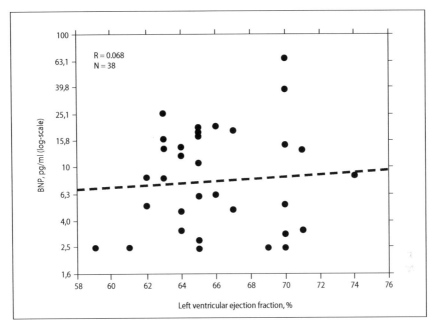

Fig. 5.6. No correlation (R = 0.068, p >> 0.1) between the log transformation of plasma BNP concentration, measured with an IRMA method, and left ventricular ejection fraction values, assessed by echocardiography, in 38 healthy adult subjects (mean age ± SD = 57.3 ± 9.4 years, range 35-78 years). A *dotted line* indicates the hypothetical linear regression. Data obtained in the author's laboratory

Unfortunately, using echocardiography as the unique reference standard may lead to misinterpretations when evaluating the diagnostic accuracy of the CNH assay. A systematic review of clinical studies in patient populations with a prevalence of HF ranging from 3.8% to 51% to determine the diagnostic accuracy of BNP assays found that the sensitivity (ranging from 90 to 97%) was much less variable (by 4.4-fold) than the specificity (ranging from 53 to 84%) [5]. Furthermore, in a meta-analysis [72], diagnostic accuracy of BNP assays greatly varied according not only to the group of patients studied, but also to the reference standard used (left ventricular EF <40% or <55%, diagnosis of diastolic dysfunction, diagnosis of systolic + diastolic dysfunction, or integrative clinical criteria). These data indicate that the choice of a suitable and accurate reference standard for evaluation of the diagnostic accuracy of the BNP assay in patients with HF may be a problem that is actually underestimated in the literature. For a proper definition of diagnostic accuracy, tested individuals should be grouped into those with and without disease, by means of an independent clinical judgment, considering both the CNH assay and echocardiographic data.

Careful echocardiographic examinations usually show slightly better or even similar diagnostic accuracy than the BNP assay in patients with cardiac diseases [73,74]. On the other hand, the CNH assay may have some advantages compared to echocardiographic examinations alone in specific clinical settings. For example, Williams et al.

suggested that in patients with chronic HF, the NT-proBNP assay reflects functional cardiac impairment and decreased exercise capacity (measured by peak exercise oxygen consumption) better than the left ventricular EF [75].

Several studies indicate that BNP and NT-proBNP are powerful and independent risk markers of cardiovascular events (especially mortality) not only in patients with HF, but also in those with acute coronary syndrome, as reported in recent and systematic reviews [5, 76-78]. Some studies also suggested that the cardiovascular risk increases progressively to CNH concentration [77-79]; that is, there is no threshold that actually identifies patients with null risk.

Diagnostic sensitivity of BNP/NT-proBNP assays in detecting left ventricular systolic dysfunction could be suboptimal in asymptomatic or low-risk individuals, especially in women [9]. Specificity of BNP assays in patients with HF ranged from 53 to 84% and positive predictive values from 3 to 85% in several studies [5]. These data indicate that CNH assays can produce a relatively large number of false-positive results. Consequently, many individuals, actually without HF (about 15-60% of those with positive CNH tests), might undergo expensive and/or harmful investigations to rule out the disease, or even be inappropriately labeled as cardiac patients [5].

Several false-positive results can be observed in patients with various clinical diagnoses, as reported in Table 5.1. In these patients, increased plasma BNP may predict, even in the presence of a normal echocardiographic examination, an increased risk of mortality or major cardiac events, including pulmonary embolism [80-82] and hypertension [83], renal failure [84, 85], septic shock [86], some chronic inflammatory diseases (such as amyloidosis and sarcoidosis) [87, 88], and diabetes mellitus [89].

On the other hand, false-negative results could be found in patients on treatment with anti-adrenergic agents, diuretics and/or ACE inhibitors, all drugs that can reduce CNH levels [5]. As shown in Figure 5.7, a large number of patients with only mild HF (NYHA classes I and II) may have values slightly above or even under the 99th percentile of distribution values of BNP concentration in healthy subjects (about 50 ng/l, measured by an IRMA method). In these patients, successful treatment and consequent improvement in cardiac function and exercise capacity, and reduction in filling pressure and cardiac volumes, is usually associated with a marked fall in CNH levels: thus, a larger number of patients could have BNP values within the reference range values [5, 90]. However, at matched echocardiographic alterations, patients in whom BNP levels drop in response to therapy have a reduced rate of major cardiac events or mortality, compared to untreated hypertensive patients, who could have similar echocardiographic abnormalities. This represents the rationale for using the CNH assay for therapy decision making and for monitoring HF patients [5, 61-65].

In populations with a higher prevalence of cardiac diseases, including only individuals with a clinical suspicion of HF, the diagnostic sensitivity of BNP can improve up to 95%, or even more, as long as appropriate cut-off values are selected [5, 72]. In this case, a strategy called "SnNout", which maximizes test sensitivity, could be used to rule out the presence of HF [91]. Furthermore, CNH assay also shows high (>95%) negative predictive values [5, 20], which can help to confirm the absence of HF. This is the rationale for choosing the CNH assay as the first step for an algorithm for the diagnosis of HF [69, 70]. Such a clinical strategy has proved successful in some recent studies evaluating the cost-effectiveness of using plasma BNP measurements for screening of cardiac dysfunction in the general population [92-94].

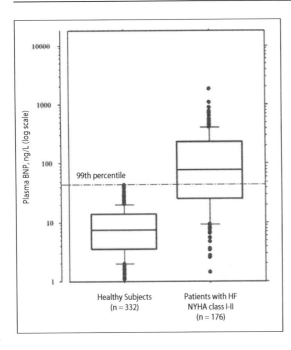

Fig. 5.7. Plasma BNP values (measured with an IRMA method) in adult healthy subjects and patients with mild heart failure (NYHA class I-II). The number of subjects included in each group is indicated within brackets. The *dotted line* shows the 99th percentile of normal distribution. The results are expressed as boxes with five horizontal lines, displaying the 10th, 25th, 50th (median), 75th, and 90th percentiles of the variable. All values above the 90th percentile and below the 10th percentile (outliers) are plotted separately (as *circles*). Data obtained in the author's laboratory

5.1.5 Biological Variation of Plasma BNP: a Problem or a Clinical Resource?

The variability of measured plasma concentrations of many substances is due to three different sources: pre-analytical, analytical and inherent biological variation. The latter is usually described as a random variation around a homeostatic setting point, and defined as the intra-individual or within-subject biological variation [95]. Several physiological parameters and endogenous substances are closely regulated by complex biological mechanisms in such a way as to vary little. If a random variation is assumed for an analyte, the effect of imprecision on dispersion can be taken into consideration for setting generally applicable quality specifications for assay performance in order to indicate an acceptable (or desirable) degree of assay precision. Accordingly, the desirable assay imprecision should be equal to or less than half of the intra-individual biological variation [96,97].

In order to achieve a correct interpretation of serial test results that are collected for follow-up or tailored treatment of HF patients, several studies [97-101] recently evaluated the biological variation of BNP and its related peptides, in both healthy subjects and cardiac patients.

Due to secretory bursts and its rapid turnover (half-life about 15-20 min) [1, 102] (see Chapter 3, section 3.6.2 for more details), it is not surprising that intra-individual biological variations of plasma BNP levels were found to be very large, in both healthy subjects and patients with heart failure (ranging from 30 to 50%) [97,99-101]. Assuming a random variation around a homeostatic setting point, the calculated reference change values at 95% confidence interval ranged from 99 to 130% for BNP in healthy subjects and patients [97, 99-101]. According to this estimated confidence interval, only a decrease of more than 50% or a more than 2-fold increase in plasma BNP should be assumed to be statistically significant in an individual patient.

In contrast with this assumption, a recent clinical trial [90] has suggested that a BNP decrease inferior to this calculated reference change could be clinically relevant in patients with heart failure. In this study, only the group of patients treated with the β-blocker agent carvedilol, who respond on average with a decrease of only 38% in plasma BNP, showed a clinical improvement [90]. Furthermore, several studies have demonstrated that cardiovascular risk (mortality or major cardiovascular events) increases continuously and progressively throughout the whole range of BNP concentrations in patients with cardiovascular diseases [5, 77-79].

In order to explain these conflicting findings, it should be taken into account that BNP secretion is closely regulated by specific pathophysiological mechanisms. Thus, changes in plasma hormone levels cannot be interpreted as random variations around a setting point, but as strictly determined by the activation level of the counter-regulatory system and by changes in hemodynamics. The clinician should look at the intra-individual variation in BNP as a mirror of variation in neuro-endocrine network activity.

According to this hypothesis, it was suggested to consider all changes in BNP concentration as potentially clinically relevant, even when narrower than the calculated intra-individual biological variation [103]. In other words, BNP variations should be interpreted and considered by physicians, as the variability of heart rhythm and blood pressure, by taking into account clinical history and examination, comprehensive of the response to specific treatments, as well as of laboratory and instrumental test findings.

There is another important practical consequence of this approach. According to an intra-individual biological variation of about 30%, the estimated imprecision goal for BNP immunoassays should be 15% (i.e., equal to half of the intra-individual variation) [95, 96]. On the contrary, we suggest that all the measured variations of plasma BNP greater than two to three times the analytical imprecision of assay used should be potentially considered as clinically relevant. Following this approach, the assay imprecision of BNP immunoassays should be as low as possible.

Of course, the great number of pathophysiological mechanisms affecting the CNH system makes it sometimes difficult for clinicians to recognize the cause(s) of variations in its activity. However, we believe that the BNP assay should be considered as an intellectual spur for the search for an explanation of variations in hormone concentrations, which should always be related to pathophysiological stimuli and/or pharmacological interventions. In this sense, the assessment of BNP time-course concentrations is a novel, meaningful diagnostic tool for the follow-up of patients with cardiac disease.

5.2 CNH Assay as Diagnostic and Prognostic Tool in Cardiac Diseases

In this second part of the Chapter 5, we will review the clinical relevance of CNH assay (especially of BNP and NT-proBNP). There has been an explosion of clinical researches and trials concerning the routinary use of CNH (especially BNP) assay in the diagnosis and risk stratification of patients with cardiovascular diseases in the first years of the new century (see Chapter 1, section 1.2, and Figs. 1.2 and 1.3). It is clearly impossible to cover all these scientific contributes. In order to reduce the number of references without reducing the efficacy and objectiveness, we have used systematic reviews and meta-analyses, when available.

First, we will review the clinical relevance of CNH assay in the screening and classification of patients with cardiac dysfunction, divided according to the severity of disesae and age, or associated to some particular clinical conditions (such as myocardial infarction or treatment with cardiotoxic drugs) (sections from 5.2.2 to 5.2.6). Moreover, we will discuss the diagnostic accuracy and clinical relevance of assay in coronary artery disease (section 5.2.7), where more recently BNP and NT-proBNP are increasingly frequently assayed with (almost in part) unexpected results. Finally, the diagnostic accuracy of CNH assay will be compared to that of other clinical tests, such as ECG, echocardiogram and chest radiogram (section 5.3).

The last part of the Chapter is dedicated to prognostic relevance of CNH assay in cardiac diseases and general population (sections from 5.4.1 to 5.4.3), to relevance of measurement of CNH in tailoring the therapy (section 5.5.1), and to its cost-effectiveness (section 5.5.2) in patients with HF.

5.2.1 Use of CNH Assay in the Screening and Classification of Patients with Cardiac Dysfunction

The diagnosis of HF can often be difficult, mainly in primary care settings, where patients may present with non-specific symptoms and signs, such as dyspnea, fatigue, and ankle swelling [68-70]. In several population-based studies, fewer than 40% of patients with a suspected diagnosis of HF in primary care had this diagnosis confirmed by more specific and accurate clinical investigations, which are often expensive, time-consuming and demanding for the patient [68-70, 104, 105]. As a result, a relatively simple and inexpensive biochemical test (such as the CNH assay) may be very useful to confirm the clinical suspicion of HF in this clinical setting [5, 34, 35].

The aim of the following paragraphs will be to discuss the diagnostic accuracy of CNH assays (especially BNP/NT-proBNP assays) following the principal recommendations of evidence-based laboratory medicine principles [71, 106, 107].

5.2.2 Diagnostic Accuracy of CNH Assay in Asymptomatic, Mild Ventricular Systolic Dysfunction

Patients with asymptomatic left ventricular systolic dysfunction are likely to have lower plasma BNP than those with overt HF [2-5, 34, 35, 62-66, 72], as shown in Fig. 3.13.

Two large studies [9, 66] evaluated the diagnostic accuracy of the CNH assay as a screening method in a general population. The first study analyzed the Framingham Heart Study cohort (3,177 individuals) using BNP and NT-proANP in the evaluation of left ventricular hypertrophy and systolic dysfunction in a community population [9]. The presence of the disease was evaluated by using echocardiographic findings (the prevalence of left ventricular systolic dysfunction was 9.3% in the 1,470 men and 2.5% in the 1,707 women tested, respectively). The area under the curve (AUC) of receiver operating characteristic (ROC) analysis for CNH assay for identifying both left ventricular hypertrophy and systolic dysfunction was on average about 0.75, with a good specificity (assumed 95% both for men and women) and negative predictive value (NPV, on average ranging from 92% to 97% in men, and from 91% to 98% in women), but a poor sensitivity (i.e., ranging from 27% to 28% in men, and from 13% to 40% in women) and positive predictive value (PPV, from 22% to 38% in men, and from 5% to 40% in women), using gender-related BNP cut-off values [9].

The aim of the second study was to examine the validity of plasma BNP measurement (with the same IRMA method as the other study) for detection of various cardiac abnormalities in a rural Japanese population (1,098 subjects, 693 men and 405 women), with a low prevalence of coronary heart disease and left ventricular systolic dysfunction (i.e., only 37 participants, corresponding to 3.0%, showed an EF <30%) [66]. The diagnosis was carried out by two independent cardiologists based on a medical questionnaire, chest radiogram, electrocardiogram (ECG), and echocardiographic report. The optimal threshold for identification of disease was a BNP concentration of 50 ng/l (14.4 pmol/l), with an area under the ROC curve of 0.970, a sensitivity of 89.7%, a specificity of 95.7%, PPV of 44.3%, and NPV of 99.6%, respectively.

The conclusions of these two studies, though similar in aim, as well as in clinical and experimental protocols, were strongly conflicting. The Japanese study suggested that the BNP assay is a very efficient and cost-effective mass screening technique for identifying patients with various cardiac abnormalities regardless of etiology and degree of left ventricular systolic dysfunction [66], while the Framingham study suggested only limited usefulness of the CNH assay as a mass screening tool for this clinical condition, especially in women [9].

This discrepancy may be due to the different gold standard used for the diagnosis of heart failure adopted in the two studies, as discussed in a previous paragraph (section 5.1.5, "Diagnostic accuracy of CNH assay in plasma from patients with cardiac diseases"). However, these two studies, taken as a whole, indicate that the CNH assay may have only a limited usefulness as a screening method for HF in a general population, owing to the poor sensitivity and PPV. However, both studies also found good specificity and NPV, thus suggesting that the CNH assay may be used to rule out HF in an asymptomatic (or pauci-symptomatic) individual.

5.2.3 Diagnostic Accuracy of CNH Assay in Patients with Suspected HF

Many studies [92, 108-128] have suggested that the CNH assay could be useful as a screening method and/or for the differential diagnosis in patients suspected of HF in different clinical settings: a) randomly selected high-risk community populations; b) primary-care patients with a new diagnosis of HF; c) patients with acute dyspnea in the emergency department; d) consecutive unselected hospital inpatients; e) patients admitted to the intensive care unit.

The studies concerning the diagnostic accuracy of the CNH assay in patients with HF have also been analyzed by two recent systematic reviews [5, 72]; unfortunately, these studies showed quite heterogeneous data, thus introducing some bias in the statistical analysis. In particular, even some high-quality studies were not designed with the primary goal of evaluating the diagnostic accuracy of the CNH assay. Indeed, this aim was considered only at a post-hoc analysis and retrospectively assessed in blood samples collected for different original purposes, some years before the actual evaluation of diagnostic accuracy. This may introduce a significant bias, although its true clinical relevance is difficult to assess [5].

The second most important cause of heterogeneous data is the different reference (gold) standard used to evaluate the diagnostic accuracy of the CNH assay. In some studies, the patients studied were stratified and grouped according to clinical severity, as described by functional classification (usually NYHA classification). In other studies, only echocardiographic measurements were used as "gold standard" for the accuracy of the CNH assay for the diagnosis of left ventricular dysfunction (and not for the clinical diagnosis of HF) [5, 72].

Furthermore, comparison of studies concerning the diagnostic accuracy of CNH assay is also difficult because different populations were enrolled and different immunoassays were used. Indeed, diagnostic accuracy (especially predictive values) is strictly dependent on disease prevalence (pre-test probability), which greatly varies according to the clinical setting considered (i.e., screening for general population, out-patients seen by a general practitioner, or in primary care, emergency department, coronary care unit, and so on). In particular, the prevalence of HF in the populations studied varied from less than 5% (in studies of screening of asymptomatic population) to more than 50% (in studies including patients referred to hospital with suspicion of HF) [5]. Another factor, often underestimated, is that the "gold standard" (which is not an objective rule, but a clinical synthesis or another diagnostic test) could vary with the disease prevalence, sometimes in a different manner than the CNH assay.

Finally, recent data reported in the literature suggested that diagnostic accuracy may vary significantly in relation with the specific cardiac peptide measured and/or immunoassay used [5, 19, 21, 72, 129-131]. At the present time, the different BNP immunoassays also show greatly different imprecision [132]. Consequently, it is not clear whether the observed significant variation in diagnostic accuracy is due to a difference in pathophysiological behavior of measured peptides and/or in assay performance [5]. Unfortunately, some studies do not clearly indicate the type of immunoassay used to measure CNH, while the majority do not report the assay performance (and often even the reference values) evaluated in their own laboratory.

Taking all studies as a whole, a recent meta-analysis showed that the odds ratio for diagnostic accuracy of BNP assay in different groups of patients with suspected HF is highly significant [72]. In particular, the pooled diagnostic odds ratio, when clinical criteria were used as gold standard for HF, was 30.9 (95% confidence interval 27.0-35.4), while it fell to 11.9 (8.4-16.1) when a value $\leq$40% of left ventricular EF, estimated by echocardiography, was used as reference standard [72].

Diastolic dyfunction can play a major role in determining signs and symptoms in patients with congestive HF [65, 120, 121]. Although Doppler echocardiography is currently used to examine the left ventricular diastolic filling dynamics, the limitations of this technique suggest the need for other objective measures [122]. Despite these limitations, several studies indicated that the CNH assay, in particular the BNP assay, may be useful for the diagnosis of left ventricular diastolic dysfunction [123, 125, 126]. However, some conflicting results have been reported, probably due to the different cause of and/or mechanisms responsible for cardiac dysfunction [127, 128]. In a recent meta-analysis, including data of three studies comparing the diagnostic accuracy of BNP assay in patients with diastolic dysfunction, the pooled odds ratio was 28.3 (95% confidence interval 2.66-300.5) [72]. However, a bias may affect these studies, as suggested by the significant test of heterogeneity ($c^2 = 128.4, p < 0.001$) [72].

Finally, Wright et al. [133] evaluated the effect of NT-proBNP assay on the clinical diagnostic accuracy of HF in primary care by means of a prospective, randomized controlled trial in 305 patients. Each patient was randomized in two groups, one in which the general practioner had at their disposal the NT-proBNP assay results (NT-proBNP assay group), while the other did not (control group). The diagnostic accuracy improved by 21% in the NT-proBNP assay group and by 8% in the control group ($p = 0.002$). This study indicates that NT-proBNP measurement significantly improves the clinical diagnostic accuracy of HF in general practice [133].

5.2.4 Diagnostic Accuracy of CNH Assay in Patients with Acute Myocardial Infarction

Circulating levels of CNH increase after acute myocardial infarction (AMI); the extent of the increase is related to the size of the infarct [134-137]. Patients with smaller infarcts tend to have a monophasic increase in plasma BNP, peaking at 20 hours after the onset of symptoms; on the other hand, those with larger infarcts, lower EF, and clinical signs of HF may present a further peak at 5 days after admission [135]. Other studies are less convincing regarding the ability of the CNH assay to identify patients with significant myocardial dysfunction after AMI [138, 139]. These conflicting results could be due to the differences in sample collection time, type of CNH (ANP, BNP, or NT-proBNP) measured, type of assay (competitive vs non-competitive), and inclusion criteria adopted. However, persisting elevation of CNH levels at 1 or 2 months after AMI usually suggests a high risk of adverse remodeling and subsequent HF [5], although this finding should be confirmed by further specifically addressed studies.

The diagnostic accuracy of the BNP assay in patients with myocardial infarction was evaluated in a recent meta-analysis [72] taking into account only two studies [140,141], fitting the inclusion criteria of this analysis; the pooled odds ratio was 9.4 (95% confidence interval 4.5-19.4).

5.2.5 Diagnostic Accuracy of CNH Assay in Elderly People

Heart failure is primarily a disease of old age; chronic HF increases in prevalence with aging from <1% in people aged <65 years to >5% in those >65 years of age, and this clinical condition is the first cause of morbidity and mortality in older people [68-70, 142]. A recent study demonstrated that elderly patients present with more advanced HF, as evidenced by their higher morbidity and mortality rate along with greater neurohormonal activation [142]. According to these findings, elderly people should be considered to be a population with high risk for developing HF and so the BNP/NT-proBNP assay may be useful as a screening test for HF in older age. Indeed, several studies reported that the BNP/NT-proBNP assay could be clinically useful in elderly people suspected to have HF [16, 142-147].

Two studies compared the diagnostic accuracy of the BNP assay and that of ECG in elderly people screened for HF. A prospective cohort study specifically evaluated the diagnostic accuracy for HF of BNP assay in 299 consecutive patients (mean age 79 years, 65% women) attending day-hospital over a period of 13 months [143]. This study suggested that both BNP assay and ECG were sensitive in detecting left ventricular systolic dysfunction, but lacked specificity (but the combination of the two tests improved diagnostic accuracy) [143]. The other study reported that both the ECG and the plasma concentration of BNP were highly efficient in excluding left ventricular systolic dysfunction in 407 75-year-old subjects [144]. However, compared with the BNP, the ECG yields a lower number of false-positive cases. Therefore, this study suggested that in screening for left ventricular systolic dysfunction in elderly people, the BNP assay has a diagnostic value in addition to the ECG, but only in individuals with abnormal ECG [144].

Another study indicated that the BNP assay may be particularly useful in ederly patients, especially in differentiating cardiogenic pulmonary edema from respiratory causes of dyspnea [146]. Screening of populations with more than 1% prevalence of HF (such as people with age more than 60 years) with BNP followed by echocardiography should provide a health benefit at a cost that is comparable to or less than other accepted health interventions [145]. Finally, the NT-proBNP assay was demonstrated to be useful for detecting HF among people living in elderly nursing homes [147].

5.2.6 Detection of Drug Cardiotoxicity by means of BNP Assay

Another example of the clinical relevance of BNP assay is the possibility of identifying HF caused by drug cardiotoxicity [148-153]. Cardiotoxicity is a potential side-effect of some chemotherapeutic agents [154]. The anthracycline class of cytotoxic antibiotics are the most famous, but other chemotherapeutic agents can also cause serious cardiotoxicity and are not so well recognized (including cyclophosphamide, ifosfamide, mitomycin and fluorouracil) [154]. In a large retrospective study of more than 4,000 patients, an incidence of clinical chronic HF of 2.2% was found [155]. However, a more recent study suggests that about 20% of patients treated with anthracycline show a decrease in ventricular function below the normal limits, if followed with serial measurements of left ventricular EF, assessed by an accurate radionuclide method [156]. This supports the recommendations of monitoring cardiac function in anthracycline-treated patients with accurate and suitable methods.

Experimental studies in rats indicated that plasma BNP and serum cardiac troponin T (cTnT) significantly increased from 6 to 12 weeks after adriamycin administration with deterioration of cardiac function, as assessed by echocardiography [157]. However, in this study the increase in cTnT was antecedent to the increase in BNP and the deterioration of cardiac function [157].

Several studies demonstrated that the release pattern of cardiac-specific troponin I (cTnI) after high-dose chemotherapy is a sensitive and reliable marker of acute minor myocardial damage and is able to identify patients at different risks of cardiac events 3 years later [158-160]. On the other hand, several studies demonstrated that the BNP assay may also be a marker of chemotherapy cardiotoxicity [148-152]. In particular, two recent studies [161, 162] also suggested that BNP/NT-proBNP assay is a predictive marker of cardiac dysfunction in patients affected by aggressive malignancies and treated with high-dose chemotherapy. The acute release of circulating levels of troponin should be only a mirror of the death of myocardiocytes, while the persistent increase in BNP, after several days or weeks from the administration of cardiotoxic drug, should be specifically related to ventricular remodeling and myocardial dysfunction. Further studies are necessary to confirm these data, and to evaluate the respective diagnostic accuracy and clinical relevance of troponin and BNP assays in the follow-up of patients treated with potentially cardiotoxic drugs.

5.2.7 Diagnostic Accuracy of CNH Assay in Coronary Artery Disease

Two very recent studies suggested that the BNP assay could be a reliable marker of ischemia in patients with coronary artery disease [163, 164]. Exercise electrocardiography is the most widely used non-invasive method to detect the presence of coronary artery disease; however, its usefulness is limited by relatively modest sensitivity and specificity [165-167]. Other more accurate non-invasive tests, such as exercise echocardiography and exercise testing with radionuclide imaging, are less widely available and considerably more expensive.

It could be hypothesized that exercise-induced ischemia results in increased wall stress and triggers release of CNH from myocardiocytes. According to this hypothesis, Foote et al. [163] measured NT-proBNP and BNP in blood samples from a group of normal volunteers, and two groups of patients, one with and the other without coronary artery disease, before and after maximal exercise. Post-exercise increases in NT-proBNP and BNP were approximately 4-fold higher in the ischemic group than in the non-ischemic group; while in volunteers, the increase was almost identical to that of the non-ischemic patient group. At equal specificity to the ECG (58.8%), the sensitivities of the BNP/NT-proBNP assay in detecting ischemia were 90 and 80%, respectively; in contrast, the sensitivity of the exercise ECG was only 37.5%.

In the study by Sabatine et al. [164], transient myocardial ischemia was associated with an immediate rise in circulating BNP levels, and the magnitude of the rise was proportional to the severity of ischemia. These findings demonstrate an important link between the severity of an acute ischemic insult and the circulating levels of BNP. However, further studies are necessary to evaluate the relevance of the BNP/NT-proBNP assay.

5.3 Comparison between the Diagnostic Accuracy of CNH Assay and that of Other Tests and Clinical Investigations

Signs and symptoms correlate poorly with the presence of HF, for this reason diagnosis relies on clinical judgment based on a combination of history, physical examination and appropriate investigation [65, 69, 70, 168].

Davie et al. [169] found that left ventricular systolic dysfunction was virtually never present if the ECG was normal (sensitivity 94%, NPV 98%), and a screening ECG reduced the need for echocardiograms by 50%. However, several studies demonstrate that CNH assay can improve the diagnostic accuracy of history, ECG, and chest radiography [167-174].

Cowie et al. [110] reported that ROC curves for BNP (AUC = 0.96), ANP (0.93), and NT-proANP (0.89) were better than that for cardiothoracic ratio on chest radiogram (0.79) in screening for patients likely to have HF and requiring further clinical assessment. Nielsen et al. [92] found that BNP assay showed a diagnostic accuracy better than ECG in a random sample of 1,257 community subjects. Another study suggested that BNP assay together with the presence of major ECG abnormalities and history reduced by a factor of six (in comparison to consideration of BNP assay in isolation) the number of subjects requiring echocardiography to detect one case of myocardial dysfunction in a large population screening (1,360 patients tested) [171].

Several studies have compared the diagnostic accuracy of BNP assay and ECG in the elderly population. In 75-year-old subjects both the ECG and the plasma concentration of BNP are highly efficient in excluding left ventricular systolic dysfunction, as recently suggested [173]. In another study, several types of structural heart disease, in particular valvular heart disease, could be identified exclusively by BNP testing, suggesting that BNP measurement can make a significant contribution to screening for CHF precursors when used in combination with ECG in elderly populations (856 subjects enrolled, with age ≥65 years) [174]. However, compared with the BNP assay, the ECG yielded a lower number of false-positive cases in another study [172]. In screening for left ventricular systolic dysfunction, the BNP has a diagnostic value in addition to the ECG, but only in individuals with abnormal ECG [172].

NT-proBNP alone was a better predictor of left ventricular dysfunction than any other single or combination of factors, while the ECG had a poor predictive value for left ventricular systolic dysfunction in identifying patients with left ventricular systolic dysfunction in a high-risk population (243 patients, 129 men, median age 73 years, range 20-94) [173].

Another study [170] compared the diagnostic accuracy of BNP assay, ECG, chest radiography and echocardiography; the results of this study confirmed that sensitivity, specificity and accuracy of BNP assay and echocardiography were significantly better than those of ECG and chest radiography [170].

A huge number of studies have compared the diagnostic accuracy of BNP assay and echocardiography in patients with acute or chronic HF [5, 62-65, 72, 175]. According to the guidelines for the diagnosis of heart failure proposed by the Task Force on Heart Failure of the European Society of Cardiology [69], echocardiography is recommended as the most practical tool to demonstrate cardiac dysfunction. However, a recent epidemiological study [176] suggested that the diagnosis of HF might be better defined in terms of symptoms, elevated neuro-hormones and impaired cardiac workload.

In more than 50% of the clinical studies, the echocardiographic investigation has been considered as the gold standard (more exactly the reference standard method) for the evaluation of diagnostic accuracy of CNH assay in patients with heart failure [5, 72]. When we use the echocardiography investigation as reference method, we assume that BNP assay cannot theoretically have a better diagnostic accuracy than it. Indeed, conflicting results were found when different clinical settings (patient's selection) and/or gold standard were used [5, 72]. Choy et al. [177] showed that in post-AMI patients plasma BNP is superior to all clinical indices of left ventricular systolic dysfunction (EF <40%), including signs and symptoms and a clinical score (Peel Index). Dokainish et al. [178] found that BNP assay and comprehensive Doppler echocardiography have similar diagnostic accuracy for congestive HF, although echo-Doppler trended toward higher specificity than BNP for congestive HF. Moreover, serial BNP measurements during the treatment of acute HF provide incremental prognostic information over clinical presentation and repetitive echocardiographic examination [179]. Mak et al. [180] suggested that both BNP assay and a complete echocardiographic examination do not have adequate discriminatory power to be used in isolation in the evaluation of left ventricular diastolic function. Therefore, all available information, including systolic function, chamber dimensions and all Doppler variables must be considered in the analysis of individual patients [180]. Steg et al. [181] recently assessed the diagnostic performance of BNP testing and echocardiographic assessment of left ventricular systolic function, separately and combined, for the identification of congestive HF in 1,586 patients presenting to the emergency department with acute dyspnea. The proportions of patients who were correctly classified were 67% for BNP alone, 55% for EF alone, 82% for the two variables together, and 97.3% when clinical, ECG, and chest radiograph data were added. This study suggested that BNP measurement was superior to two-dimensional echocardiographic determination of left ventricular EF in identifying congestive HF, regardless of the threshold value. The two methods combined have marked additive diagnostic value [181].

Some recent studies indicated that BNP/NT-proBNP levels do not accurately predict serial hemodynamic changes and consequently do not obviate the need for pulmonary artery catheterization in patients requiring invasive hemodynamic monitoring [182-184].

In conclusion, BNP assay shows significantly higher predictive characteristics than ECG and chest radiography, and a cost-benefit value significantly greater than that of echocardiography [92, 170]. BNP measurement may exclude normal heart with high probability owing to its high degree of sensitivity and NPV when used in screening high-risk populations, therefore reducing the echocardiographic diagnostic burden; this is the rationale for considering the BNP assay in the first step of an algorithm for the differential diagnosis of heart failure [37, 65, 69, 70, 168, 175].

5.4 Use of CNH Assay as Prognostic Marker in Cardiovascular Diseases

Several well-designed and conducted studies suggested that the CNH assay may be useful as a prognostic marker mainly in two clinical conditions: HF and acute coronary artery syndromes (ACS), as also demonstrated by systematic reviews [5, 76, 184, 185].

5.4.1 Prognosis in HF

The prognostic role of CNH assay (especially NT-proANP, BNP and NT-proBNP) in patients with HF is well demonstrated by a huge number of studies [16, 147, 186-199]. In all these studies, CNH concentrations were always found to be independent risk markers for morbidity (increased future major cardiovascular events and/or hospitalization) and/or mortality in patients with acute or chronic HF [5]. In some studies CNH levels were stronger predictors of mortality and/or major cardiovascular events than left ventricular EF, NYHA class, and/or presence of diabetes or hypertension, as well as sex and age in patients with chronic HF [188, 189, 192, 194-196, 198, 199]. In some recent studies [197, 199], NT-proANP was shown to be a more powerful predictor than BNP and NT-proBNP, but these differences may be due to the analytical performance of methods used rather than a true specific characteristic of peptide measured in the study. Further studies are necessary to clarify whether there is a true difference among the NT-proANP, BNP and NT-proBNP as predictor markers in patients with HF.

A continuous relationship was generally found between BNP levels and mortality [194], thus suggesting that it is not possible to observe a threshold for the risk. On average, a systematic analysis of the most important studies suggested an odds ratio of about 2 for the risk of mortality in patients with BNP values above the cut-off [5].

Further evaluation needs the clinical relevance of combined use of CNH assay with other functional parameters (such as peak oxygen consumption) [90, 201, 202], neurohormones [203-206], and markers of fibrinolysis [207] or cardiac necrosis [208, 209]. Some studies suggest that the combination of BNP assay with the assessment of peak oxygen consumption [202] or with specific markers of cardiac necrosis [209] improves risk stratification of patients with HF.

Sereral studies reported that some neuro-effectors, hormones (including peptide, thyroid and steroid hormones), and cytokines are increased in patients with HF, as recently reviewed [2, 5, 210-220] (see also Chapter 3, section 3.5, for a more complete discussion on this field). In general, BNP assay was found to be the most powerful indicator for poor outcome compared to other neuro-effectors and hormones, at least in the largest studies [5, 204, 206]. However, more data on the clinical relevance of combination of two or more neuro-hormones in risk stratification of HF are necessary.

5.4.2 Prognosis in ACS

Acute coronary artery syndrome encompasses a continuum of cardiac ischemic events, ranging from unstable angina pectoris, with no biochemical evidence of myocardial necrosis, to ST-elevation AMI [221, 222]. The prognosis of patients with ACS varies widely, and several clinical, electrocardiographic, and biochemical markers have been used to identify high-risk individuals in need of aggressive intervention [222].

Several studies reported that CNH assay (in particular BNP and NT-proBNP) provides valuable prognostic information in patients with ACS [117, 138, 223-231]. A recent meta-analysis confirmed the powerful prognostic value of BNP/NT-proBNP in patients with ACS for death both in the short term (<50 days, mean odds ratio 3.38, CI 95% 2.44-4.68) and long term (>10 months, mean odds ratio 4.31, 3.77-4.94) [76].

As for the prognostic role of BNP assay in patients with HF, more data on the clinical relevance of combination with other markers in risk stratification of HF are necessary. However, some studies suggest that BNP levels improve a simple risk score in patients with unstable angina and non-ST-elevation myocardial infarction [239] as well as the risk-assessment performance obtained with the cTnI and hs-CRP assays in patients with ST-segment elevation myocardial infarction [234]. These data suggest the utility of a "multimarker strategy" or biomarker profile to characterize patients with ACS [78].

A recent study [240] reported that there may be clear differences among the profiles of individual natriuretic peptide levels in the 2 years after AMI. Similar profiles were found with BNP and NT-proBNP plasma concetrations, while those of NT-proANP and CNP differed significantly in a cohort of 236 patients with AMI complicated by clinical, radiologic or echocardiographic evidence of left ventricular dysfunction. Moreover, a single measurement of plasma natriuretic peptide levels during the hospital admission provides limited prognostic information, while NT-proBNP measured by an ELISA method in the 30 days after AMI identifies a cohort of patients at increased risk of adverse outcome thereafter [240].

Two recent studies reported that in patients with clinically stable, angiographically documented coronary artery disease, plasma BNP [241] or NT-proBNP [242] levels are independently related to long-term survival in a multivariate model. These studies suggested that BNP and NT-proBNP are markers of long-term mortality even in patients with stable coronary disease and add prognostic information above and beyond that provided by conventional cardiovascular risk factors and the degree of left ventricular systolic dysfunction [241, 242].

In order to explain these clinical findings, it is important to note that experimental studies in animals reported that myocardial ischemia or even hypoxia *per se* could induce the synthesis/secretion of CNH (in particular BNP) from the intact heart *in vivo* as well as ventricular cells in culture [243-244]. Furthermore, these experimental data are also in accordance with recent clinical studies indicating that transient myocardial ischemia in patients with stable coronary artery disease is associated with an immediate rise in circulating BNP levels, and that the magnitude of rise is proportional to the severity of ischemia [163, 164, 246].

5.4.3 Prognostic Relevance of CNH Assay in the General Population

While measurement of plasma BNP concentration has been shown to be useful in the diagnosis of HF (especially acute HF), its role as a screening test for detection of preclinical ventricular remodeling or dysfunction in the general population has not been established [5, 246, 247]. However, some studies evaluated the prognostic relevance of CNH assay in the general population, especially in high-risk populations, such as elderly people [16, 187, 224, 244-248]. These studies demonstrated that CNH (and especially BNP/NT-proBNP) levels are a sensitive and accurate biochemical marker of an increased risk of cardiac morbidity and total mortality in very elderly persons [16, 147, 188, 227, 248, 249]. However, in a community-based study (mean age 56 years) there were no significant trends of increasing incidence of hypertension across BNP categories in men or women, while higher plasma BNP levels were associated with increased risk of BP progression in men but not women [250]. The differences between the results of this study [250] and those of others [16, 185, 227, 248, 249] may be due to the different age and gender of subjects studied. Probably, the prognostic power of BNP assay increases progressively with age and may be gender-dependent.

Additional investigations are warranted to confirm the powerful prognostic value of BNP assay in elderly people and to elucidate the basis for these gender-related differences [246, 247].

5.5 CNH Assay in Management of Patients with HF

5.5.1 Clinical Relevance of CNH Assay in Tailoring the Therapy of HF

Medical therapy for HF is based on improving the symptoms and signs of fluid retention (change in dyspnea, edemas, and body weight are the usual markers of response to treatment) and titrating the dosage of drugs (such as diuretics, ACE inhibitors, β-blockers, and spironolactone) following the evidence from randomized clinical trials [65, 68-70]. Currently, there is no specific surrogate end-point for treating patients with HF that can be used to fine-tune therapy [65, 68-70].

Many authors have suggested that the results of CNH assay (especially BNP/NT-proBNP assay) may be useful in monitoring and tailoring the medical therapy in HF patients, and in providing a practical objective indicator of optimal therapy [61-65, 68-

70, 85, 90, 168, 252-265], including patients subjected to cardiac transplantation [266]. CNH usually respond to effective treatment with drugs [5, 61-65] or left ventricular assist device [267, 268] with a prompt reduction of their circulating levels. Indeed, ACE inhibitors, valsartan, diuretics, nitrates, and endothelin receptor antagonists have been shown to reduce plasma CNH levels in parallel with hemodynamic and clinical improvement [62, 63, 252, 258, 271-277].

More variable effects on plasma CNH levels have been reported after therapy with β-blockers [90, 278-292]. Some authors suggested that these variable effects may be at least in part attributable to different specificities or to ancillary properties of β-blockers [62]. Ohta et al. [293] reported that both high and low doses of carvedilol have the effect of increasing plasma ANP and BNP levels in rats. This effect was closely related to the upregulation of ANP and BNP mRNA expression, and the down-regulation of NPR-C mRNA expression in the heart [293]. According to these data, we could assume that an acute administration of β-blockers causes an early rise in plasma CNH, while sustained treatment, significantly improving cardiac function and clinical conditions, induces a significant fall in hormone levels [90, 284, 287, 289, 290].

Despite this huge number of studies suggesting the clinical relevance of monitoring patients with HF by means of CNH assay, at present only two studies [252, 253] have been designed specifically to evaluate the clinical use of CNH assay in monitoring and tailoring the medical therapy in patients with HF.

Murdoch et al. [252] studied 20 patients with mild to moderate chronic HF and receiving stable conventional therapy, who were randomly assigned to titration of ACE-inhibitor dosage, according to serial measurement of plasma BNP or to optimal empirical ACE-inhibitor therapy for 8 weeks. Only the BNP-driven approach was associated with a significant reduction in plasma BNP concentration throughout the duration of the study and a significantly greater suppression when compared with empiric therapy after 4 weeks (mean reduction in BNP group -42.1%, 95% CI -58.2, -19.7; mean reduction in empiric therapy group -12.0%, 95% CI CI -31.8, 13.8; P= 0.03) [252].

Troughton et al. [253] studied 69 patients with impaired systolic function (EF <40%) and symptomatic HF (NYHA class II-IV), who were randomized to receive treatment guided by either plasma NT-proBNP concentration or standardized clinical assessment. During the follow-up (minimum 6 months, median 9.5 months), there were fewer total cardiovascular events (death, hospital admission, or HF decompensation) in the NT-proBNP-guided group than in the clinical group (19 vs 54, $p = 0.02$). At 6 months, 27% of patients in the NT-proBNP-guided group and 53% in the clinical group had experienced a first cardiovascular event ($p = 0.034$). Changes in left ventricular function, quality of life, renal function, and adverse events were similar in both groups [253].

Morimoto et al. [263] conducted a cost-effectiveness analysis of regular BNP measurement in the outpatient setting. The target population was symptomatic CHF patients aged 35-85 years, recently discharged from the hospital. Intervention was BNP measurement once every 3 months (BNP group) or no BNP measurement (clinical group). The baseline analysis during the 9-month period after hospitalization suggested that the introduction of BNP measurement in heart failure management is not only cost-effective by reducing hospitalization, but also improves the outcome of patients, as assessed by (quality-adjusted life year) analysis [263].

A recent randomized clinical trial compared the titration of β-blocker therapy with bisoprolol according to plasma levels of BNP wih empiric clinical therapy based on signs and symptoms [294]. Forty-one patients with heart failure were randomized into a clinical trial. The clinical group had β-blocker dosage increased according to standard care, whereas the BNP group had β-blocker dosage up-titrated according to plasma BNP levels plus standard care. The primary outcome was mean β-blocker dose achieved after 3 months. BNP-guided up-titration of β-blocker in ambulatory patients with heart failure did not result significantly different doses of β-blocker at the end of 3 months. However, 45% of patients in the clinical group were on the maximum dose of β-blocker vs. only 19% of patients in the BNP group, although left ventricular ejection fraction was significantly improved in both groups by 7.3%. The slightly lower doses in the BNP group were possibly better tolerated than the doses achieved in the clinical group. Furthermore, a trend toward better quality of life was seen in the BNP group [294].

Accurate diagnosis of clinical deterioration in heart failure can be difficult [68,69]. To prevent development into overt congestion, which often requires hospitalization, early diagnosis is of paramount importance. There is a need for objective measurements to aid early diagnosis in a setting where symptoms may be non-specific and abnormalities on physical examination often subtle and minor [295]. Heart failure guidelines recommend the use of weight gain monitoring to help in this task, with the added advantage that patient self-care is encouraged [68,69]. It is advised that an increase of 2 Kg over stable body weight over a period of 48-72 h should initiate contact with medical or nursing personnel [68,69,295]. However, Lewin et al. recently suggested that neither weight gain nor increase in BNP are adequately sensitive as a screen for clinical deterioration in patients with established heart failure (34 clinically stable and other 43 with clinical deterioration of heart failure status) [295]. In particular, weight gain is very insensitive, though an increase of 2 Kg demonstrates high specificity for clinical deterioration. On the other hand, BNP change appears to provide better sensitivity than weight change, but it has poor specificity in an established heart failure population [295].

In conclusion, all the clinical trials reported above have several limitations, such as the relatively low number of patients enrolled (usually less than 100), the limitation due to the fact that the study was performed in a single center, and/or the non-complete group randomization. Therefore, further larger randomized, multicenter clinical trias are necessary to definitevely demonstrate the usefulness of CNH assay in monitoring and tailoring the medical therapy in patients with heart failure, as also indicated in a recent conseusus conference [296]. Indeed, at the time of writing this review, some multicenter randomized clinical trials were in progress. Preliminary results of one of these clinical trials [297] were recently presented an international meeting. This study suggested that the use of BNP plasma levels to guide medical therapy reduced the death and hospital admission for heart failure as well as the delayed time to first event compared with clinically guided treatment [297].

5.5.2 Cost-Effectiveness of CNH Assay in Management of Patients with Acute or Chronic HF

Several studies suggested that BNP assay may reduce the need for cardiac investigations [65,69,145,147,175]. Indeed, ruling out suspicion of HF by CNH test would make it unnecessary to carry out other investigations, which are often time-consuming, expensive, invasive, and sometimes potentially harmful for the patient [65,69]. Some studies have been designed to test this possibility [92-94,147,263-265].

Nielsen et al. [92] sought to assess the cost-effectiveness of using plasma BNP as a pre-echocardiographic screening test for left ventricular systolic dysfunction in the general population. Screening high-risk subjects by BNP before echocardiography could reduce the cost per detected case of left ventricular systolic dysfunction by 26% for the cost ratio of 1/20 (BNP/echocardiogram). Greater reduced costs (up to 50%) can be predicted for the group of low-risk subjects [92]. Other studies reported similar results [93,145], including a study on old people living in nursing homes [147].

Mueller et al. [265] conducted a prospective, randomized, controlled study of 452 patients who presented to the emergency department with acute dyspnea: 225 patients were randomly assigned to a diagnostic strategy involving the measurement of BNP, and 227 were assessed in a standard manner. This study indicated that BNP assay improved the evaluation and treatment of patients with acute dyspnea and thereby reduced the time to discharge and the total cost of treatment in the emergency department [265]. Other studies suggested that BNP testing can also reduce the cost for hospitalization in patients with heart failure [263, 264], including old people living in nursing homes [147].

However, the cost-effectiveness analysis strongly depends on the relative cost of the BNP test compared to that of echocardiograms and/or hospitalization, as well as on the prevalence of HF in the population screened. Unfortunately, these parameters can vary considerably among departments, countries, and health-care systems; so that each laboratory/clinical department should analyze the cost-effectiveness in its own economical framework. Furthermore, cost-effectiveness analysis is also dependent on the sensitivity of BNP assay for detecting HF. Cost-effectiveness will improve if more specific assays are used: this would decrease the number of subjects with false-positive results, and consequently the number of further useless investigations. However, further larger and randomized clinical trials are necessary to confirm the clinical relevance and cost-effectiveness of BNP assay in the follow-up of patients with HF.

5.6 Summary and Conclusion

Several recent experimental and clinical studies strongly suggest that the circulating CNH should be better considered as an index of activation of the neuro-endocrine system, rather than a marker of myocardial dysfunction, as recently reviewed [298]. The activation or deactivation of the CNH system is almost always the resultant of one or more physiological or pathological changes. For this reason, the results of CNH assays must be interpreted by taking into account clinical history and examination, as well as all laboratory and instrumental tests. Of course, the great number of pathophysiological mechanisms that can affect the CNH system render sometimes difficult for clinicians to recognize the cause(s) of variations in its activity. CNH assays should be considered as an intellectual spur for the search of pathophysiological mechanisms that can satisfactorily explain the measured variations in hormone concentrations. On the other hand, CNH measurements add a complementary information to other instrumental and investigative tests [296].

The clinical relevance of CNH measurement (especially BNP and NT-proBNP assay) as diagnostic and prognostic marker in patients with cardiac disease have been recently confirmed [5, 72, 76, 186, 296, 299, 300]. In populations with higher prevalence of cardiac diseases, including only individuals with clinical suspicion of HF, the diagnostic sensitivity and negative prediective value of BNP/NT-proBNP assay are both 95%, or even more, as long as appropriate cut-off values are selected [5, 72, 296]. This is the rationale for choosing the BNP/NT-proBNP assay as the first step for an algorithm for the diagnosis of HF together with ECG and/or chest radiography [69, 70, 296, 299, 300]. Such a clinical strategy has been proved successful in some recent studies evaluating the cost-effectiveness of using plasma BNP measurements for screening of cardiac dysfunction in the general population [92-94].

The prognostic value of CNH assay for cardiac and non-cardiac death or major cardiovascular events is now well demonstrated in patients with acute or chronic HF [5, 72, 76, 186, 296, 299, 300], as well as with stable artery coronary disease or ACS [5, 76, 117, 138, 223-242]. An increasing number of studies indicate that BNP/NT-proBNP concentration is also an independent risk factor for mortality (cardiac and/or total) in non-cardiac disease, including pulmonary embolism and hypertension, renal failure, septic shock, amyloidosis, sarcoidosis and diabetes mellitus (see also Chapter 7 for more details), as recently reviewed [298]. Increased CNH levels in these non-cardiac diseases are a useful indication for the clinician that the heart is "under stress".

Despite this huge number of studies suggesting the clinical relevance of monitoring patients with HF by means of CNH assay [5], at present, only two studies [252, 253] were designed to specifically evaluate the clinical use of CNH assay in monitoring and tailoring the medical therapy in patients with HF. We hope that the results of larger randomized, multicenter clinical trias, now in progress, are able to confirm the usefulness of CNH assay in monitoring and tailoring the medical therapy in patients with heart failure [296]. Indeed, preliminary results of a multicenter, randomized clinical trial [297] have recently suggested that the use of BNP plasma levels to guide medical therapy reduced the death and hospital admission for heart failure as well as the delayed time to first event compared with clinically guided treatment.

References

1. De Bold AJ, Ma KKY, Zhang Y et al (2001) The physiological and pathophysiological modulation of the endocrine function of the heart. (Review) Can J Physiol Pharmacol 79:705-714
2. Clerico A (2002) Pathophysiological and clinical relevance of circulating levels of cardiac natriuretic hormones: is their assay merely a marker of cardiac disease? (Opinion Article) Clin Chem Lab Med 40:752-760
3. Ruskoaho H (2003) Cardiac hormones as diagnostic tools in heart failure. (Review) Endocr Rev 24:341-356
4. de Lemos JA, McGuire DK, Drazner MH (2003) B-type natriuretic peptide in cardiovascular disease. (Review) Lancet 362:316-322
5. Clerico A, Emdin M (2004) Diagnostic accuracy and prognostic relevance of the measurement of the cardiac natriuretic peptides: a review. (Review) Clin Chem 50:33-50
6. Goetze JP (2004) Biochemistry of pro-B-type natriuretic peptide-derived peptides: the endocrine heart revisited. (Review) Clin Chem 9:1503-1510
7. Clerico A, Del Ry S, Maffei S et al (2002) Circulating levels of cardiac natriuretic hormones in healthy adult subjects: effects of aging and sex. Clin Chem Lab Med 40:371-377
8. Redfield MM, Rodeheffer RJ, Jacobsen SJ et al (2002) Plasma brain natriuretic peptide concentration: impact of age and gender. J Am Coll Cardiol 40:976-982
9. Vasan RS, Benjamin EJ, Larson MG et al (2002) Plasma natriuretic peptides for community screening for left ventricular hypertrophy and systolic dysfunction. JAMA 288:1252-1259

10. Wang TJ, Larson MG, Levy D et al (2002) Impact of age and sex on plasma natriuretic peptide levels in healthy adults. Am J Cardiol 90:254-258

11. Friesinger GC (1999) Cardiovascular disease in the elderly. (Review) Cardiol Clin 17:35-49

12. De Bold AJ, Bruneau BG, Kuroski de Bold ML (1996) Mechanical and neuroendocrine regulation of the endocrine heart. (Review) Cardiovasc Res 31:7-18

13. Kuroski de Bold ML (1999) Estrogen, natriuretic peptides and the renin-angiotensin system. (Review) Cardiovasc Res 41:524-531

14. Maffei S, Del Ry S, Prontera C, Clerico A (2001) Increase in circulating levels of cardiac natriuretic peptides after hormone replacement therapy in postmenopausal women. Clin Sci 101:447-453

15. Sayama H, Nakamura Y, Saito N, Kinoshita M (1999) Why is the concentration of plasma brain natriuretic peptide in elderly inpatients greater than normal? Coron Artery Dis 10:537-540

16. Ueda R, Yokouchi M, Suzuki T et al (2003) Prognostic value of high plasma brain natriuretic peptide concentrations in very elderly persons. Am J Med 114:266-270

17. Giannessi D, Andreassi MG, Del Ry S et al (2001) Possibility of age regulation of the natriuretic peptide C-receptor in human platelets. J Endocrinol Invest 24:8-16

18. Clerico A, Del Ry S, Giannessi D (2000) Measurement of natriuretic cardiac hormones (ANP, BNP, and related peptides) in clinical practice: the need for a new generation of immunoassay methods. (Review) Clin Chem 46:1529-1534

19. Hammerer-Lercher A, Neubauer E, Muller S et al (2001) Head-to-head comparison of N-terminal pro-brain natriuretic peptide, brain natriuretic peptide and N-terminal pro-atrial natriuretic peptide in diagnosing left ventricular dysfunction. Clin Chim Acta 310:193-197

20. Prontera C, Emdin M, Zucchelli GC et al (2003) Fully-automated NT-proBNP and IRMA methods for BNP and ANP in heart failure and healthy subjects. (Letter) Clin Chem 49:1552-1554

21. Clerico A, Prontera C, Emdin M et al (2005) Analytical performance and diagnostic accuracy of immunometric assays for the measurement of plasma BNP and NT-proBNP concentrations. Clin Chem 51:445-447

22. Clerico A, Caprioli R, Del Ry S, Giannessi D (2001) Clinical relevance of cardiac natriuretic peptides measured by means of competitive and non-competitive immunoassay methods in patients with renal failure on chronic hemodialysis. J Endocrinol Invest 24:24-30

23. Ylitalo K, Uusimaa P, Vuolteenaho O et al (1999) Vasoactive peptide release in relation to hemodynamic and metabolic changes during rapid ventricular pacing. Pacing Clin Electrophysiol 22:1064-1070

24. Clerico A, Iervasi G (1995) Alterations in metabolic clearance of atrial natriuretic peptides in heart failure: how do they relate to the resistance to atrial natriuretic peptides? (Review) J Card Fail 1:323-328

25. Charloux A, Piquard F, Doutreleau S et al (2003) Mechanisms of renal hyporesponsiveness to ANP in heart failure. (Review) Eur J Clin Invest 33:769-778

26. Clerico A, Iervasi G, Pilo A (2000) Turnover studies on cardiac natriuretic peptides: methodological, pathophysiological and therapeutical considerations. (Review) Curr Drug Metab 1:85-105

27. Clerico A, Iervasi G (1995) Alterations in metabolic clearance of atrial natriuretic peptides in heart failure: how do they relate to the resistance to atrial natriuretic peptides? J Card Fail 1:323-328

28. Cody RJ, Atlas SA, Laragh JH et al (1986) Atrial natriuretic factor in normal subjects and heart failure patients: plasma levels and renal, hormonal and hemodynamic responses to peptide infusion. J Clin Invest 78:1362-1374

29. Saito Y, Nakao K, Nishimura K et al (1987) Clinical application of atrial natriuretic polypeptide in patients with congestive heart failure: beneficial effects on left ventricular function. Circulation 76:115-124

30. Komeichi H, Moreau R, Cailmail S et al (1995) Blunted natriuresis and abnormal systemic hemodynamic responses to C-type and brain natriuretic peptides in rats with cirrhosis. J Hepatol 22:319-325

31. Zeidel ML (2000) Physiological responses to natriuretic hormones. In: Fray JCS, Goodman HM (eds) Handbook of physiology, Section 7, The endocrine system, Volume III: Endocrine

regulation of water and electrolyte balance. Oxford University Press, New York, pp 410-435

32. Iervasi G, Clerico A, Berti S et al (1995) Altered tissue degradation and distribution of atrial natriuretic peptide in patients with idiopathic dilated cardiomyopathy and its relationship with clinical severity of the disease and sodium handling. Circulation 91:2018-2027

33. Clerico A, Iervasi G, Pilo A (2005) Turnover studies on cardiac natriuretic peptides: methodological, pathophysiological and therapeutical considerations. Curr Drug Metab 1:85-105

34. Apple FS, Panteghini M, Ravkilde J et al (2005) Quality specifications for B-type natriuretic peptide assays. Clin Chem 51:486-493

35. Panteghini M, Clerico A (2004) Understanding the clinical biochemistry of N-terminal pro-B-type natriuretic peptide: the prerequisite for its optimal clinical use. (Review) Clin Lab 50:325-331

36. Belenky A, Smith A, Zhang B et al (2004) The effect of class-specific protease inhibitors on the stabilization of B-type natriuretic peptide in human plasma. Clin Chim Acta 340:163-172

37. Shimizu H, Masuta K, Aono K et al (2002) Molecular forms of human brain natriuretic peptide in plasma. Clin Chim Acta 316:129-135

38. Shimizu H, Masuta K, Asada H et al (2003) Characterization of molecular forms of probrain natriuretic peptide in human plasma. Clin Chim Acta 334:233-239

39. Trindade PT, Rouleau JL (2001) Vasopeptidase inhibitors: potential role in the treatment of heart failure. (Review) Heart Fail Monit 2:2-7

40. Sagnella GA (2002) Vasopeptidase inhibitors. (Review) J Renin Angiotensin Aldosterone Syst 3:90-95

41. Dawson A, Struthers AD (2002) Vasopeptidase inhibitors in heart failure. (Review) J Renin Angiotensin Aldosterone Syst 3:156-159

42. Floras JS (2002) Vasopeptidase inhibition: a novel approach to cardiovascular therapy. (Review) Can J Cardiol 18:177-182

43. Andreassi MG, Del Ry S, Palmieri C et al (2001) Up-regulation of 'clearance' receptors in patients with chronic heart failure: a possible explanation for the resistance to biological effects of cardiac natriuretic hormones. Eur J Heart Fail 3:407-414

44. Tsunoda K, Mendelsoohn FAO, Sexton PM et al (1988) Decreased atrial natriuretic peptide binding in renal medulla in rats with chronic heart failure. Circ Res 62:155-161

45. Tsutamoto T, Kanamory T, Morigami N et al (1993) Possibility of downregulation of atrial natriuretic peptide receptor coupled to guanylate cyclase in peripheral vascular beds of patients with chronic severe heart failure. Circulation 87:70-75

46. Mukkaddam-Daher S, Tremblay J, Fujio N et al (1996) Alteration of lung atrial natriuretic peptide receptors in genetic cardiomyopathy. Am J Physiol 271:138-145

47. Kuhn M, Voss M, Mitko D et al (2004) Left ventricular assist device support reverses altered cardiac expression and function of natriuretic peptides and receptors in end-stage heart failure. Cardiovasc Res 64:308-314

48. Fan D, Bryan PM, Antos LK et al (2004) Downregulation does not mediate natriuretic peptide-dependent desensitization of NPR-A or NPR-B: guanylyl cyclase-linked natriuretic peptide receptors do not internalize. Mol Pharmacol (printed online Sept 30, 2004)

49. Bryan PM, Potter LR (2002) The atrial natriuretic peptide receptor (NPR-A/GC-A) is dephosphorylated by distinct microcystin-sensitive and magnesium-dependent protein phosphatases. J Biol Chem 277:16041-16047

50. Potter LR, Hunter T (1998) Phosphorylation of the kinase homology domain is essential for activation of the A-type natriuretic peptide receptor. Mol Cell Biol 18:2164-2172

51. Dessi-Fulgheri P, Sarzani R, Rappelli A (1998) The natriuretic peptide system in obesity-related hypertension: new pathophysiological aspects. J Nephrol 11:296-299

52. Sarzani R, Strazzullo P, Salvi F et al (2004) Natriuretic peptide clearance receptor alleles and susceptibility to abdominal adiposity. Obes Res 12:351-356

53. Mehra MR, Uber PA, Park MH et al (2004) Obesity and suppressed B-type natriuretic peptide levels in heart failure. J Am Coll Cardiol 43:1590-1595

54. Wang TJ, Larson MG, Levy D et al (2004) Impact of obesity on plasma natriuretic peptide levels. Circulation 109:594-600

55. Ahluwalia A, MacAllister RJ, Hobbs AJ (2004) Vascular actions of natriuretic peptides. Cyclic GMP-dependent and -independent mechanisms. Basic Res Cardiol 99:83-89

56. Drewett JG, Ziegler RJ, Trachte GJ (1990) Neuromodulatory effects of atrial natriuretic factor are independent of guanylate cyclase in adrenergic neuronal pheochromocytoma cells. J Pharmacol Exp Ther 255:497-503

57. Anand-Srivastava MB, Sairam MR, Cantin M (1988) Ring-deleted analogs of atrial natriuretic factor inhibit adenylate cyclase/cAMP system. Possible coupling of clearance atrial natriuretic factor receptors to adenylate cyclase/cAMP signal transduction system. J Biol Chem 265:8566-8572

58. Packer M (1992) The neurohormonal hypothesis: a theory to explain the mechanisms of disease progression in heart failure. (Review) J Am Coll Cardiol 20:248-254

59. Benedict CR (1994) Neurohormonal aspects of congestive heart failure. (Review) Cardiol Clin 12:9-23

60. Emdin M, Passino C, Prontera C et al (2004) Cardiac natriuretic hormones, neuro-hormones, thyroid hormones and cytokines in normal subjects and patients with heart failure. Clin Chem Lab Med 42:627-636

61. Richards AM, Lainchbury JG, Nicholls MG et al (2002) BNP in hormone-guided treatment of heart failure. (Review) Trends Endocrinol Metab 13:151-155

62. Latini R, Masson S, De Angelis N, Anand I (2002) Role of brain natriuretic peptide in the diagnosis and management of heart failure: current concepts. (Review) J Card Fail 8:288-299

63. Richards M, Troughton RW (2004) NT-proBNP in heart failure: therapy decisions and monitoring. (Review) Eur J Heart Fail 6:351-354

64. Bettencourt P (2004) NT-proBNP and BNP: biomarkers for heart failure management. (Review) Eur J Heart Fail 6:359-363

65. Cowie MR, Mendez GF (2002) BNP and congestive heart failure. (Review) Prog Cardiovasc Dis 44:293-321

66. Nakamura M, Endo H, Nasu M et al (2002) Value of plasma B type natriuretic peptide measurement for heart disease screening in a Japanese population. Heart 87:131-135

67. Kawai K, Hata K, Tanaka K et al (2004) Attenuation of biological compensatory action of cardiac natriuretic peptide system with aging. Am J Cardiol 93:719-723

68. A report of the American College of Cardiology (2001) American Heart Association Task Force on Practice Guidelines. Evaluation and management of chronic heart failure in the adult. ACC/AHA Practice Guidelines

69. Remme WJ, Swedberg K (2001) Task Force Report. Guidelines for the diagnosis and treatment of chronic heart failure. Eur Heart J 22:1527-1560

70. NICE (2003) Clinical Guideline 5. Chronic heart failure. Management of chronic heart failure in adults in primary and secondary care. London, pp 1-44

71. Bossuyt PM (2003) Study design and quality of evidence. In: Price CP, Christenson RH (eds) Evidence-based laboratory medicine. From principles to outcome. AACC Press, Washington DC, pp 75-92

72. Doust JA, Glasziou PP, Pietrzak E, Dobson AJ (2004) A systematic review of the diagnostic accuracy of natriuretic peptides for heart failure. (Review) Arch Intern Med 164:1978-1984

73. Logeart D, Saudubray C, Beyne P et al (2002) Comparative values of Doppler echocardiography and B-type natriuretic peptide assay in the etiologic diagnosis of acute dyspnea. J Am Col Cardiol 40:1794-1800

74. Dokainish H, Zoghbi WA, Lakkis NM et al (2004) Comparative accuracy of B-type natriuretic peptide and tissue Doppler echocardiography in the diagnosis of congestive heart failure. Am J Cardiol 93:1130-1135

75. Williams SG, Ng LL, O'Brien RJ et al (2004) Comparison of plasma N-brain natriuretic peptide, peak oxygen consumption, and left ventricular ejection fraction for severity of chronic heart failure. Am J Cardiol 93:1560-1561

76. Galvani M, Ferrini D, Ottani T (2004) Natriuretic peptides for risk stratification of patients with acute coronary syndromes. (Review) Eur J Heart Fail 6:327-333

77. Jernberg T, James S, Lindahl B et al (2004) Natriuretic peptides in unstable coronary artery disease. (Review) Eur Heart J 25:1486-1493
78. Wiviott SD, de Lemos JA, Morrow DA (2004) Pathophysiology, prognostic significance and clinical utility of B-type natriuretic peptide in acute coronary syndromes. (Review) Clin Chim Acta 346:119-128
79. Kellett J (2004) Prediction of in-hospital mortality by brain natriuretic peptide levels and other independent variables in acutely ill patients with suspected heart disease. Can J Cardiol 20:686-690
80. Kruger S, Graf J, Merx MW et al (2004) Brain natriuretic peptide predicts right heart failure in patients with acute pulmonary embolism. Am Heart J 147:60-65
81. Kucher N, Printzen G, Goldhaber SZ (2003) Prognostic role of brain natriuretic peptide in acute pulmonary embolism. Circulation 107:2545-2547
82. ten Wolde M, Tulevski II, Mulder JW et al (2003) Brain natriuretic peptide as a predictor of adverse outcome in patients with pulmonary embolism. Circulation 107:2082-2084
83. Nagaya N, Nishikimi T, Uematsu M et al (2000) Plasma brain natriuretic peptide as a prognostic indicator in patients with primary pulmonary hypertension. Circulation 102:865-870
84. Vesely DL (2003) Natriuretic peptides and acute renal failure. (Review) Am J Physiol Renal Physiol 285:F167-177
85. McCullough PA, Kuncheria J, Mathur VS (2004) Diagnostic and therapeutic utility of B-type natriuretic peptide in patients with renal insufficiency and decompensated heart failure. (Review) Rev Cardiovasc Med 5:16-25
86. Castillo JR, Zagler A, Carrillo-Jimenez R, Hennekens CH (2004) Brain natriuretic peptide: a potential marker for mortality in septic shock. Int J Infect Dis 8:271-274
87. Palladini G, Campana C, Klersy C et al (2003) Serum N-terminal pro-brain natriuretic peptide is a sensitive marker of myocardial dysfunction in AL amyloidosis. Circulation 107:2440-2445
88. Yasutake H, Seino Y, Kashiwagi M et al (2005) Detection of cardiac sarcoidosis using cardiac markers and myocardial integrated backscatter. Int J Cardiol 102:259-268
89. Bhalla MA, Chiang A, Epshteyn VA et al (2004) Prognostic role of B-type natriuretic peptide levels in patients with type 2 diabetes mellitus. J Am Coll Cardiol 44:1047-1052
90. Takeda Y, Fukutomi T, Suzuki S et al (2004) Effects of carvedilol on plasma B-type natriuretic peptide concentration and symptoms in patients with heart failure and preserved ejection fraction. Am J Cardiol 94:448-453
91. Sackett DL, Haynes RB (2002) The architecture of diagnostic research. Br Med J 324:539-541
92. Nielsen OW, McDonagh TA, Robb SD, Dargie HJ (2003) Retrospective analysis of the cost-effectiveness of using plasma brain natriuretic peptide in screening for left ventricular systolic dysfunction in the general population. J Am Coll Cardiol 41:113-120
93. Sim V, Hampton D, Phillips C et al (2003) The use of brain natriuretic peptide as a screening test for left ventricular systolic dysfunction - cost-effectiveness in relation to open access echocardiography. Fam Pract 20:570-574
94. Ng LL, Loke I, Davies JE et al (2003) Identification of previously undiagnosed left ventricular systolic dysfunction: community screening using natriuretic peptides and electrocardiography. Eur J Heart Fail 5:775-782
95. Fraser CG (2004) Inherent biological variation and reference values. (Review) Clin Chem Lab Med 42:758-764
96. Cotlove E, Harris EK, Williams GZ (1970) Biological and analytic components of variation in long-term studies of serum constituents in normal subjects. 3. Physiological and medical implications. Clin Chem 16:1028-1032
97. Pagani F, Stefini F, Panteghini M (2003) Biological variation in serum concentrations of N-terminal pro-brain natriuretic peptide (NT-proBNP). (Abstract) Clin Chem 49:A34
98. Melzi d'Eril GV, Tagnochetti T, Nauti A et al (2003) Biological variation of N-terminal pro-brain natriuretic peptide in healthy individuals. Clin Chem 49:1554-1555
99. Wu AH, Smith A, Wieczorek S et al (2003) Biological variation for N-terminal pro- and B-type natriuretic peptides and implications for therapeutic monitoring of patients with congestive heart failure. Am J Cardiol 92:628-631

100. Wu AHB, Smith A (2004) Biological variation of the natriuretic peptides and their role in monitoring patients with heart failure. Eur J Heart Fail 6:355-358

101. Bruins S, Fokkema MR, Romer JW et al (2004) High intraindividual variation of B-type natriuretic peptide (BNP) and amino-terminal proBNP in patients with stable chronic heart failure. Clin Chem 50:2052-2058

102. Vanderheyden M, Bartunek J, Goethals M (2004) Brain and other natriuretic peptides: molecular aspects. Eur J Heart Fail 6:261-268

103. Clerico A, Zucchelli GC, Pilo A, Emdin M (2005) Clinical relevance of biological variation of B-Type natriuretic peptide. (Letter) Clin Chem 51:925-926

104. Remes J, Miettinen H, Reunanen A, Pyorala K (1991) Validity of clinical diagnosis of heart failure in primary health care. Eur Heart J 12:315-321

105. Fox KF, Cowie MR, Wood DA et al (2001) Coronary artery disease as the cause of incident heart failure in the population. Eur Heart J 22:228-236

106. McQueen MJ (2001) Overview of evidence-based medicine: challenges for evidence-based laboratory medicine. (Review) Clin Chem 47:1536-1546

107. Bossuyt PM, Reitsma JB, Bruns DE et al (2003) Towards complete and accurate reporting of studies of diagnostic accuracy: the STARD initiative. Clin Chem 49:1-6

108. Omland T, Aakvaag A, Vik-Mo H (1996) Plasma cardiac natriuretic peptide determination as a screening test for the detection of patients with mild left ventricular impairment. Heart 76:232-237

109. Hobbs FDR, Davis RC, Roalfe AK et al (2002) Reliability of N-terminal pro-brain natriuretic peptide assay in diagnosis of heart failure: cohort study in representative and high risk community populations. Br Med J 324:1498-1500

110. Cowie MR, Struthers AD, Wood DA et al (1997) Value of natriuretic peptides in assessment of patients with possible new heart failure in primary care. Lancet 350:1349-1353

111. Maisel AS, Krishnaswamy P, Nowak RM et al (2002) Rapid measurement of B-type natriuretic peptide in the emergency diagnosis of heart failure. N Engl J Med 347:161-167

112. Maisel AS, McCord J, Nowak RM et al (2003) Bedside B-type natriuretic peptide in the emergency diagnosis of heart failure with reduced or preserved ejection fraction. Results from the Breathing Not Properly Multinational Study. J Am Coll Cardiol 41:2010-2017

113. Fisher Y, Filzmaier K, Stiegler H et al (2001) Evaluation of a new, rapid bedside test for qualitative determination of B-type natriuretic peptide. Clin Chem 47:591-594

114. Apple FS, Trinity E, Steen J et al (2003) BNP test utilization for CHF in community hospital practice. Clin Chim Acta 328:191-193

115. Bay M, Kirk V, Parner J et al (2003) NT-proBNP: a new diagnostic screening tool to differentiate between patients with normal and reduced left ventricular systolic function. Heart 89:150-154

116. McLean AS, Tang B, Nalos M et al (2003) Increased B-type natriuretic peptide (BNP) level is a strong predictor for cardiac dysfunction in intensive care unit patients. Anaesth Intensive Care 31:21-27

117. Richards AM, Nicholls MG, Yandle TG et al (1998) Plasma N-terminal pro-brain natriuretic peptide and adrenomedullin: new neurohormonal predictors of left ventricular function and prognosis after myocardial infarction. Circulation 97:1921-1929

118. Yasue H, Yoshimura M, Sumida H et al (1994) Localization and mechanism of secretion of B-type natriuretic peptide in comparison with those of A-type natriuretic peptide in normal subjects and patients with heart failure. Circulation 90:195-203

119. Nakagawa O, Ogawa Y, Itoh H et al (1995) Rapid transcriptional activation and early mRNA turnover of brain natriuretic peptide in cardiocyte hypertrophy. Evidence for brain natriuretic peptide as an "emergency" cardiac hormone against ventricular overload. J Clin Invest 96:1280-1287

120. Vasan RS, Benjamin EJ, Levy D (1995) Prevalence, clinical features and prognosis of diastolic heart failure: an epidemiologic perspective. J Am Coll Cardiol 26:1565-1574

121. Bonow R, Udelson JE (1992) Left ventricular diastolic dysfunction as a cause of congestive heart failure. Ann Intern Med 117:502-510

122. Grodecki PV, Klein AL (1993) Pitfalls in the echo-Doppler assessment of diastolic dysfunction. Echocardiography 10:213-234

123. Suzuki T, Yamaoki K, Nakajima O et al (2000) Screening for cardiac dysfunction in asymptomatic patients by measuring B-type natriuretic peptide levels. Jpn Heart J 41:205-214
124. Maisel AS, Koon J, Krishnaswamy P et al (2001) Utility of B-natriuretic peptide as a rapid, point-of-care test for screening patients undergoing echocardiography to determine left ventricular dysfunction. Am Heart J 141:367-374
125. Lubien E, DeMaria A, Krishnaswamy P et al (2002) Utility of B-natriuretic peptide in detecting diastolic dysfunction: comparison with Doppler velocity recordings. Circulation 105:595-601
126. Vanderheyden M, Goethals M, Verstreken S et al (2004) Wall stress modulates brain natriuretic peptide production in pressure overload cardiomyopathy. J Am Coll Cardiol 44:2349-2354
127. Hayakawa H, Komada Y, Hirayama M et al (2001) Plasma levels of natriuretic peptides in relation to doxorubicin-induced cardiotoxicity and cardiac function in children with cancer. Med Pediatr Oncol 37:4-9
128. Ono M, Tanabe K, Asanuma T et al (2001) Doppler echocardiography-derived index of myocardial performance (TEI index): comparison with brain natriuretic peptide levels in various heart diseases. Jpn Circ J 65:637-642
129. Prontera C, Emdin M, Zucchelli GC et al (2004) Analytical performance and diagnostic accuracy of a fully-automated electrochemiluminescent assay of the N-terminal fragment of brain natriuretic peptide in patients with cardiomyopathy: comparison with immunoradiometric assay methods for brain natriuretic peptide and atrial natriuretic peptide. Clin Chem Lab Med 42:37-44
130. Panteghini M, Clerico A (2004) Understanding the clinical biochemistry of N-terminal pro-B-type natriuretic peptide: the prerequisite for its optimal clinical use. Clin Lab 50:325-331
131. Apple S, Panteghini M, Ravkilde J et al (2005) Quality specifications for B-type natriuretic peptide assays. Clin Chem 51:486-493
132. Clerico A, Prontera C, Emdin M et al (2005) Analytical performance and diagnostic accuracy of immunometric assays for the measurement of plasma BNP and NT-proBNP concentrations. Clin Chem 51:445-447
133. Wright SP, Doughty RN, Pearl A et al (2003) Plasma amino-terminal pro-brain natriuretic peptide and accuracy of heart-failure diagnosis in primary care: a randomized, controlled trial. J Am Coll Cardiol 42:1793-1800
134. Horio T, Shimada K, Kohno M et al (1993) Serial changes in atrial and brain natriuretic peptides in patients with acute myocardial infarction treated with early coronary angioplasty. Am Heart J 126:293-299
135. Morita E, Yasue H, Yoshimura M et al (1993) Increased plasma levels of brain natriuretic peptide in patients with acute myocardial infarction. Circulation 88:82-91
136. Arakawa N, Nakamura M, Aoki H, Hiramori K (1994) Relationship between plasma level of brain natriuretic peptide and myocardial infarct size. Cardiology 85:334-340
137. Uusimaa P, Ruskoaho H, Vuolteenaho O et al (1999) Plasma vasoactive peptides after acute myocardial infarction in relation to left ventricular dysfunction. Int J Cardiol 69:5-14
138. Omland T, Aakvaag A, Bonarjee VV et al (1996) Plasma brain natriuretic peptide as an indicator of left ventricular systolic function and long-term survival after acute myocardial infarction. Comparison with plasma atrial natriuretic peptide and N-terminal proatrial natriuretic peptide. Circulation 93:1963-1969
139. Panteghini M, Cuccia C, Bonetti G et al (2003) Rapid determination of brain natriuretic peptide in patients with acute myocardial infarction. Clin Chem Lab Med 41:164-168
140. Bettencourt P, Ferreira A, Pardal-Oliveira N et al (2000) Clinical significance of brain natriuretic peptide in patients with postmyocardial infarction. Clin Cardiol 23:921-927
141. Choy AM, Darbar D, Lang CC et al (1994) Detection of left ventricular dysfunction after acute myocardial infarction: comparison of clinical, echocardiographic, and neurohormonal methods. Br Heart J 72:16-22
142. Baruch L, Glazer RD, Aknay N et al (2004) Morbidity, mortality, physiologic and functional parameters in elderly and non-elderly patients in the Valsartan Heart Failure Trial (Val-HeFT). Am Heart J 148:951-957

143. Hutcheon SD, Gillespie ND, Struthers AD, McMurdo ME (2002) B-type natriuretic peptide in the diagnosis of elderly day hospital patients. Age Ageing 31:295-301

144. Hedberg P, Lonnberg I, Jonason T et al (2004) Electrocardiogram and B-type natriuretic peptide as screening tools for left ventricular systolic dysfunction in a population-based sample of 75-year-old men and women. Am Heart J 148:524-529

145. Heidenreich PA, Gubens MA, Fonarow GC et al (2004) Cost-effectiveness of screening with B-type natriuretic peptide to identify patients with reduced left ventricular ejection fraction. J Am Coll Cardiol 43:1019-1026

146. Ray P, Arthaud M, Lefort Y et al (2004) Usefulness of B-type natriuretic peptide in elderly patients with acute dyspnea. Intensive Care Med 30:2230-2236

147. Valle R, Aspromonte N, Barro S et al (2005) The NT-proBNP assay identifies very elderly nursing home residents suffering from pre-clinical heart failure. Eur J Heart Fail 7:542-551

148. Suzuki T, Hayashi D, Yamazaki T et al (1998) Elevated B-type natriuretic peptide levels after anthracycline administration. Am Heart J 136:362-363

149. Nousiainen T, Jantunen E, Vanninen E et al (1998) Acute neurohumoral and cardiovascular effects of idarubicin in leukemia patients. Eur J Haematol 61:347-353

150. Nousiainen T, Jantunen E, Vanninen E et al (1999) Natriuretic peptides as markers of cardiotoxicity during doxorubicin treatment for non-Hodgkin's lymphoma. Eur J Haematol 62:135-141

151. Okumura H, Iuchi K, Yoshida T et al (2000) Brain natriuretic peptide is a predictor of anthracycline-induced cardiotoxicity. Acta Haematol 104:158-163

152. Hayakawa H, Komada Y, Hirayama M et al (2001) Plasma levels of natriuretic peptides in relation to doxorubicin-induced cardiotoxicity and cardiac function in children with cancer. Med Pediatr Oncol 37:4-9

153. Pinarli FG, Oguz A, Sedef Tunaoglu SF et al (2005) Late cardiac evaluation of children with solid tumors after anthracycline chemotherapy. Pediatr Blood Cancer 44:370-377

154. Gharib MI, Burnett AK (2002) Chemotherapy-induced cardiotoxicity: current practice and prospects of prophylaxis. (Review) Eur J Heart Fail 4:235-242

155. Von Hoff DD, Layard MW, Basa P et al (1979) Risk factors for doxorubicin-induced congestive heart failure. Ann Intern Med 91:710-717

156. Daugaard G, Lassen U, Bie P et al (2005) Natriuretic peptides in the monitoring of anthracycline induced reduction in left ventricular ejection fraction. Eur J Heart Fail 7:87-93

157. Koh E, Nakamura T, Takahashi H (2004) Troponin-T and brain natriuretic peptide as predictors for adriamycin-induced cardiomyopathy in rats. Circ J 68:163-167

158. Cardinale D, Sandri MT, Martinoni A et al (2000) Left ventricular dysfunction predicted by early troponin I release after high-dose chemotherapy. J Am Coll Cardiol 36:517-522

159. Sandri MT, Cardinale D, Zorzino L et al (2003) Minor increases in plasma troponin I predict decreased left ventricular ejection fraction after high-dose chemotherapy. Clin Chem 49:248-252

160. Cardinale D, Sandri MT, Colombo A et al (2004) Prognostic value of troponin I in cardiac risk stratification of cancer patients undergoing high-dose chemotherapy. Circulation 109:2749-2754

161. Pichon MF, Cvitkovic F, Hacene K et al (2005) Drug-induced cardiotoxicity studied by longitudinal B-type natriuretic peptide assays and radionuclide ventriculography. In vivo 19:567-576

162. Sandri MT, Salvatici M, Cardinale D et al (2005) N-Terminal pro-B-type natriuretic peptide after high-dose chemotherapy: a marker predictive of cardiac dysfunction? Clin Chem 51:1405-1410

163. Foote RS, Pearlman JD, Siegel AH, Yeo KT (2004) Detection of exercise-induced ischemia by changes in B-type natriuretic peptide. J Am Coll Cardiol 44:1980-1987

164. Sabatine MS, Morrow DA, de Lemos JA et al (2004) TIMI Study Group. Acute changes in circulating natriuretic peptide levels in relation to myocardial ischemia. J Am Coll Cardiol 44:1988-1995

165. Gianrossi R, Detrano R, Mulvihill D et al (1989) Exercise-induced ST depression in the diagnosis of coronary artery disease: a meta-analysis. Circulation 80:87-98

166. Froelicher VF, Lehmann KG, Thomas R et al (1998) The electrocardiographic exercise test

in a population with reduced workup bias: diagnostic performance, computerized interpretation, and multivariable prediction: Veterans Affairs Cooperative Study in Health Services #016 (QUEXTA) Study Group. Quantitative exercise testing and angiography. Ann Intern Med 128:965-974

167. Morise AP, Diamond GA (1995) Comparison of the sensitivity and specificity of exercise electrocardiography in biased and unbiased populations of men and women. Am Heart J 130:741-747

168. Cardarelli R, Lumicao TG (2003) B-type natriuretic peptide: a review of its diagnostic, prognostic, and therapeutic monitoring value in heart failure for primary care physicians. (Review) J Am Board Fam Pract 16:327-333

169. Davie AP, Francis CM, Love MP et al (1996) Value of the electrocardiogram in identifying heart failure due to left ventricular systolic dysfunction. Br Med J 312:222

170. Ogawa K, Oida A, Sugimura H et al (2002) Clinical significance of blood brain natriuretic peptide level measurement in the detection of heart disease in untreated outpatients: comparison of electrocardiography, chest radiography and echocardiography. Circ J 66:122-126

171. Ng LL, Loke I, Davies JE et al (2003) Identification of previously undiagnosed left ventricular systolic dysfunction: community screening using natriuretic peptides and electrocardiography. Eur J Heart Fail 5:775-782

172. Hedberg P, Lonnberg I, Jonason T et al (2004) Electrocardiogram and B-type natriuretic peptide as screening tools for left ventricular systolic dysfunction in a population-based sample of 75-year-old men and women. Am Heart J 148:524-529

173. Talwar S, Squire IB, Davies JE et al (1999) Plasma N-terminal pro-brain natriuretic peptide and the ECG in the assessment of left-ventricular systolic dysfunction in a high risk population. Eur Heart J 20:1736-1744

174. Nakamura M, Sakai T, Osawa M et al (2005) Comparison of positive cases for B-type natriuretic peptide and ECG testing for identification of precursor forms of heart failure in an elderly population. Int Heart J 46:477-487

175. Struthers AD (1993) Plasma concentrations of brain natriuretic peptide: will this new test reduce the need for cardiac investigations? (Editorial) Br Heart J 70:397-398

176. Thomas MD, Fox KF, Coats AJ, Sutton GC (2004) The epidemiological enigma of heart failure with preserved systolic function. Eur J Heart Fail 6:125-136

177. Choy AM, Darbar D, Lang CC et al (1994) Detection of left ventricular dysfunction after acute myocardial infarction: comparison of clinical, echocardiographic, and neurohormonal methods. Br Heart J 72:16-22

178. Dokainish H, Zoghbi WA, Lakkis NM et al (2004) Comparative accuracy of B-type natriuretic peptide and tissue Doppler echocardiography in the diagnosis of congestive heart failure. Am J Cardiol 93:1130-1151

179. Gackowski A, Isnard R, Golmard JL et al (2004) Comparison of echocardiography and plasma B-type natriuretic peptide for monitoring the response to treatment in acute heart failure. Eur Heart J 25:1788-1796

180. Mak GS, DeMaria A, Clopton P, Maisel AS (2004) Utility of B-natriuretic peptide in the evaluation of left ventricular diastolic function: comparison with tissue Doppler imaging recordings. Am Heart J 148:895-902

181. Steg PG, Joubin L, McCord J et al (2005) B-type natriuretic peptide and echocardiographic determination of ejection fraction in the diagnosis of congestive heart failure in patients with acute dyspnea. Chest 128:21-29

182. Forfia PR, Watkins SP, Rame JE et al (2005) Relationship between B-type natriuretic peptides and pulmonary capillary wedge pressure in the intensive care unit. J Am Coll Cardiol 45:1667-1671

183. O'Neill JO, Bott-Silverman CE, McRae AT 3rd et al (2005) B-type natriuretic peptide levels are not a surrogate marker for invasive hemodynamics during management of patients with severe heart failure. Am Heart J 149:363-369

184. Parsonage WA, Galbraith AJ, Koerbin GL, Potter JM (2005) Value of B-type natriuretic peptide for identifying significantly elevated pulmonary artery wedge pressure in patients treat-

ed for established chronic heart failure secondary to ischemic or idiopathic dilated cardiomyopathy. Am J Cardiol 95:883-885

185. Rodeheffer RJ (2004) Measuring plasma B-type natriuretic peptide in heart failure: good to go in 2004? (Review) J Am Coll Cardiol 44:740-749

186. Doust JA, Pietrzak E, Dobson A, Glasziou P (2005) How well does B-type natriuretic peptide predict death and cardiac events in patients with heart failure: systematic review. (Review) BMJ 330:625-633

187. Benedict CR, Shelton B, Johnstone DE et al (1996) Prognostic significance of plasma norepinephrine in patients with asymptomatic left ventricular dysfunction. SOLVD Investigators. Circulation 94:690-697

188. Wallen T, Landahl S, Hedner T et al (1997) Brain natriuretic peptide predicts mortality in the elderly. Heart 77:264-267

189. Tsutamoto T, Wada A, Maeda K et al (1999) Plasma brain natriuretic peptide level as a biochemical marker of morbidity and mortality in patients with asymptomatic or minimally symptomatic left ventricular dysfunction. Comparison with plasma angiotensin II and endothelin-1. Eur Heart J 20:1799-1807

190. Stanek B, Frey B, Hulsmann M et al (2001) Prognostic evaluation of neurohumoral plasma levels before and during beta-blocker therapy in advanced left ventricular dysfunction. J Am Coll Cardiol 38:436-442

191. Anand IS, Fisher LD, Chiang YT et al (2003) Val-HeFT Investigators. Changes in brain natriuretic peptide and norepinephrine over time and mortality and morbidity in the Valsartan Heart Failure Trial (Val-HeFT). Circulation 107:1278-1283

192. Gardner RS, Ozalp F, Murday AJ et al (2003) N-terminal pro-brain natriuretic peptide. A new gold standard in predicting mortality in patients with advanced heart failure. Eur Heart J 24:1735-1743

193. Baruch L, Glazer RD, Aknay N et al (2004) Morbidity, mortality, physiologic and functional parameters in elderly and non-elderly patients in the Valsartan Heart Failure Trial (Val-HeFT). Am Heart J 148:951-957

194. Kellett J (2004) Prediction of in-hospital mortality by brain natriuretic peptide levels and other independent variables in acutely ill patients with suspected heart disease. Can J Cardiol 20:686-690

195. Kirk V, Bay M, Parner J et al (2004) N-terminal proBNP and mortality in hospitalised patients with heart failure and preserved vs. reduced systolic function: data from the prospective Copenhagen Hospital Heart Failure Study (CHHF). Eur J Heart Fail 6:335-341

196. Berger R, Huelsmann M, Strecker K et al (2005) Neurohormonal risk stratification for sudden death and death owing to progressive heart failure in chronic heart failure. Eur J Clin Invest 35:24-31

197. Hulsmann M, Berger R, Mortl D et al (2005) Incidence of normal values of natriuretic peptides in patients with chronic heart failure and impact on survival: a direct comparison of N-terminal atrial natriuretic peptide, N-terminal brain natriuretic peptide and brain natriuretic peptide. Eur J Heart Fail 7:552-556

198. Segawa T, Nakamura M, Itai K et al (2005) Plasma B-type natriuretic peptide levels and risk factors for congestive heart failure in a Japanese general population. Int Heart J 46:465-475

199. Stanton E, Hansen M, Wijeysundera HC et al (2005) A direct comparison of the natriuretic peptides and their relationship to survival in chronic heart failure of a presumed non-ischaemic origin. Eur J Heart Fail 7:557-565

200. Bertinchant JP, Combes N, Polge A et al (2005) Prognostic value of cardiac troponin T in patients with both acute and chronic stable congestive heart failure: comparison with atrial natriuretic peptide, brain natriuretic peptide and plasma norepinephrine. Clin Chim Acta 352:143-153

201. Isnard R, Pousset F, Chafirovskaia O et al (2003) Combination of B-type natriuretic peptide and peak oxygen consumption improves risk stratification in outpatients with chronic heart failure. Am Heart J 146:729-735

202. de Groote P, Dagorn J, Soudan B et al (2004) B-type natriuretic peptide and peak exercise

oxygen consumption provide independent information for risk stratification in patients with stable congestive heart failure. J Am Coll Cardiol 43:1584-1589

203. Kyuma M, Nakata T, Hashimoto A et al (2004) Incremental prognostic implications of brain natriuretic peptide, cardiac sympathetic nerve innervation, and noncardiac disorders in patients with heart failure. J Nucl Med 45:155-163

204. Latini R, Masson S, Anand I et al (2004) The comparative prognostic value of plasma neuro-hormones at baseline in patients with heart failure enrolled in Val-HeFT. Eur Heart J 25:292-299

205. Van Beneden R, Gurne O, Selvais PL et al (2004) Superiority of big endothelin-1 and endothe-lin-1 over natriuretic peptides in predicting survival in severe congestive heart failure: a 7-year follow-up study. J Card Fail 10:490-495

206. Berger R, Huelsmann M, Strecker K et al (2005) Neurohormonal risk stratification for sud-den death and death owing to progressive heart failure in chronic heart failure. Eur J Clin Invest 35:24-31

207. Alehagen U, Dahlstrom U, Lindahl TL (2004) Elevated D-dimer level is an independent risk factor for cardiovascular death in out-patients with symptoms compatible with heart failure. Thromb Haemost 92:1250-1258

208. Ishii J, Cui W, Kitagawa F et al (2003) Prognostic value of combination of cardiac troponin T and B-type natriuretic peptide after initiation of treatment in patients with chronic heart failure. Clin Chem 49:2020-2026

209. Fonarow GC, Horwich TB (2003) Combining natriuretic peptides and necrosis markers in determining prognosis in heart failure. (Review) Rev Cardiovasc Med 4(suppl 4):S20-28

210. De Mello WC (2004) Heart failure: how important is cellular sequestration? The role of the renin-angiotensin-aldosterone system. (Review) J Mol Cell Cardiol 37:431-438

211. Sekiguchi K, Li X, Coker M et al (2004) Cross-regulation between the renin-angiotensin sys-tem and inflammatory mediators in cardiac hypertrophy and failure. (Review) Cardiovasc Res 63:433-442

212. Nian M, Lee P, Khaper N, Liu P (2004) Inflammatory cytokines and postmyocardial infarc-tion remodeling. (Review) Circ Res 94:1543-1553

213. Kanda T, Takahashi T (2004) Interleukin-6 and cardiovascular diseases. (Review) Jpn Heart J 45:183-193

214. von Haehling S, Jankowska EA, Anker SD (2004) Tumour necrosis factor-alpha and the failing heart - pathophysiology and therapeutic implications. (Review) Basic Res Cardiol 99:18-28

215. Moe GW, Rouleau JL, Nguyen QT et al (2003) Role of endothelins in congestive heart fail-ure. (Review) Can J Physiol Pharmacol 81:588-597

216. Boerrigter G, Burnett JC (2003) Endothelin in neurohormonal activation in heart failure. (Review) Coron Artery Dis 14:495-500

217. Floras JS (2003) Sympathetic activation in human heart failure: diverse mechanisms, thera-peutic opportunities. (Review) Acta Physiol Scand 177:391-398

218. Piano MR, Prasun M (2003) Neurohormone activation. (Review) Crit Care Nurs Clin North Am 15:413-421

219. Ascheim DD, Hryniewicz K (2002) Thyroid hormone metabolism in patients with congestive heart failure: the low triiodothyronine state. Thyroid 12:511-515

220. Danzi S, Klein I (2004) Thyroid hormone and the cardiovascular system. (Review) Minerva Endocrinol 29:139-150

221. Myocardial infarction redefined (2000) - a consensus document of the Joint European Soci-ety of Cardiology/American College of Cardiology committee for the redefinition of myocar-dial infarction. J Am Coll Cardiol 36:959-969

222. ACC/AHA 2002 guideline update for the management of patients with unstable angina and non-ST-segment elevation myocardial infarction (2002) A report of the American College of Cardiology/American Heart Association task force on practice guidelines (committee on the management of patients with unstable angina). American College of Cardiology and the American Heart Association, Inc, pp 1-95

223. Omland T, Persson A, Ng L et al (2002) N-terminal pro-B-type natriuretic peptide and long-term mortality in acute coronary syndromes. Circulation 106:2913-2918

224. Arakawa N, Nakamura M, Aoki H, Hiramori K (1996) Plasma brain natriuretic peptide concentrations predict survival after acute myocardial infarction. J Am Coll Cardiol 27:1656-1661

225. Darbar D, Davidson NC, Gillespie N et al (1996) Diagnostic value of B-type natriuretic peptide concentrations in patients with acute myocardial infarction. Am J Cardiol 78:284-287

226. Crilley JG, Farrer M (2001) Left ventricular remodelling and brain natriuretic peptide after first myocardial infarction. Heart 86:638-642

227. McDonagh TA, Cunningham AD, Morrison CE et al (2001) Left ventricular dysfunction, natriuretic peptides, and mortality in an urban population. Heart 86:21-26

228. Richards AM, Doughty R, Nicholls MG et al (2001) Plasma N-terminal pro-brain natriuretic peptide and adrenomedullin: prognostic utility and prediction of benefit from carvedilol in chronic ischemic left ventricular dysfunction. Australia-New Zealand Heart Failure Group. J Am Coll Cardiol 37:1781-1787

229. Inoue T, Sakuma M, Yaguchi I et al (2002) Early recanalization and plasma brain natriuretic peptide as an indicator of left ventricular function after acute myocardial infarction. Am Heart J 143:790-796

230. Sabatine MS, Morrow DA, de Lemos JA et al (2002) Multimarker approach to risk stratification in non-ST elevation acute coronary syndromes: simultaneous assessment of troponin I, C-reactive protein, and B-type natriuretic peptide. Circulation 105:1760-1763

231. Jernberg T, Stridsberg M, Lindahl B (2002) Usefulness of plasma N-terminal proatrial natriuretic peptide (proANP) as an early predictor of outcome in unstable angina pectoris or non-ST-elevation acute myocardial infarction. Am J Cardiol 89:64-66

232. Jernberg T, Stridsberg M, Venge P, Lindahl B (2002) N-terminal pro brain natriuretic peptide on admission for early risk stratification of patients with chest pain and no ST-segment elevation. J Am Coll Cardiol 40:437-445

233. Heeschen C, Hamm CW, Mitrovic V et al (2004) Platelet Receptor Inhibition in Ischemic Syndrome Management (PRISM) Investigators. N-terminal pro-B-type natriuretic peptide levels for dynamic risk stratification of patients with acute coronary syndromes. Circulation 110:3206-3212

234. Jernberg T, James S, Lindahl B et al (2004) NT-proBNP in unstable coronary artery disease - experiences from the FAST, GUSTO IV and FRISC II trials. Eur J Heart Fail 6:319-325

235. Mega JL, Morrow DA, De Lemos JA et al (2004) B-type natriuretic peptide at presentation and prognosis in patients with ST-segment elevation myocardial infarction: an ENTIRE-TIMI-23 substudy. J Am Coll Cardiol 44:335-339

236. Palazzuoli A, Calabria P, Vecchiato L et al (2004) Plasma brain natriuretic peptide levels in coronary heart disease with preserved systolic function. Clin Exp Med 4:44-49

237. Squire IB, O'Brien RJ, Demme B et al (2004) N-terminal pro-atrial natriuretic peptide (N-ANP) and N-terminal pro-B-type natriuretic peptide (N-BNP) in the prediction of death and heart failure in unselected patients following acute myocardial infarction. Clin Sci 107:309-316

238. Suzuki S, Yoshimura M, Nakayama M et al (2004) Plasma level of B-type natriuretic peptide as a prognostic marker after acute myocardial infarction: a long-term follow-up analysis. Circulation 110:1387-1391

239. Wylie JV, Murphy SA, Morrow DA et al (2004) Validated risk score predicts the development of congestive heart failure after presentation with unstable angina or non-ST-elevation myocardial infarction: results from OPUS-TIMI 16 and TACTICS-TIMI 18. Am Heart J 148:173-180

240. Squire IB, Orn S, Ng LL et al (2005) Plasma natriuretic peptides up to 2 years after acute myocardial infarction and relation to orognosis: an OPTIMAAL substudy. J Card Fail 11:492-497

241. Omland T, Richards AM, Wergeland R, Vik-Mo H (2005) B-type natriuretic peptide and long-term survival in patients with stable coronary artery disease. Am J Cardiol 95:24-28

242. Kragelund C, Gronning B, Kober L et al (2005) N-terminal pro-B-type natriuretic peptide and long-term mortality in stable coronary heart disease. N Engl J Med 352:666-675

243. Hama N, Itoh H, Shirakami G et al (1995) Rapid ventricular induction of brain natriuretic peptide gene expression in experimental acute myocardial infarction. Circulation 92:1158-1164

244. Toth M, Vuorinen KH, Vuolteenaho O et al (1994) Hypoxia stimulates release of ANP and BNP from perfused rat ventricular myocardium. Am J Physiol 266(4 Pt 2):H1572-1580
245. Goetze JP, Gore A, Moller CH et al (2004) Acute myocardial hypoxia increases BNP gene expression. FASEB J 18:1928-1930
246. Marumoto K, Hamada M, Hiwada K (1995) Increased secretion of atrial and brain natriuretic peptides during acute myocardial ischaemia induced by dynamic exercise in patients with angina pectoris. Clin Sci 88:551-556
247. Dyrbye LN, Redfield MM (2003) The role of brain natriuretic peptide in population screening. Heart Fail Rev 8:349-354
248. Freitag MH, Vasan RS (2003) Screening for left ventricular systolic dysfunction: the use of B-type natriuretic peptide. Heart Fail Monit 4:38-44
249. Davis KM, Fish LC, Elahi D et al (1992) Atrial natriuretic peptide levels in the prediction of congestive heart failure risk in frail elderly. JAMA 267:2625-2629
250. Knight EL, Fish LC, Kiely DK et al (1999) Atrial natriuretic peptide and the development of congestive heart failure in the oldest old: a seven-year prospective study. J Am Geriatr Soc 47:407-411
251. Freitag MH, Larson MG, Levy D et al (2003) Plasma brain natriuretic peptide levels and blood pressure tracking in the Framingham Heart Study. Hypertension 41:978-983
252. Murdoch DR, McDonagh TA, Byrne J et al (1999) Titration of vasodilator therapy in chronic heart failure according to plasma brain natriuretic peptide concentration: randomized comparison of the hemodynamic and neuroendocrine effects of tailored versus empirical therapy. Am Heart J 138:1126-1132
253. Troughton RW, Frampton CM, Yandle TG et al (2000) Treatment of heart failure guided by plasma aminoterminal brain natriuretic peptide (N-BNP) concentrations. Lancet 355:1126-1130
254. Kawai K, Hata K, Takaoka H et al (2001) Plasma brain natriuretic peptide as a novel therapeutic indicator in idiopathic dilated cardiomyopathy during beta-blocker therapy: a potential of hormone-guided treatment. Am Heart J 141:925-932
255. Maisel AS (2001) B-type natriuretic peptide (BNP) levels: diagnostic and therapeutic potential. (Review) Rev Cardiovasc Med 2(suppl 2):S13-18
256. Nicholls MG, Lainchbury JG, Richards AM et al (2001) Brain natriuretic peptide-guided therapy for heart failure. Ann Med 33:422-427
257. Troughton RW, Richards AM, Nicholls MG (2001) Individualized treatment of heart failure. Intern Med J 31:138-141
258. McGeoch G, Lainchbury J, Town GI et al (2002) Plasma brain natriuretic peptide after long-term treatment for heart failure in general practice. Eur J Heart Fail 4:479-483
259. Mueller C, Buser P (2002) B-type natriuretic peptide (BNP): can it improve our management of patients with congestive heart failure? (Review) Swiss Med Wkly 132:618-622
260. Hobbs RE (2003) Using BNP to diagnose, manage, and treat heart failure. (Review) Cleve Clin J Med 70:333-336
261. Richards M (2003) Outpatient management of heart failure. (Review) Heart Fail Rev 8:345-348
262. Maisel A, Hollander JE, Guss D et al (2004) Rapid Emergency Department Heart Failure Outpatient Trial investigators. Primary results of the Rapid Emergency Department Heart Failure Outpatient Trial (REDHOT). A multicenter study of B-type natriuretic peptide levels, emergency department decision making, and outcomes in patients presenting with shortness of breath. J Am Coll Cardiol 44:1328-1333
263. Morimoto T, Hayashino Y, Shimbo T et al (2004) Is B-type natriuretic peptide-guided heart failure management cost-effective? Int J Cardiol 96:177-181
264. Wu AH, Harrison A, Maisel AS (2004) Reduced readmission rate for alternating diagnoses of heart failure and pulmonary disease after implementation of B-type natriuretic peptide testing. Eur J Heart Fail 6:309-312
265. Mueller C, Scholer A, Laule-Kilian K et al (2004) Use of B-type natriuretic peptide in the evaluation and management of acute dyspnea. N Engl J Med 350:647-654
266. Kirchhoff WCh, Gradaus R, Stypmann J et al (2004) Vasoactive peptides during long-term follow-up of patients after cardiac transplantation. J Heart Lung Transplant 23:284-288

267. Kemperman H, van den Berg M, Kirkels H, de Jonge N (2004) B-type natriuretic peptide (BNP) and N-terminal proBNP in patients with end-stage heart failure supported by a left ventricular assist device. Clin Chem 50:1670-1672

268. Thompson LO, Skrabal CA, Loebe M et al (2005) Plasma neurohormone levels correlate with left ventricular functional and morphological improvement in LVAD patients. J Surg Res 123:25-32

269. Crozier IG, Nicholls MG, Ikram H et al (1989) Atrial natriuretic peptide levels in congestive heart failure in man before and during converting enzyme inhibition. Clin Exp Pharmacol Physiol 16:417-424

270. Yoshimura M, Yasue H, Tanaka H et al (1994) Responses of plasma concentrations of A type natriuretic peptide and B type natriuretic peptide to alacepril, an angiotensin-converting enzyme inhibitor, in patients with congestive heart failure. Br Heart J 72:528-533

271. Davidson NC, Coutie WJ, Webb DJ, Struthers AD (1996) Hormonal and renal differences between low dose and high dose angiotensin converting enzyme inhibitor treatment in patients with chronic heart failure. Heart 75:576-581

272. Nishikimi T, Matsuoka H, Ishikawa K et al (1996) Antihypertensive therapy reduces increased plasma levels of adrenomedullin and brain natriuretic peptide concomitant with regression of left ventricular hypertrophy in a patient with malignant hypertension. Hypertens Res 19:97-101

273. Missouris CG, Grouzmann E, Buckley MG et al (1998) How does treatment influence endocrine mechanisms in acute severe heart failure? Effects on cardiac natriuretic peptides, the renin system, neuropeptide Y and catecholamines. Clin Sci 94:591-599

274. Hara Y, Hamada M, Shigematsu Y et al (2000) Effect of beta-blocker on left ventricular function and natriuretic peptides in patients with chronic heart failure treated with angiotensin-converting enzyme inhibitor. Jpn Circ J 64:365-369

275. Tsutamoto T, Wada A, Maeda K et al (2001) Effect of spironolactone on plasma brain natriuretic peptide and left ventricular remodeling in patients with congestive heart failure. J Am Coll Cardiol 37:1228-1233

276. Johnson W, Omland T, Hall C et al (2002) Neurohormonal activation rapidly decreases after intravenous therapy with diuretics and vasodilators for class IV heart failure. J Am Coll Cardiol 39:1623-1629

277. Cotter G, Kaluski E, Stangl K et al (2004) The hemodynamic and neurohormonal effects of low doses of tezosentan (an endothelin A/B receptor antagonist) in patients with acute heart failure. Eur J Heart Fail 6:601-609

278. Bouissou P, Galen FX, Richalet JP et al (1989) Effects of propranolol and pindolol on plasma ANP levels in humans at rest and during exercise. Am J Physiol 257:R259-264

279. Colantonio D, Casale R, Desiati P et al (1991) Short-term effects of atenolol and nifedipine on atrial natriuretic peptide, plasma renin activity, and plasma aldosterone in patients with essential hypertension. J Clin Pharmacol 31:238-242

280. Yoshimura M, Yasue H, Tanaka H et al (1994) Responses of plasma concentrations of A type natriuretic peptide and B type natriuretic peptide to alacepril, an angiotensin-converting enzyme inhibitor, in patients with congestive heart failure. Br Heart J 72:528-533

281. Sanderson JE, Chan WW, Hung YT et al (1995) Effect of low dose beta blockers on atrial and ventricular (B type) natriuretic factor in heart failure: a double blind, randomised comparison of metoprolol and a third generation vasodilating beta blocker. Br Heart J 74:502-507

282. Luchner A, Burnett JC Jr, Jougasaki M et al (1998) Augmentation of the cardiac natriuretic peptides by beta-receptor antagonism: evidence from a population-based study. J Am Coll Cardiol 32:1839-1844

283. Fujimura M, Yasumura Y, Ishida Y et al (2000) Improvement in left ventricular function in response to carvedilol is accompanied by attenuation of neurohumoral activation in patients with dilated cardiomyopathy. J Card Fail 6:3-10

284. Hara Y, Hamada M, Shigematsu Y et al (2000) Effect of beta-blocker on left ventricular function and natriuretic peptides in patients with chronic heart failure treated with angiotensin-converting enzyme inhibitor. Jpn Circ J 64:365-369

285. Hirooka K, Yasumura Y, Ishida Y et al (2001) Comparative left ventricular functional and neurohumoral effects of chronic treatment with carvedilol versus metoprolol in patients with dilated cardiomyopathy. Jpn Circ J 65:931-936

286. Kawai K, Hata K, Takaoka H et al (2001) Plasma brain natriuretic peptide as a novel therapeutic indicator in idiopathic dilated cardiomyopathy during beta-blocker therapy: a potential of hormone-guided treatment. Am Heart J 141:925-932

287. Hara Y, Hamada M, Ohtsuka T et al (2002) Comparison of treatment effects of bevantolol and metoprolol on cardiac function and natriuretic peptides in patients with dilated cardiomyopathy. Heart Vessels 17:53-56

288. Persson H, Andreasson K, Kahan T et al (2002) Neurohormonal activation in heart failure after acute myocardial infarction treated with beta-receptor antagonists. Eur J Heart Fail 4:73-82

289. Fung JW, Yu CM, Yip G et al (2003) Effect of beta blockade (carvedilol or metoprolol) on activation of the renin-angiotensin-aldosterone system and natriuretic peptides in chronic heart failure. Am J Cardiol 92:406-410

290. Konishi H, Nishio S, Tsutamoto T et al (2003) Serum carvedilol concentration and its relation to change in plasma brain natriuretic peptide level in the treatment of heart failure: a preliminary study. Int J Clin Pharmacol Ther 41:578-586

291. van den Meiracker AH, Lameris TW, van de Ven LL, Boomsma F (2003) Increased plasma concentration of natriuretic peptides by selective beta1-blocker bisoprolol. J Cardiovasc Pharmacol 42:462-468

292. Yoshizawa A, Yoshikawa T, Nakamura I et al (2004) Brain natriuretic peptide response is heterogeneous during beta-blocker therapy for congestive heart failure. J Card Fail 10:310-315

293. Ohta Y, Watanabe K, Nakazawa M et al (2000) Carvedilol enhances atrial and brain natriuretic peptide mRNA expression and release in rat heart. J Cardiovasc Pharmacol 36(suppl 2):S19-23

294. Beck-da-Silva L, de Bold A, Fraser M et al (2005) BNP-guided therapy not better than expert's clinical assessment for beta-blocker titration in patients with heart failure. Congest Heart Fail 11:248-253

295. Lewin J, Ledwidge M, O'loughlin C et al (2005) Clinical deterioration in established heart failure: What is the value of BNP and weight gain in aiding diagnosis? Eur J Heart Fail 7:953-957

296. Emdin M, Clerico A, Clemenza F et al (2005) Recommendations for the clinical use of cardiac natriuretic peptides. Ital Heart J 6:430-446

297. Jourdain P, Gueffet P, Le Helloco J et al (2005) STARS-BNP Investigators on behalf of the working group on Heart failure of the French Society of Cardiology. Benefit of BNP plasma levels for optimising therapy in patients with systolic heart failure. Supported by STARS-BNP multicenter randomised study. Eur J Heart Failure 4(suppl 1):120

298. Clerico A, Recchia FA, Passino C, Emdin M (2006) Cardiac endocrine function is an essential component of the homeostatic regulation network: physiological and clinical implications. Am J Physiol Heart Circ Physiol 290:H17-29

299. Nieminen MS, Bohm M, Cowie MR et al (2005) Executive summary of the guidelines on the diagnosis and treatment of acute heart failure: the Task Force on Acute Heart Failure of the European Society of Cardiology. Eur Heart J 26:384-416

300. Swedberg K, Cleland J, Dargie H et al (2005) Guidelines for the diagnosis and treatment of chronic heart failure: executive summary (update 2005): The Task Force for the Diagnosis and Treatment of Chronic Heart Failure of the European Society of Cardiology. Eur Heart J 26:1115-1140

Chapter 6

Clinical Applications in Extra-Cardiac Diseases

Aldo Clerico • Claudio Passino • Michele Emdin

6.1 Introduction

The CNH assay may be clinically useful in many other conditions besides cardiovascular diseases [1, 2]. The list of clinical conditions with altered (increased or decreased compared to normal range) circulating levels of CNH must be continuously updated because of the huge amount of data accumulating in this field every day (see Table 5.1).

In this chapter, some extra-cardiac diseases that are characterized by an altered CNH system will be discussed in detail. In these diseases, activation of the CNH system indicates that the heart is under "stress"; this observation holds great clinical relevance [1-12] (Fig. 6.1). Indeed, several studies have demonstrated that the increase in circulating levels of CNH is an independent and strong risk factor for future major cardiovascular complications and/or death, even in extra-cardiac diseases [1-12]. In particular, we will discuss in detail the pathophysiological mechanisms that are thought to activate the

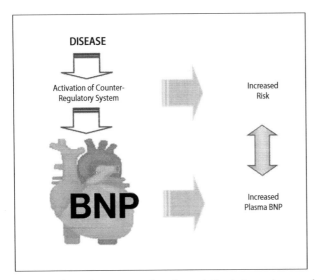

Fig. 6.1. Schematic representation of association between increased plasma BNP and cardiovascular risk. All the extra-cardiac clinical conditions able to activate the counter-regulatory system (including the adrenergic system, renin-angiotensin-aldosterone system, endothelins, cytokines, and some growth factors) also activate the CNH system and in turn an increase in plasma BNP. The activation of counter-regulatory systems, especially if longstanding and powerful, increases the risk of major cardiovascular events and death. As a result, plasma BNP should be considered as a biological marker of cardiovascular risk

CNH system for each specific disease (or group of diseases). Theoretically speaking, these mechanisms should work in many clinical conditions; this explains the increasing number of diseases in which the CNH system was found to be altered. Furthermore, clinicians should be on the look-out for an unexplained increase in CNH levels in extra-cardiac diseases. It is important to note that CNH levels can be altered in very common diseases (such as pulmonary, renal, hepatic and inflammatory diseases).

Due to the great number of clinical conditions in which the circulating levels of CNH can be altered (see Table 5.1), we will discuss in detail only the more frequent diseases or those with more (and consistent) data available in the literature. In other words, the aim of this chapter is not only to focus on the inter-relationships between the CNH system and the other synergic or counter-regulatory systems, but also to discuss more generally the complex relationships between the heart and the other organs.

6.2 Pulmonary Diseases

Several studies have evaluated the diagnostic and prognostic relevance of CNH in acute and/or chronic pulmonary diseases [4-6, 13-25]. The rationale for this clinical evaluation is that circulating levels of CNH could increase in these clinical conditions with the degree of hypoxia [26] and right heart overload [4, 18, 27-30] (see also Chapter 3, section 3.3, for a more detailed discussion of this topic).

On average, plasma BNP is greatly increased in hypoxemic chronic obstructive pulmonary disease (COPD) compared to healthy subjects [14]. BNP levels are higher among patients with *cor pulmonale* when compared to patients with only chronic respiratory disease (pulmonary fibrosis or COPD); furthermore, patients with chronic respiratory failure complicated by *cor pulmonale* show higher BNP levels than those without *cor pulmonale* [16]. In patients with chronic respiratory disease, plasma BNP was higher in those with pulmonary hypertension than in those without [17]. Several studies evaluated the diagnostic accuracy of BNP assay in the differential diagnosis of dyspnea in the emergency department [20,31-36]. In particular, the study by Morrison et al. [34] was specifically designed to determine if a point-of-care testing assay of BNP could accurately differentiate heart failure from dyspnea of pulmonary etiology in 321 patients presenting to the emergency department. Patients with right heart failure from *cor pulmonale* had BNP levels ($n = 134, 758.5 \pm 798$ ng/l) significantly higher than the group of patients with a final diagnosis of pulmonary disease ($n = 85, 61 \pm 10$ ng/l). A breakdown of patients with pulmonary disease revealed: COPD 54 ± 71 ng/l ($n = 42$); asthma 27 ± 40 ng/l ($n = 11$); acute bronchitis 44 ± 112 ng/l ($n = 14$); pneumonia 55 ± 76 ng/l ($n = 8$); tuberculosis 93 ± 54 ng/l ($n = 2$); lung cancer 120 ± 120 ng/l ($n = 4$); and acute pulmonary embolism 207 ± 272 ng/l ($n = 3$). The AUC of ROC analysis was 0.97 (0.96-0.99), and sensitivity and specificity values were 86 and 98% (accuracy 91%), respectively, according to a cut-off value of 94 ng/l in separating cardiac from pulmonary diseases [34, 37]. These data have been confirmed by the results found in larger clinical trials reported by the Breathing Not Properly Multinational Study Group [13, 20, 31, 32, 36] (Fig. 6.2). In particular, the proportions of patients presenting to the emergency department with acute dyspnea, who were correctly classified, were 67% for BNP test alone, 55% for left ventricular ejection fraction alone, 82% for the two variables together, and 97.3% when clinical, ECG, and chest radiograph data were added [13]. This study suggested that

BNP measurement was superior to two-dimensional echocardiographic determination of left ventricular ejection fraction in identifying congestive heart failure, regardless of the threshold value. The two methods combined have marked additive diagnostic value [13]. However, some recent studies indicated that BNP/NT-proBNP levels do not accurately predict serial hemodynamic changes and consequently do not obviate the need for pulmonary artery catheterization in patients requiring invasive hemodynamic monitoring [38-40], including critically ill patients with respiratory failure [41].

These studies, taken as a whole, strongly indicate that the BNP assay in the emergency department should help to differentiate pulmonary from cardiac etiologies of dyspnea, but also that it is not useful to differentiate among pulmonary etiologies [20, 31, 32, 36, 37]. However, BNP levels are usually greatly increased in patients with right ventricular pressure overload caused by primary pulmonary hypertension or pulmonary embolism [4, 27, 37], thus suggesting that BNP assay should be useful in these clinical conditions [29, 30].

Several studies reported that BNP assay shows a relevant prognostic value in pulmonary diseases [4-6, 14, 15, 17]. During a follow-up period of more than 12 months, plasma BNP was found to be an independent predictor of end-stage chronic respirato-

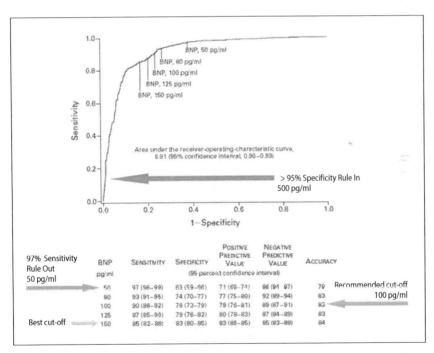

Fig. 6.2. Diagnostic accuracy of a point-of-care testing method for the BNP assay in 1,586 patients who came to the emergency department with acute dyspnea (Breathing Not Properly Multinational Study). Values for sensitivity and specificity calculated by means of ROC curve analysis are reported. Patients with BNP values below 50 pg/ml (corresponding to 50 ng/l) should be ruled out for the diagnosis of heart failure, while patients with values above 500 pg/ml (500 ng/l) have a very high probability of having heart failure (modified from Maisel et al. [31])

ry disease death in 31 consecutive patients with chronic respiratory disease [20]. Nagaya et al. [6] reported that baseline plasma BNP was an independent predictor of mortality in 60 patients with primary pulmonary hypertension at diagnostic catheterization. Survival was strikingly worse for patients with a supramedian value of follow-up BNP (≥180 ng/l) than for those with an inframedian value; in addition, ROC analysis indicated that its prognostic power was comparable or even superior to hemodynamic evaluation [6]. Finally, BNP assay was demonstrated to be an independent and powerful predictor of fatal events in patients with pulmonary embolism [3-5].

6.3 Kidney Diseases

It is well known that cardiovascular events are the major prognostic determinants in patients with end-stage renal disease (ESRD). Cardiovascular deaths represent more than 50% of total mortality. In these patients, creatinine levels are associated with increased risk of mortality, cardiovascular disease, and chronic heart failure [42, 43]. Circulating levels of CNH are greatly increased in renal failure: several studies tested their diagnostic accuracy and prognostic risk for cardiovascular events in ESRD patients [44-55].

In particular, Ishii et al. [49] prospectively compared the predictive value of myocardial necrosis markers (cTnT and cTnI) and CNH (ANP and BNP, both measured by IRMA methods) in 100 consecutive outpatients on chronic dialysis without acute coronary artery syndrome. In a stepwise multivariate Cox regression analysis, only cTnT and a history of heart failure requiring hospitalization were independent predictors of both all-cause and cardiac mortality after a 2-year follow-up [49]. Cataliotti et al. [50] examined the relationship of CNH assay to cardiac mortality in 112 dialysis patients without clinical evidence of congestive heart failure. BNP levels were significantly associated with greater risk of cardiovascular death in Cox regression analysis, as were ANP levels. Goto et al. [51] investigated whether increased plasma levels of ANP or BNP predict future cardiac events in 53 patients undergoing chronic hemodialysis without clinical symptoms suggestive of cardiac disorders and followed for 11.3 ± 0.2 months. Using the Kaplan-Meier method, the incidence of cardiac events was significantly greater in patients with higher levels of ANP or BNP. Naganuma et al. [52] evaluated the risk of cardiac mortality for 36 months in 164 hemodialysis patients and 14 healthy volunteers by stepwise multivariate Cox proportional hazards analysis. BNP, left ventricular mass index, and C-reactive protein (CRP) were found to be independent predictors of cardiac death, compared to other biochemical and clinical parameters. Apple et al. [54] confirmed that plasma NT-proBNP, CRP, cTnT, and cTnI were all independently predictive of subsequent death in ESRD patients.

Further studies are necessary to confirm the clinical relevance of CNH assay in the stratification risk for cardiac or total mortality in ESRD patients, as suggested by the conflicting results reported above [44-54]. However, the most recent and largest studies all confirmed the prognostic value of BNP/NT-proBNP assay in ESRD patients for future cardiovascular events [44-54]. Moreover, the predictive power of BNP assay is independent from that of other biomarkers of inflammation or endothelial dysfunction (such as CRP and asymmetric dimethyl arginine) [56].

The usefulness of the CNH assay as a diagnostic marker of cardiac function in patients with end-stage renal disease is also doubtful, especially when taking into account the different behavior of CNH and their N-terminal pro-peptides, and when comparing the assay with other biomarkers and/or hemodynamic parameters [1, 2, 57]. While only a few data are available on the NT-proBNP assay, the BNP assay seems to show better diagnostic accuracy and clinical performance as a prognostic marker of cardiac involvement and mortality than the ANP assay.

These conflicting results reported on diagnostic accuracy and prognostic cardiac morbidity and mortality of CNH assay in ESRD patients could be due to the relatively small number of patients studied, when compared to the larger number of patients in studies concerning heart failure or acute coronary artery syndrome. Moreover, only studies with long follow-up periods in a large population allow an accurate determination of a sound number of clinically significant events [58, 59]. Furthermore, renal failure can be considered to be the end-stage of all renal diseases, so that patients with chronic renal failure studied by different groups could have very different clinical history and characteristics, pharmacological treatment, and cardiovascular risk background. Whereas glomerulonephritis was the leading cause of chronic renal failure in the past, diabetic and hypertensive nephropathy are now more frequent [60]. Patients with diabetes mellitus and systemic arterial hypertension are also at high risk for major cardiovascular events: consequently, the prevalence of hypertension and/or diabetes can greatly influence the evaluation of the diagnostic accuracy and the risk power for a CNH assay in patients with renal failure.

Differences in degradation pathways may also affect the clinical results, especially when biologically active peptides (i.e., ANP and BNP) are compared to inactive ones (such as NT-proANP and NT-proBNP). Biologically active peptides are degraded by both receptor-mediated and enzymatic processes, while the inactive peptides are degraded only by an enzymatic process. Furthermore, it is possible that enzymes responsible for the degradation of different peptides are also different. However, the per cent extraction by the human kidney of BNP and NT-proBNP is very similar (about 20%), while that of ANP is much higher (about 70%), as suggested by data reported in Table 6.1. These data indicate that renal impairment may affect circulating levels of ANP more than those of BNP and NT-proBNP.

Table 6.1. Extraction of BNP and NT-proBNP by kidney. The concentration of ANP, BNP and NT-proBNP were measured in 10 subjects submitted to catheterization of renal vessels by means of accurate, non-competitive sandwich immunoassay methods. All these subjects showed a normal renal function. Data obtained in the authors' laboratory

Peptide (assay method)	Renal artery concentration (ng/l)	Renal vein concentration (ng/l)	Per cent extraction (%)
ANP (IRMA)	128.2 ± 59.5	40.4 ± 23.5	69.7 ± 4.4
BNP (MEIA, AxSYM system)	107.7 ± 81.9	84.7 ± 59.8	19.8 ± 4.8
NT-proBNP (ECLIA, Elecsys system)	480.0 ± 617.1	363.5 ± 446.6	20.4 ± 11.6

6.4 Acute and Chronic Inflammatory Diseases

Increased levels of CNH were frequently reported in severe sepsis, including septic shock [9, 61-66], as well as in some chronic inflammatory diseases, such as amyloidosis [10, 67] and sarcoidosis [11].

Myocardial depression is well recognized as an early feature of human septic shock, causing absence of appropriate oxygen supply to peripheral tissues and subsequent death. Early systolic dysfunction has been identified in these patients and seems to be related to mortality [9]. A significant increase in CNH (including ANP, BNP and CNP) was found in patients with septic shock or severe sepsis [9, 61-66]; in particular, BNP values reflected left ventricular dysfunction, while ANP values were related to IL-6 production, rather than to cardiovascular dysfunction [65]. These studies suggest the hypothesis that BNP/NT-proBNP assay is a marker for mortality in septic shock-associated myocardial dysfunction [9] or severe sepsis [64, 66]. If, in the future, a body of evidence emerges to support this hypothesis, utilization of BNP as a marker for mortality in septic shock would have major clinical and public health implications.

Amyloidoses are disorders of protein conformation and metabolism that result in tissue deposition of insoluble fibrils, organ dysfunction, and death. Half of patients present with various degrees of cardiac amyloidosis at diagnosis, but virtually all eventually die of cardiac-related death [10]. Expression of ANP and BNP and their genes was augmented in the ventricular myocytes of patients with cardiac amyloidosis [68]. Furthermore, BNP/NT-proBNP was found to be the most sensitive index of myocardial dysfunction and the most powerful prognostic determinant of death in primary systemic amyloidosis [10, 67] (Fig. 6.3). The multivariate model including NT-proBNP could discriminate prognostic groups better than the models including increased interventricular septum thickness, or clinical judgment of heart involvement, or even a score accounting for relevant echocardiographic and clinical evidence of heart involvement [10]. The BNP/NT-proBNP assay can add prognostic information for newly diagnosed patients more effectively than echocardiography, and can be useful in designing therapeutic strategies and monitoring response [10, 67].

It is interesting to note that the CNH increase in many patients with systemic amyloidosis before treatment may actually reflect the cardiotoxicity of the amyloidogenic light chains [10]. These patients may have severe myocardial infiltration but minimal heart failure; thus indicating that the increased secretion of CNH by cardiomyocytes may be dependent, at least in the early phase of the disease, on local inflammatory processes rather than on hemodynamic changes (including an increase in the wall stress) [10, 67]. This may explain the greater sensitivity of the BNP/NT-proBNP assay compared to echocardiography in patients with cardiac amyloidosis [10, 67]. In conclusion, BNP levels (and those of its related peptides) seem to be elevated in cardiac amyloidosis, regardless of the presence or absence of clinical evidence of heart failure [67].

Sarcoidosis is a systemic granulomatous disease of unknown etiology, which commonly affects the lungs, eyes, or skin, with a favorable prognosis [69]. However, once the heart is involved, unfavorable cardiac complications occur in many patients [70]. These complications include high-degree atrioventricular block, ventricular tachyarrhythmias, and congestive heart failure, which often result in sudden death. Accordingly, earlier detection of cardiac involvement is essential to reduce such cardiac com-

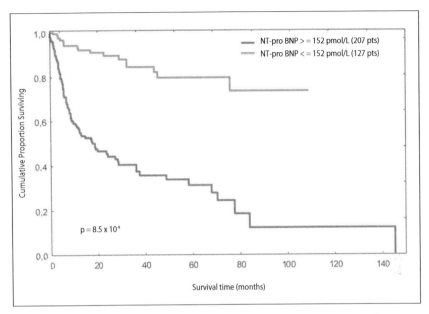

Fig. 6.3. Survival of 334 patients with AL amyloidosis divided into two groups according to NT-proBNP cut-off value (152 pmol/l, corresponding to 1,285 ng/l) at diagnosis. The death rate for patients with NT-proBNP values above the cut-off was about 10-fold higher than that for patients with values below the calculated cut-off value. The best cut-off value (152 pmol/l) was calculated by ROC curve analysis for the detection for heart involvement corresponding to a sensitivity of 93%, a specificity of 90% and an accuracy of 92%. (Data kindly supplied by Giampaolo Merlini, MD, Department of Biochemistry, University Hospital "IRCCS Policlinico S. Matteo", University of Pavia, modified from [10])

plications because the disease is treatable with corticosteroids and other immunosuppressive agents [11, 70]. Holter monitoring, two-dimensional echocardiography, and radionuclide myocardial imaging are generally used to detect cardiac involvement, but the cardiac lesions are still often overlooked because of their subclinical disease progression [11, 70]. Yasutake et al. [11] recently suggested that both ANP and BNP are useful markers for identifying patients with sarcoidosis and cardiac complication(s) and that they are also useful predictors for cardiac events in patients with cardiac sarcoidosis.

6.5 CNH Assay in Cerebrovascular Disease

Hyponatremia, commonly associated with diuresis and natriuresis, is frequent in patients with subarachnoid hemorrhage (SAH). Several authors have investigated whether CNH are related to such hyponatremia in SAH. Indeed, CNH (including ANP, BNP and CNP) levels were frequently found to be increased in patients with SAH [71-84]. In a recent study, increasing serum BNP levels were independently associated with hyponatremia, and they significantly increased during the first 24 hours after onset of delayed ischemic neurological deficits and showed a predictive power similar to the 2-week Glasgow Coma Scale score [81].

As the increase in CNH (especially BNP) is well documented in patients with SAH [71-84], its pathophysiological role in this clinical condition is not clear. Some studies reported that the increase in plasma hormones is unrelated to severity, stress hormone activation, or markers of cardiac injury [78, 79]. On the other hand, other authors have suggested that BNP secretion in SAH patients is closely related to the bleeding intensity and vasospasm severity, as well as to development of delayed ischemic neurological deficits [83]. According to this hypothesis, BNP might play a role in the pathophysiology of cerebral vasospasm, through its systemic effects on blood pressure and plasma volume [83], or of focal edema [80, 82].

Furthermore, the origin of CNH found in plasma of SAH patients is not clear. In the absence of evidence for activation of natriuretic peptides within the brain, some authors suggested that the prompt and consistent increase in both ANP and BNP supports the view that the heart is the source of increased natriuretic peptide secretion after acute SAH [75, 76, 79], even if the mechanism relating the brain (especially hypothalamic) insult to the secretion of CNH by the heart is not known [83].

Since CNH do not cross the blood-brain barrier [85], the release of CNH from the heart into the peripheral circulatory system does not explain the higher cerebrospinal fluid concentrations of CNH found in patients with SAH [71]. Consequently, these data suggest that an increased CNH production takes place also in the hypothalamus in patients with SAH. Two possible mechanisms should be considered: the release secondary to humoral and/or paracrine signals and the response to hypoxia due to vasospasm [83]. Since ANP, BNP and CNP are produced in the brain (in particular in the hypothalamus) and their production is mediated and induced by triggers such as catecholamines [86], endothelin [87] and arginine vasopressin [88], a paracrine loop should be considered as a possible mechanism by which CNH is produced extensively in SAH within the hypothalamus [83]. On the other hand, BNP could be released from hypoxic tissue and produced in the brain in response to ischemia secondary to cerebral vasospasm [75, 86]. According to this hypothesis, the enhanced CNH secretion takes part in a counter-mechanism, which protects the brain against ischemic insult caused by vasospasm [72, 83].

A recent study [89] reported that elevated values of plasma NT-proANP and NT-proBNP in the acute phase of stroke indicate an increased risk of future mortality. High plasma levels of peptides predicted mortality after stroke better than any other risk variable, with the risk of death being 4-fold among the patients with high peptide values. Another recent study [90] reported that NT-proBNP and renin, but not CRP, are independent predictors of risk of developing myocardial infarction after stroke or transient ischemic attack, providing information additional to that provided by classic risk factors, and may enable more effective targeting of prevention strategies for myocardial infarction.

In conclusion, circulating levels of CNH are often elevated in patients with acute cerebrovascular disorders. The pathophysiological mechanism(s) and tissue(s) responsible for the increase in production/secretion of CNH are not well known. However, recent studies suggest that CNH levels may be independent predictors of death or non-fatal cardiac events in patients with stroke or transient ischemic attack.

6.6 Liver Diseases

It is well known that cardiac dysfunction may be present in patients with liver cirrhosis. Many experimental [91, 92] and clinical studies [93-108] have documented the increase in CNH circulating levels in patients with liver cirrhosis. In particular, a recent study reported that plasma BNP levels are significantly increased even in non-alcoholic cirrhotic patients with left ventricular ejection fraction in the normal range and also correlated with the Child-Pugh score, a clinical classification that strongly predicts survival in liver cirrhosis [108]. These data suggest that an insidious cardiac dysfunction may be present in cirrhotic patients [108].

Elevated circulating levels of CNH in patients with cirrhosis most likely reflect increased cardiac ventricular secretion of these peptides. Elevation of circulating levels of ANP with cirrhosis was associated with increased ventricular steady-state ANP messenger RNA concentrations in rats [109]. Some authors suggested that the increased ANP gene expression in cirrhosis may involve a novel mechanism not related to myocardial stretch because neither increased ventricular pressure nor dilatation was present [109].

To clarify the involvement in the pathogenesis and also to evaluate the potential therapeutic effects of CNH in liver cirrhosis, several authors infused CNH (especially ANP and BNP) or their synthetic analogs [110-124]. A blunted natriuretic response to CNH infusion was usually found in patients [113-115, 120-124], as well as in experimental animals with liver cirrhosis [92, 125]. It is conceivable that the overactivity of the counter-regulatory system was of major importance in determining the blunted renal response to CNH in patients with liver cirrhosis [122], in a similar manner as demonstrated in patients with heart failure without liver cirrhosis. However, other mechanisms acting at the pre-receptor and receptor level may also play a role in inducing the resistance to natriuretic effects of CNH, as also suggested by other authors [106] (see Chapter 5, section 5.1.5, for more details).

6.7 Thyroid Diseases

The heart is highly sensitive to the effects of thyroid hormones. Thyroid hormone is an important regulator of cardiac function and cardiovascular hemodynamics. Triiodothyronine (T3), the physiologically active form of thyroid hormone, binds to nuclear receptor proteins and mediates the expression of several important cardiac genes, inducing transcription of the positively regulated genes, including α-myosin heavy chain (MHC) and the sarcoplasmic reticulum calcium ATPase [126]. Negatively regulated genes include β-MHC and phospholamban, which are down-regulated in the presence of normal serum levels of thyroid hormone. T3-mediated effects on the systemic vasculature include relaxation of vascular smooth muscle, resulting in decreased arterial resistance and diastolic blood pressure. Moreover, T3 increases heart rate, cardiac contractility, and cardiac output by means of both direct (on cardiomyocytes) and indirect effects (via hemodynamic changes) [126] (Fig. 6.4, Table 6.2).

Pathological states associated with either hypo- or hyperthyroidism display abnormalities in cardiac function that frequently contribute to the morbidity and mortality associated with these disorders [126]. T3 has also been shown to activate growth in cardiac myocytes *in vitro* [127-129] and *in vivo* [130, 131], through a combination of direct and indirect effects, leading to increased cell size, protein synthesis, and changes in gene expression.

Furthermore, thyroid hormones regulate a number of genes in the heart, including those encoding ANP and BNP, and in this way increase the secretion and genetic expression of CNH *in vivo* and *in vitro* [132-135]. T3-dependent effects appear to be unique from those associated with so-called pathological hypertrophy (e.g. that due to hemodynamic overload *in vivo*) in that T3 treatment of the pathologically hypertrophied myocardium produces a shift in the gene expression profile away from that which is typically identified with pathological hypertrophy alone [136] and toward a profile more closely resembling the physiological hypertrophy associated with exercise training [129].

Several experimental [137] and clinical studies [138-147] indicated that the CNH system is affected in thyroid disease. In particular, CNH (especially ANP) circulating levels are altered in the hyperthyroid state (reaching the circulating levels usually found in mild heart failure) and return within the normal range after appropriate treatment, which restores euthyroidism [139-141]. On the other hand, conflicting results have been found in hypothyroid patients, although most studies have found decreased levels of CNH [138, 144-146]. These experimental and clinical studies, taken as a whole, demonstrate that production/secretion and circulating levels of CNH are strongly influenced by thyroid function. Furthermore, treatment of the dysthyroid state resulted in a significant increase in circulating levels of CNH in hypothyroid patients and a decrease in hyperthyroid patients.

Dysthyroidism greatly affects cardiac function. Hyperthyroid patients (especially the youngest and those with only mild disease) have raised pulse rate, increased cardiac output and ejection fraction associated with reduced total peripheral resistance, and hypothyroid patients have the reverse [126, 148-150] (Table 6.2). Furthermore, isovolumetric relaxation time, an index of diastolic function, is usually increased in hypothyroid patients and decreased in hyperthyroid patients [126, 150]. From a theoretical point of view, taking into account only the cardiac functional parameters, we would expect increased CNH

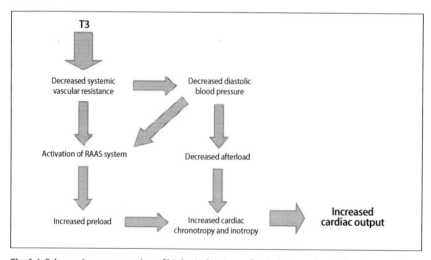

Fig. 6.4. Schematic representation of biological actions of tri-iodothyronine (T3) on heart and cardiovascular system

levels in hypothyroid patients (who usually have a depressed cardiac function), but not in hyperthyroid patients (who on average have normal or even increased left ventricular ejection fraction, cardiac output and isovolumetric relaxation time values); that is the complete reverse of the condition actually observed (i.e., increased levels in hyperthyroidism and decreased levels in hypothyroidism). As a result, changes in cardiac function parameters cannot alone explain all changes in circulating CNH associated with thyroid disease. However, blood volume as well as the preload can be increased in hyperthyroidism and decreased in hypothyroidism (Table 6.2, Fig. 6.4) [126, 150]; these findings can in part explain the altered circulating CNH levels (especially for plasma ANP).

On the other hand, several experimental studies [132-135] indicate that thyroid hormones *per se* exert a direct, positive stimulation on CNH expression and secretion. This direct stimulatory effect may be considered an important mechanism in explaining the variations of CNH in dysthyroid states. Another factor that might contribute to variation of CNH levels in some hyperthyroid patients is the increase in circulating products formed by the precursor peptide degradation, due to increased activation of aminopeptidases (such as BNP and NT-proBNP peptides produced from the intact proBNP) [144].

The inter-relationships between thyroid and heart are complex and in part not well known: not only thyroid disease can affect cardiac function, but also thyroid function can be altered in severe heart disease [126]. Indeed, a typical pattern of altered thyroid hormone metabolism characterized by low T3 circulating levels has been described in patients with acute or chronic heart disease (such as acute myocardial infarction and severe heart failure) [126, 150-153] and after cardiothoracic surgery [154-156]. Indeed, low thyroid hormone concentrations, in particular low serum T3 concentrations (the so-called low-T3 syndrome), are common in patients with non-thyroidal illnesses, including cardiac disorders [126, 157-159]. From a clinical point of view, it is important to note that HF patients with low-T3 syndrome have greatly increased CNH levels, while in hypothyroid patients without myocardial dysfunction the circulating levels of CNH are in the normal range or even slightly increased (see Table 5.4).

The principal pathophysiological mechanism underlying low circulating T3 is the reduced enzyme activity of 5-monodeiodinase responsible for converting thyroxine into T3 in peripheral tissues [157, 158]. This low-T3 syndrome has commonly been interpreted by the medical community as a euthyroid sick syndrome, an adaptive compensatory and thus beneficial response that decreases energy consumption in diseased states [157, 158]. This interpretation, however, has recently been questioned because some studies documented the benefit gained from treating patients with synthetic thyroid hormones [126, 160-166]. Indeed, low-T3 syndrome is a strong and independent predictor of mortality in cardiac patients, especially those with heart failure [167, 168]. However, further studies are mandatory in order to confirm the beneficial effects of treatment with thyroid hormones in heart failure and especially to establish and standardize the therapeutic protocols.

6.8 Diabetes Mellitus

Cardiovascular disease is the leading cause of morbidity and mortality in diabetic subjects [169, 170]. The commonest cardiovascular complications are ischemic cardiomyopathy and left ventricular dysfunction. Some studies have demonstrated that diabetes mellitus is associated with increased left ventricular wall thickness and mass, independently of blood pressure levels and body mass index [171]. Diabetes mellitus is also associated with heart failure, mainly through its association with hypertension and coronary artery disease [169, 170]. In addition, the existence of a primary myocardial disease, "diabetic cardiomyopathy", has been proposed as evidence has accumulated for the presence of myocardial dysfunction in diabetic patients in the absence of ischemic, valvular or hypertensive heart disease [169]. Thus, diabetes mellitus, independently of the mechanism, is associated with an increased risk of left ventricular hypertrophy, left ventricular dysfunction and coronary artery disease [169-171]. Taking these issues into account, several studies have evaluated a possible pathophysiological role of the CNH system in diabetes mellitus.

In experimental animals (rats and pigs) with streptozotocin-induced diabetes [172-176] and in Zucker diabetic fatty rats [177], mRNA expression and content of ANP and/or BNP are usually increased in cardiac [172-177] and renal [178-180] tissue. Furthermore, increased circulating levels of CNH (especially ANP) have usually been found in diabetic experimental aminals [173, 178, 180-183] and in plasma of rat fetuses with diabetic mothers [184].

Increased circulating levels of CNH have been reported frequently in patients with both type 1 [185, 186] and type 2 [187-191] diabetes mellitus, especially in patients with microalbuminuria or cardiovascular complications [12, 191]. Furthermore, BNP was demonstrated to be a reliable predictor of future cardiac and all-cause mortality in patients with diabetes mellitus [12]. However, BNP and NT-proBNP levels were also found to be elevated in some type 2 diabetes mellitus patients without overt cardio-vascular disease and macroalbuminuria [189, 191]. These data suggest that diabetes *per se* could be affecting the CNH system. Indeed, a recent study demonstrated that insulin significantly increased protein synthesis and stimulated ANP secretion and gene expression in primary culture of neonatal rat cardiac myocytes, while exposure to high glucose had no effect [192]. These findings are in accordance with other studies demonstrating that insulin has mitogenic and metabolic effects in most cell types, including cardiac tissue [193, 194]. Furthermore, a clinical study reported that acute hyperinsulinemia (induced by glucose clamp or glucose challenge test) can increase ANP (but not BNP) concentration in patients with type 2 diabetes mellitus [195]. However, a recent study reported that BNP levels in 223 type 2 diabetes mellitus patients increased only by the progression of cardiovascular diseases, such as coronary artery disease, but not by the current diabetic control [191].

Assay of BNP may be an alternative way of identifying subjects who have a high total cardiovascular risk score. Dawson et al. [196] compared the BNP level with Framingham 10-year risk scores for coronary heart disease and stroke and New Zealand cardiovas-cular risk scores in 231 patients who had type 2 diabetes and no pre-existing coronary heart disease or stroke. There was a significant correlation between log BNP and 10-year risk for coronary heart disease and stroke, and there were significantly higher BNP levels in those who had high cardiovascular risk as assessed by the New Zealand risk score. This study suggested that BNP may be a useful way of measuring total cardio-vascular risk, thus having the potential to target the most aggressive primary preven-tive therapies toward the most needy [196].

Diabetic nephropathy results from the interaction of genetic factors with chronic hyperglycemia [197]. ANP may affect the course of diabetic nephropathy by inducing afferent arteriolar dilatation and efferent constriction within the glomerulus [179,

198, 199]. In subjects with type 1 diabetes mellitus, high glomerular filtration rate and ANP concentration correlated with each other [200], and ANP infusion increased glomerular filtration rate, filtration fraction, and albuminuria [201]. Moreover, ANP favors diabetic hyperfiltration [181, 198, 199]. Thus, the ANP gene (PND) is a candidate gene for diabetic nephropathy, but investigations [197, 202-206] on this topic have been controversial.

The first study [202] investigated ANP gene polymorphisms (C708 versus T708 and ScaI) and type 1 diabetic nephropathy from 454 patients with type 1 diabetes mellitus from an Italian population. This study suggested a significant association of C708T polymorphism with microalbuminuria in long-term diabetes and with both lower plasma ANP levels and widespread albumin leakage, and also a strong association between ScaI polymorphism and both diabetic nephropathy and plasma ANP concentrations. These results were confirmed by another study concerning the general population of Mexico City; both polymorphisms of ANP were associated with albuminuria independently of hypertension, and were suggested to play a role in protecting subjects against development of albuminuria [203]. Another polymorphism, named Hpa II, does not seem to play a major role in the development of diabetic nephropathy in either type 1 or type 2 diabetes mellitus [202, 205].

Several ANP gene polymorphisms (G663A, C708T, T2238C, G2311T, and T2332C) were evaluated in a more recent cross-sectional study with a 6-year follow-up [197]. In this study [197], none of the genotypes or haplotypes was significantly associated with the disease in the case-control study. In the follow-up, C708T and T2238C showed a weak association with disease progression, but T2238C was strongly associated with progression in poorly controlled subjects. The raw effect of the 2238C allele (hazard risk ratio 1.93, 95% CI 1.15-3.24; $p = 0.012$) was further confirmed by the haplotype analysis, suggesting that the 2238C allele of PND may affect the course of nephropathy in inadequately controlled type 1 diabetic patients [197]. Moreover, another study [204] found no association between ANP T2238C polymorphism and ANP levels in Japanese subjects. Finally, the functional effect of ANP T2238C polymorphism was evaluated three times after low-salt, normal, and high-salt diets in 105 Polish subjects. Following all three diets, plasma ANP levels were strongly associated with T2238C polymorphism and were lowest in TT subjects [197]. The reasons for these discrepancies are unclear. Survival bias and population stratification cannot be ruled out in case-control studies; differences in study design were probably a major cause of the differences in the results obtained. Therefore, functional significance and clinical relevance of this polymorphism, as well as of all the other PND (ANP gene) polymorphisms, remain to be determined.

In conclusion, CNH levels can be above the reference limits in patients with diabetes mellitus, and increase further if renal and/or cardiovascular complications are present. The CNH assay can be useful for cardiovascular risk stratification in patients with diabetes mellitus [12]; however, screening approaches, including BNP assay, do not appear to be sufficiently sensitive to identify subclinical dysfunction in patients with diabetes mellitus, which requires sophisticated echocardiographic analysis [207]. Further studies are necessary to evaluate whether CNH assay may also be useful in the early detection of myocardial dysfunction, as well as to demonstrate the functional and clinical relevance of polymorphisms of some CNH genes in patients with diabetes mellitus.

6.9 Obesity

Obesity is a major risk factor for hypertension and hypertension-related disorders such as left ventricular hypertrophy [208, 209]. The mechanisms linking obesity to the development of hypertension have not been established, although it has been suggested that renal sodium and water retention [210] and increased activation of the sympathetic and rennin-angiotensin systems [211] may contribute. Because the natriuretic peptide system plays a key role in the regulation of these processes, it has been speculated that obese individuals have an impaired natriuretic peptide response, and the phrase "natriuretic handicap" has been used to describe this phenomenon [212]. The existence of such a handicap has not been proven, although limited experimental data suggest that ANP levels fail to rise appropriately in obese subjects after a saline load [213]. Furthermore, some recent studies reported that CNH levels (BNP and NT-proANP) are inversely related to body mass index (BMI) in patients with heart failure [214, 215], as well as in the general population [216], thus supporting the concept of a natriuretic handicap.

Obesity is associated with salt retention and increased cardiac output [217], which would be expected to produce elevated natriuretic peptide levels. That obesity seems to have the opposite effect is counterintuitive and presumably attributable to non-hemodynamic factors. Natriuretic peptide clearance receptors (NPR-C) are abundant in adipose tissue, suggesting that adipocytes participate in the removal of natriuretic peptides from the circulation [218, 219]. In experimental animals, caloric deprivation through fasting results in dramatic decreases in NPR-C gene expression and increased circulating ANP levels [220]. Elevated NPR-C gene expression has been documented in the adipose tissue of humans with obesity and hypertension [213] and allelic variants of this gene have been associated with lower plasma natriuretic peptide levels [221].

However, another study [222] found that in normotensive and hypertensive obese subjects, the relationships of ANP and BNP levels follow the same trend as in lean hypertensives, with ANP mainly influenced by diastolic dysfunction and BNP influenced by both left ventricular hypertrophy and diastolic dysfunction. Moreover, NT-proBNP, which does not bind to the NPR-C, also shows an inverse relationship with BMI in healthy subjects [223] and patients with acute dyspnea [224]. In a very recent study, low BNP and NT-proBNP levels are more closely (and inversely) related to lean mass rather than fat mass, as assessed by direct dual-energy X-ray absorptiometry in a probability-based random large sample of Dallas County residents (2,971 subjects aged 30-65 years) [224]. These data suggest that subjects with increased BMI probably have a decreased production/secretion of CNH rather than a reduced clearance. Therefore, further studies are necessary to clarify the pathophysiological mechanism(s) that play(s) a role in decreasing the CNH levels in patients with higher BMI values.

On the other hand, there is recent evidence that the CNH system promotes adipose tissue lipolysis in primates [225]. This effect is mediated by the interaction of CNH with its active receptors through guanylyl cyclase activation and cGMP production.

In conclusion, several data suggest that there is a close inter-relationship between the CNH system and fat cells. However, the pathophysiological mechanisms relating the CNH system to the adipose tissue are complex and not well known at present. Therefore, further studies are needed to clarify the role of the CNH system and its pathophysiological revelance in obesity and hypertension-related disorders.

6.10 Adrenal Gland Diseases

The interactions between the CNH system and adrenal gland are very close and complex. In this context, some specific considerations should be taken into account:

1. The biological actions of CNH (including vasorelaxation, diuresis and natriuresis, suppression of aldosterone, vasopressin release, and thirst) are the opposite of those of the renin-angiotensin-aldosterone system (RAAS), so that the effectors of these two systems should be considered as endogenous antagonists [226]. This close relationship is further strengthened by the complementary localization of the specific receptors of these two systems in several organs (including brain, adrenal gland, vasculature, heart, and kidney). These two opposing systems allow fine-tuning of volume and pressure by the body [226, 227].

2. Several studies have demonstrated that angiotensin II and some steroid hormones (especially corticosteroids and estrogens) can stimulate the production/secretion of CNH [227-239] as well as that of their NPR-A and NPR-B receptors [240, 241] in many mammalian organs and tissues (see Chap. 3 for more details). On the other hand, CNH inhibit steroidogenesis (including cortisol and aldosterone genesis) as well as renin and angiotensin production in mammalian adrenal gland [242-248] and other tissues (especially cardiac and vasal tissues) [249, 250]. As a result, CNH and RAAS systems are linked by means of a negative feedback mechanism.

3. Adrenal normal and tumor cells synthesize CNH (ANP, BNP and CNP), both in fasciculata and medullary cells [251-255]. These findings indicate that CNH can regulate steroidogenesis in both a paracrine and endocrine manner.

4. Adrenal cells of the "zona glomerulosa", "zona fasciculata" and medulla share a high quantity of NPR-A, NPR-B and NPR-C receptors [256-262]. However, in rats, the three subtypes were expressed most abundantly in the zona glomerulosa [261, 262], and NPR-A was expressed more than NPR-B and NPR-C [262]. These findings suggest that, in rats, ANP and BNP should have a more powerful action than CNP on adrenal gland tissue.

According to points 1-4 mentioned above, it is not surprising that adrenal gland disease can affect the CNH system. Indeed, all clinical conditions characterized by an increased secretion of corticosteroid and/or mineralcorticoid hormones [263-268] or catecholamines [269] also show increased circulating levels of CNH. Besides the direct stimulation of steroid hormones on CNH production/secretion, the hypersecretion of steroid hormones with sodium-retention activity produces an increase in cardiac load and volume retention, which in turn stimulates the production/secretion of CNH [264, 268]. A recent study [268] indicated that ANP and BNP are suitable markers of cardiac load and volume retention in patients with primary aldosteronism. In particular, this study confirmed that ANP and BNP are elevated in patients with primary aldosteronism compared to normotensive controls, and also that these levels are reduced after adenoma resection [268]. Patients affected by Cushing's disease with increased levels of ANP also share a blunted *in vivo* response of the second-messenger cGMP to exogenous infusion of ANP [266]. This finding indicates that in Cushing's disease there is a resistance to the biological effects of CNH, although it is not possible to specify whether the resistance is at the receptor or post-receptor level [270].

Patients affected by Addison's disease usually share plasma ANP values in the lower part of the normal range; however, ANP levels may be increased in some patients with clinical conditions characterized by hypofunction of the adrenal gland [271, 272]. This effect may be due to the lack of adrenal control on ANP synthesis/secretion [271] or more frequently (and probably) to the mineralcorticoid replacement [272]. Indeed, plasma ANP was demonstrated to be a more sensitive index of mineralcorticoid over-replacement than plasma renin concentration in patients with Addison's disease [272]. As a result, increased levels of plasma ANP in patients with Addison's disease undergoing mineralcorticoid replacement strongly suggest an over-replacement.

6.11 Summary and Conclusion

Many studies have demonstrated that CNH assay may be clinically useful in many other clinical conditions besides cardiovascular diseases. The more common extra-cardiac clinical conditions with altered (increased or decreased compared to normal range) circulating levels of CNH include pulmonary diseases, renal and liver failure, acute cere-brovascular disorders, acute and chronic inflammatory diseases, and some metabolic and endocrinological diseases. In these conditions, activation of the CNH system indicates that the heart is under "stress"; this observation holds great clinical relevance (Fig. 6.1). Indeed, several studies have demonstrated that the increase in circulating levels of CNH is an independent and strong risk factor for future major cardiovascular complications and/or death, even in extra-cardiac diseases [1-12].

We have discussed in detail the pathophysiological mechanisms that are thought to activate the CNH system for each specific disease (or group of diseases). Theoretically speaking, these mechanisms should work in many clinical conditions; this explains the progressive number of diseases in which the CNH system was found to be altered. On the other hand, from a clinical point of view, clinicians should be on the look-out for an unexplained increase in CNH levels in extra-cardiac diseases.

References

1. Clerico A (2002) Pathophysiological and clinical relevance of circulating levels of cardiac natriuretic hormones: are they merely markers of cardiac disease? (Opinion Article) Clin Chem Lab Med 40:752-760
2. Clerico A, Emdin M (2004) Diagnostic accuracy and prognostic relevance of the measurement of the cardiac natriuretic peptides: a review. Clin Chem 50:33-50
3. Kruger S, Graf J, Merx MW et al (2004) Brain natriuretic peptide predicts right heart failure in patients with acute pulmonary embolism. Am Heart J 147:60-65
4. Kucher N, Printzen G, Goldhaber SZ (2003) Prognostic role of brain natriuretic peptide in acute pulmonary embolism. Circulation 107:2545-2547
5. Ten Wolde M, Tulevski II, Mulder JW et al (2003) Brain natriuretic peptide as a predictor of adverse outcome in patients with pulmonary embolism. Circulation 107:2082-2084
6. Nagaya N, Nishikimi T, Uematsu M et al (2000) Plasma brain natriuretic peptide as a prognostic indicator in patients with primary pulmonary hypertension. Circulation 102:865-870
7. Vesely DL (2003) Natriuretic peptides and acute renal failure. Am J Physiol Renal Physiol 285:F167-177
8. McCullough PA, Kuncheria J, Mathur VS (2004) Diagnostic and therapeutic utility of B-type natriuretic peptide in patients with renal insufficiency and decompensated heart failure. Rev Cardiovasc Med 5:16-25

9. Castillo JR, Zagler A, Carrillo-Jimenez R, Hennekens CH (2004) Brain natriuretic peptide: a potential marker for mortality in septic shock. Int J Infect Dis 8:271-274

10. Palladini G, Campana C, Klersy C et al (2003) Serum N-terminal pro-brain natriuretic peptide is a sensitive marker of myocardial dysfunction in AL amyloidosis. Circulation 107:2440-2445

11. Yasutake H, Seino Y, Kashiwagi M et al (2005) Detection of cardiac sarcoidosis using cardiac markers and myocardial integrated backscatter. Int J Cardiol 102:259-268

12. Bhalla MA, Chiang A, Epshteyn VA et al (2004) Prognostic role of B-type natriuretic peptide levels in patients with type 2 diabetes mellitus. J Am Coll Cardiol 44:1047-1052

13. Steg PG, Joubin L, McCord J et al (2005) B-type natriuretic peptide and echocardiographic determination of ejection fraction in the diagnosis of congestive heart failure in patients with acute dyspnea. Chest 128:21-29

14. Lang CC, Coutie WJ, Struthers AD et al (1992) Elevated levels of brain natriuretic peptide in acute hypoxaemic chronic obstructive pulmonary disease. Clin Sci 83:529-533

15. Ando T, Ogawa K, Yamaki K et al (1996) Plasma concentrations of atrial, brain, and C-type natriuretic peptides and endothelin-1 in patients with chronic respiratory diseases. Chest 110:462-468

16. Bando M, Ishii Y, Sugiyama Y, Kitamura S (1999) Elevated plasma brain natriuretic peptide levels in chronic respiratory failure with cor pulmonale. Respir Med 93:507-514

17. Ishii J, Nomura M, Ito M et al (2000) Plasma concentration of brain natriuretic peptide as a biochemical marker for the evaluation of right ventricular overload and mortality in chronic respiratory disease. Clin Chim Acta 301:19-30

18. Tulevski II, Hirsch A, Sanson BJ et al (2001) Increased brain natriuretic peptide as a marker for right ventricular dysfunction in acute pulmonary embolism. Thromb Haemost 86:1193-1196

19. Maeder M, Ammann P, Rickli H, Diethelm M (2003) Elevation of B-type natriuretic peptide levels in acute respiratory distress syndrome. Swiss Med Wkly 133:515-518

20. McCullough PA, Hollander JE, Nowak RM et al (2003) Uncovering heart failure in patients with a history of pulmonary disease: rationale for the early use of B-type natriuretic peptide in the emergency department. Acad Emerg Med 10:198-204

21. Pruszczyk P, Kostrubiec M, Bochowicz A et al (2003) N-terminal pro-brain natriuretic peptide in patients with acute pulmonary embolism. Eur Respir J 22:649-653

22. Koulouri S, Acherman RJ, Wong PC et al (2004) Utility of B-type natriuretic peptide in differentiating congestive heart failure from lung disease in pediatric patients with respiratory distress. Pediatr Cardiol 25:341-346

23. Leuchte HH, Holzapfel M, Baumgartner RA et al (2004) Clinical significance of brain natriuretic peptide in primary pulmonary hypertension. J Am Coll Cardiol 43:764-770

24. Leuchte HH, Neurohr C, Baumgartner R et al (2004) Brain natriuretic peptide and exercise capacity in lung fibrosis and pulmonary hypertension. Am J Respir Crit Care Med 170:360-365

25. Pruszczyk P, Szulc M, Kostrubiec M (2004) Potential clinical application of brain natriuretic peptides in acute pulmonary embolism. Eur Heart J 25:621

26. Goetze JP, Gore A, Moller CH et al (2004) Acute myocardial hypoxia increases BNP gene expression. FASEB J 18:1928-1930

27. Nagaya N, Nishikimi T, Okano Y et al (1998) Plasma brain natriuretic peptide levels increase in proportion to the extent of right ventricular dysfunction in pulmonary hypertension. J Am Coll Cardiol 31:202-208

28. Mariano-Goulart D, Eberle MC, Boudousq V et al (2003) Major increase in brain natriuretic peptide indicates right ventricular systolic dysfunction in patients with heart failure. Eur J Heart Fail 5:481-488

29. Yap LB, Mukerjee D, Timms PM et al (2004) Natriuretic peptides, respiratory disease, and the right heart. (Review) Chest 126:1330-1336

30. Yap LB (2004) B-type natriuretic peptide and the right heart. (Review) Heart Fail Rev 9:99-105

31. Maisel AS, Krishnaswamy P, Nowak RM et al (2002) Rapid measurement of B-type natriuretic peptide in the emergency diagnosis of heart failure. N Engl J Med 347:161-167

32. Maisel AS, McCord J, Nowak RM et al (2003) Bedside B-type natriuretic peptide in the emer-

gency diagnosis of heart failure with reduced or preserved ejection fraction. Results from the Breathing Not Properly Multinational Study. J Am Coll Cardiol 41:2010-2017

33. Maisel A, Hollander JE, Guss D et al (2004) Rapid Emergency Department Heart Failure Outpatient Trial investigators. Primary results of the Rapid Emergency Department Heart Failure Outpatient Trial (REDHOT). A multicenter study of B-type natriuretic peptide levels, emergency department decision making, and outcomes in patients presenting with shortness of breath. J Am Coll Cardiol 44:1328-1333

34. Morrison LK, Harrison A, Krishnaswamy P et al (2002) Utility of a rapid B-natriuretic peptide assay in differentiating congestive heart failure from lung disease in patients presenting with dyspnea. J Am Coll Cardiol 39:202-209

35. Knudsen CW, Omland T, Clopton P et al (2004) Diagnostic value of B-type natriuretic peptide and chest radiographic findings in patients with acute dyspnea. Am J Med 116:363-368

36. McCullough PA, Nowak RM, McCord J et al (2002) B-type natriuretic peptide and clinical judgment in emergency diagnosis of heart failure: analysis from Breathing Not Properly (BNP) Multinational Study. Circulation 106:416-422

37. Maisel AS (2001) B-type natriuretic peptide (BNP) levels: diagnostic and therapeutic potential. Rev Cardiovasc Med 2(suppl 2):S13-18

38. Forfia PR, Watkins SP, Rame JE et al (2005) Relationship between B-type natriuretic peptides and pulmonary capillary wedge pressure in the intensive care unit. J Am Coll Cardiol 45:1667-1671

39. O'Neill JO, Bott-Silverman CE, McRae AT 3rd et al (2005) B-type natriuretic peptide levels are not a surrogate marker for invasive hemodynamics during management of patients with severe heart failure. Am Heart J 149:363-369

40. Parsonage WA, Galbraith AJ, Koerbin GL, Potter JM (2005) Value of B-type natriuretic peptide for identifying significantly elevated pulmonary artery wedge pressure in patients treated for established chronic heart failure secondary to ischemic or idiopathic dilated cardiomyopathy. Am J Cardiol 95:883-885

41. Jefic D, Lee JW, Jefic D et al (2005) Utility of B-type natriuretic peptide and N-terminal pro B-type natriuretic peptide in evaluation of respiratory failure in critically ill patients. Chest 128:288-295

42. Fried LF, Shlipak MG, Crump C et al (2003) Renal insufficiency as a predictor of cardiovascular outcomes and mortality in elderly individuals. J Am Coll Cardiol 41:1364-1372

43. Collins AJ (2003) Cardiovascular mortality in end-stage renal disease. Am J Med Sci 325:163-167

44. Mallamaci F, Zoccali C, Tripepi G et al (2001) CREED Investigators. The Cardiovascular Risk Extended Evaluation. Diagnostic potential of cardiac natriuretic peptides in dialysis patients. Kidney Int 59:1559-1566

45. Osajima A, Okazaki M, Kato H et al (2001) Clinical significance of natriuretic peptides and cyclic GMP in hemodialysis patients with coronary artery disease. Am J Nephrol 21:112-119

46. Nishikimi T, Futoo Y, Tamano K et al (2001) Plasma brain natriuretic peptide levels in chronic hemodialysis patients: influence of coronary artery disease. Am J Kidney Dis 37:1201-1208

47. Zoccali C, Mallamaci F, Benedetto FA et al (2001) Creed Investigators. Cardiac natriuretic peptides are related to left ventricular mass and function and predict mortality in dialysis patients. J Am Soc Nephrol 12:1508-1515

48. Sugihara K, Fujimoto S, Motomiya Y et al (2001) Usefulness of long axis M-mode echocardiographic measurements for optimum dialysis in patients on maintenance hemodialysis: comparison with changes in plasma levels of atrial natriuretic peptide and brain natriuretic peptide. Clin Nephrol 56:140-149

49. Ishii J, Nomura M, Okuma T et al (2001) Risk stratification using serum concentrations of cardiac troponin T in patients with end-stage renal disease on chronic maintenance dialysis. Clin Chim Acta 312:69-79

50. Cataliotti A, Malatino LS, Jougasaki M et al (2001) Circulating natriuretic peptide concentrations in patients with end-stage renal disease: role of brain natriuretic peptide as a biomarker for ventricular remodeling. Mayo Clin Proc 76:1111-1119

51. Goto T, Takase H, Toriyama T et al (2002) Increased circulating levels of natriuretic peptides predict future cardiac event in patients with chronic hemodialysis. Nephron 92:610-615

52. Naganuma T, Sugimura K, Wada S et al (2002) The prognostic role of brain natriuretic peptides in hemodialysis patients. Am J Nephrol 22:437-444
53. Osajima A, Okazaki M, Tamura M et al (2002) Comparison of plasma levels of mature adrenomedullin and natriuretic peptide as markers of cardiac function in hemodialysis patients with coronary artery disease. Nephron 92:832-839
54. Apple FS, Murakami MM, Pearce LA, Herzog CA (2004) Multi-biomarker risk stratification of N-terminal pro-B-type natriuretic peptide, high-sensitivity C-reactive protein, and cardiac troponin T and I in end-stage renal disease for all-cause death. Clin Chem 50:2279-2285
55. Mueller C, Laule-Kilian K, Scholer A et al (2005) B-type natriuretic peptide for acute dyspnea in patients with kidney disease: insights from a randomized comparison. Kidney Int 67:278-284
56. Mallamaci F, Tripepi G, Cutrupi S et al (2005) Prognostic value of combined use of biomarkers of inflammation, endothelial dysfunction, and myocardiopathy in patients with ESRD. Kidney Int 67:2330-2337
57. Goetze JP (2004) Biochemistry of pro-B-type natriuretic peptide-derived peptides: the endocrine heart revisited. Clin Chem 9:1503-1510
58. Fletcher RH, Fletcher SW, Wagner EH (1996) Clinical epidemiology. The essentials, 3rd edn. Lippincot Williams & Wilkins, Phildelphia
59. Sackett DL, Haynes RB, Guyatt GH, Tugwell P (1991) Clinical epidemiology. A basic science for clinical medicine, 2nd edn. Little, Brown and Company, Boston
60. Shorecki K, Green J, Brenner BM (2005) Chronic renal failure. In: Kasper DL, Braundwald E, Fauci AS, Hauser SL, Longo DL, Jameson JL (eds) Harrison's principles of internal medicine, 16th edn. McGrawHill, New York, pp 1653-1663
61. Hama N, Itoh H, Shirakami G et al (1994) Detection of C-type natriuretic peptide in human circulation and marked increase of plasma CNP level in septic shock patients. Biochem Biophys Res Commun 198:1177-1182
62. Hartemink KJ, Groeneveld AB, de Groot MC et al (2001) Alpha-atrial natriuretic peptide, cyclic guanosine monophosphate, and endothelin in plasma as markers of myocardial depression in human septic shock. Crit Care Med 29:80-87
63. Mazul-Sunko B, Zarkovic N, Vrkic N et al (2001) Pro-atrial natriuretic peptide hormone from right atria is correlated with cardiac depression in septic patients. J Endocrinol Invest 24:RC22-24
64. Brueckmann M, Huhle G, Lang S et al (2005) Prognostic value of plasma N-terminal pro-brain natriuretic peptide in patients with severe sepsis. Circulation 112:227-234
65. Witthaut R, Busch C, Fraunberger P et al (2003) Plasma atrial natriuretic peptide and brain natriuretic peptide are increased in septic shock: impact of interleukin-6 and sepsis-associated left ventricular dysfunction. Intensive Care Med 29:1696-1702
66. Hoffmann U, Brueckmann M, Bertsch T et al (2005) Increased plasma levels of NT-proANP and NT-proBNP as markers of cardiac dysfunction in septic patients. Clin Lab 51:373-379
67. Nordlinger M, Magnani B, Skinner M, Falk RH (2005) Is elevated plasma B-natriuretic peptide in amyloidosis simply a function of the presence of heart failure? Am J Cardiol 96:982-984
68. Takemura G, Takatsu Y, Doyama K et al (1998) Expression of atrial and brain natriuretic peptides and their genes in hearts of patients with cardiac amyloidosis. J Am Coll Cardiol 31:254-265
69. Wu JJ, Schiff KR (2004) Sarcoidosis. Am Fam Physician 2004; 70: 312-22
70. Bargout R, Kelly RF (2004) Sarcoid heart disease: clinical course and treatment. Int J Cardiol 97:173-182
71. Rosenfeld JV, Barnett GH, Sila CA et al (1989) The effect of subarachnoid hemorrhage on blood and CSF atrial natriuretic factor. J Neurosurg 71:32-37
72. Isotani E, Suzuki R, Tomita K et al (1994) Alterations in plasma concentrations of natriuretic peptides and antidiuretic hormone after subarachnoid hemorrhage. Stroke 25:2198-2203
73. Berendes E, Walter M, Cullen P et al (1997) Secretion of brain natriuretic peptide in patients with aneurysmal subarachnoid haemorrhage. Lancet 349:245-249
74. Wijdicks EF, Schievink WI, Burnett JC Jr (1997) Natriuretic peptide system and endothelin in aneurysmal subarachnoid hemorrhage. J Neurosurg 87:275-280
75. Tomida M, Muraki M, Uemura K, Yamasaki K (1998) Plasma concentrations of brain natriuretic peptide in patients with subarachnoid hemorrhage. Stroke 29:1584-1587

76. Sviri GE, Feinsod M, Soustiel JF (2000) Brain natriuretic peptide and cerebral vasospasm in subarachnoid hemorrhage. Clinical and TCD correlations. Stroke 31:118-122

77. Wijdicks EF, Heublein DM, Burnett JC Jr (2001) Increase and uncoupling of adrenomedullin from the natriuretic peptide system in aneurysmal subarachnoid hemorrhage. J Neurosurg 94:252-256

78. Berendes E, Van Aken H, Raufhake C et al (2001) Differential secretion of atrial and brain natriuretic peptide in critically ill patients. Anesth Analg 93:676-682

79. Espiner EA, Leikis R, Ferch RD et al (2002) The neuro-cardio-endocrine response to acute subarachnoid haemorrhage. Clin Endocrinol 56:629-635

80. Fukui S, Nawashiro H, Otani N et al (2003) Focal brain edema and natriuretic peptides in patients with subarachnoid hemorrhage. Acta Neurochir Suppl 86:489-491

81. McGirt MJ, Blessing R, Nimjee SM et al (2004) Correlation of serum brain natriuretic peptide with hyponatremia and delayed ischemic neurological deficits after subarachnoid hemorrhage. Neurosurgery 54:1369-1373

82. Fukui S, Katoh H, Tsuzuki N et al (2004) Focal brain edema and natriuretic peptides in patients with subarachnoid hemorrhage. J Clin Neurosci 11:507-511

83. Sviri GE, Shik V, Raz B, Soustiel JF (2003) Role of brain natriuretic peptide in cerebral vasospasm. Acta Neurochir 145:851-860

84. Tsubokawa T, Shiokawa Y, Kurita H, Kaneko N (2004) High plasma concentration of brain natriuretic peptide in patients with ruptured anterior communicating artery aneurysm. Neurol Res 26:893-896

85. McKinley MJ, Allen AM, Burns P et al (1998) Interaction of circulating hormones with the brain: the roles of the subfornical organ and the organum vasculosum of the lamina terminalis. Clin Exp Pharmacol Physiol Suppl 25:S61-67

86. Huang W, Lee D, Yang Z et al (1992) Norepinephrine stimulates immunoreactive (ir) atrial natriuretic peptide (ANP) secretion and pro-ANP mRNA expression from rat hypothalamic neurons in culture: effects of alpha 2-adrenoceptors. Endocrinology 130:2426-2428

87. Levin ER, Isackson PJ, Hu RM (1991) Endothelin increases atrial natriuretic peptide production in cultured rat diencephalic neurons. Endocrinology 128:2925-2930

88. Levin ER, Hu RM, Rossi M, Pickart M (1992) Arginine vasopressin stimulates atrial natriuretic peptide gene expression and secretion from rat diencephalic neurons. Endocrinology 131:1417-1423

89. Makikallio AM, Makikallio TH, Korpelainen JT et al (2005) Natriuretic peptides and mortality after stroke. Stroke 36:1016-1020

90. Campbell DJ, Woodward M, Chalmers JP et al (2005) Prediction of myocardial infarction by N-terminal-pro-B-type natriuretic peptide, C-reactive protein, and renin in subjects with cerebrovascular disease. Circulation 112:110-116

91. Olivera A, Gutkowska J, Rodriguez-Puyol D et al (1988) Atrial natriuretic peptide in rats with experimental cirrhosis of the liver without ascites. Endocrinology 122:840-846

92. Lopez C, Jimenez W, Arroyo V et al (1989) Role of altered systemic hemodynamics in the blunted renal response to atrial natriuretic peptide in rats with cirrhosis and ascites. J Hepatol 9:217-226

93. Burghardt W, Wernze H, Diehl KL (1986) Atrial natriuretic peptide in hepatic cirrhosis: relation to stage of disease, sympathoadrenal system and renin-aldosterone axis. Klin Wochenschr 64(suppl 6):103-107

94. Henriksen JH, Schutten HJ, Bendtsen F, Warberg J (1986) Circulating atrial natriuretic peptide (ANP) and central blood volume (CBV) in cirrhosis. Liver 6:361-368

95. Nozuki M, Mouri T, Itoi K et al (1986) Plasma concentrations of atrial natriuretic peptide in various diseases. Tohoku J Exp Med 148:439-447

96. Bonkovsky HL, Hartle DK, Mellen BG et al (1988) Plasma concentrations of immunoreactive atrial natriuretic peptide in hospitalized cirrhotic and noncirrhotic patients: evidence for a role of deficient atrial natriuretic peptide in pathogenesis of cirrhotic ascites. Am J Gastroenterol 83:531-535

97. Burghardt W, Muller R, Diehl KL, Wernze H (1988) Interrelationship between atrial natriuretic peptide and plasma renin, aldosterone and catecholamines in hepatic cirrhosis: the effect of passive leg rising. Z Kardiol 77(suppl 2):104-110

98. Cernacek P, Crawhall JC, Levy M (1988) Atrial natriuretic peptide: blood levels in human disease and their measurement. Clin Biochem 21:5-17

99. Colantonio D, Casale R, Pasqualetti P (1989) Plasma levels of atrial natriuretic peptide in compensated and decompensated cirrhosis of the liver. Relationship with the renin-aldosterone system. Panminerva Med 31:166-170

100. Tesar V, Horky K, Petryl J et al (1989) Atrial natriuretic factor in liver cirrhosis - the influence of volume expansion. Horm Metab Res 21:519-522

101. Vinel JP, Denoyel P, Viossat I et al (1989) Atrial natriuretic peptide, plasma renin activity, plasma volume, systemic vascular resistance and cardiac output in patients with cirrhosis. J Gastroenterol Hepatol 4:529-535

102. Messa P, Cannella G, Mioni G et al (1993) Atrial natriuretic peptide and hemodynamic changes after concentrated ascitic fluid reinfusion in cirrhotic patients. Nephron 65:67-72

103. Chen YX, Wang SC, Zhao GN et al (1993) Plasma endothelin levels in cirrhotic patients and their correlation with atrial natriuretic peptide. Chin Med J 106:643-646

104. Parlapiano C, Labellarte A, Primi F et al (1994) ANP in the cirrhotic patient. A clinical contribution. Minerva Endocrinol 19:121-126

105. Trevisani F, Colantoni A, Sica G et al (1995) High plasma levels of atrial natriuretic peptide in preascitic cirrhosis: indirect evidence of reduced natriuretic effectiveness of the peptide. Hepatology 22:132-137

106. Tulassay T, Tulassay Z, Rascher W (1990) Atrial natriuretic peptide in patients with decompensated hepatic cirrhosis. Gastroenterol J 50:140-143

107. Henriksen JH, Gotze JP, Fuglsang S et al (2003) Increased circulating pro-brain natriuretic peptide (proBNP) and brain natriuretic peptide (BNP) in patients with cirrhosis: relation to cardiovascular dysfunction and severity of disease. Gut 52:1511-1517

108. Yildiz R, Yildirim B, Karincaoglu M et al (2005) Brain natriuretic peptide and severity of disease in non-alcoholic cirrhotic patients. J Gastroenterol Hepatol 20:1115-1120

109. Poulos JE, Gower WR, Fontanet HL et al (1995) Cirrhosis with ascites: increased atrial natriuretic peptide messenger RNA expression in rat ventricle. Gastroenterology 108:1496-1503

110. Brabant G, Juppner H, Kirschner M et al (1986) Human atrial natriuretic peptide (ANP) for the treatment of patients with liver cirrhosis and ascites. Klin Wochenschr 64(suppl 6):108-111

111. Petrillo A, Scherrer U, Gonvers JJ et al (1988) Atrial natriuretic peptide administered as intravenous infusion or bolus injection to patients with liver cirrhosis and ascites. J Cardiovasc Pharmacol 12:279-285

112. Salerno F, Badalamenti S, Incerti P et al (1988) Renal response to atrial natriuretic peptide in patients with advanced liver cirrhosis. Hepatology 8:21-26

113. Beutler JJ, Koomans HA, Rabelink TJ et al (1989) Blunted natriuretic response and low blood pressure after atrial natriuretic factor in early cirrhosis. Hepatology 10:148-153

114. Laffi G, Marra F, Pinzani M et al (1989) Effects of repeated atrial natriuretic peptide bolus injections in cirrhotic patients with refractory ascites. Liver 9:315-321

115. Laffi G, Pinzani M, Meacci E et al (1989) Renal hemodynamic and natriuretic effects of human atrial natriuretic factor infusion in cirrhosis with ascites. Gastroenterology 96:167-177

116. Fried T, Aronoff GR, Benabe JE et al (1990) Renal and hemodynamic effects of atrial natriuretic peptide in patients with cirrhosis. Am J Med Sci 299:2-9

117. Miyase S, Fujiyama S, Chikazawa H, Sato T (1990) Atrial natriuretic peptide in liver cirrhosis with mild ascites. Gastroenterol Jpn 25:356-362

118. Badalamenti S, Borroni G, Lorenzano E et al (1992) Renal effects in cirrhotic patients with avid sodium retention of atrial natriuretic factor injection during norepinephrine infusion. Hepatology 15:824-829

119. Brenard R, Moreau R, Pussard E et al (1992) Hemodynamic and sympathetic responses to human atrial natriuretic peptide infusion in patients with cirrhosis. J Hepatol 14:347-356

120. Gines P, Tito L, Arroyo V et al (1992) Renal insensitivity to atrial natriuretic peptide in patients with cirrhosis and ascites. Effect of increasing systemic arterial pressure. Gastroenterology 102:280-286

121. Abraham WT, Lauwaars ME, Kim JK et al (1995) Reversal of atrial natriuretic peptide resistance by increasing distal tubular sodium delivery in patients with decompensated cirrhosis. Hepatology 22:737-743

122. La Villa G, Riccardi D, Lazzeri C et al (1995) Blunted natriuretic response to low-dose brain natriuretic peptide infusion in nonazotemic cirrhotic patients with ascites and avid sodium retention. Hepatology 22:1745-1750

123. Jespersen B, Eiskjaer H, Jensen JD et al (1995) Effects of high dose atrial natriuretic peptide on renal haemodynamics, sodium handling and hormones in cirrhotic patients with and without ascites. Scand J Clin Lab Invest 55:273-287

124. Gadano A, Moreau R, Vachiery F et al (1997) Natriuretic response to the combination of atrial natriuretic peptide and terlipressin in patients with cirrhosis and refractory ascites. J Hepatol 26:1229-1234

125. Komeichi H, Moreau R, Cailmail S et al (1995) Blunted natriuresis and abnormal systemic hemodynamic responses to C-type and brain natriuretic peptides in rats with cirrhosis. J Hepatol 22:319-325

126. Danzi S, Klein I (2004) Thyroid hormone and the cardiovascular system. Minerva Endocrinol 29:139-150

127. Deng XF, Rokosh DG, Simpson PC (2000) Autonomous and growth factor-induced hypertrophy in cultured neonatal mouse cardiac myocytes. Comparison with rat. Circ Res 87:781-788

128. Forini F, Paolicchi A, Pizzorusso T et al (2001) 3,5,3'-Triiodothyronine deprivation affects phenotype and intracellular $[Ca2+]i$ of human cardiomyocytes in culture. Cardiovasc Res 51:322-330

129. Kinugawa K, Yonekura K, Ribeiro RC et al (2001) Regulation of thyroid hormone receptor isoforms in physiological and pathological cardiac hypertrophy. Circ Res 89:591-598

130. Basset A, Blanc J, Messas E et al (2001) Renin-angiotensin system contribution to cardiac hypertrophy in experimental hyperthyroidism: an echocardiographic study. J Cardiovasc Pharmacol 37:163-172

131. Kobori H, Ichihara A, Miyashita Y et al (1999) Local renin-angiotensin system contributes to hyperthyroidism-induced cardiac hypertrophy. J Endocrinol 160:43-47

132. Gardner DG, Gertz BJ, Hane S (1987) Thyroid hormone increases rat atrial natriuretic peptide messenger ribonucleic acid accumulation *in vivo* and *in vitro*. Mol Endocrinol 1:260-265

133. Matsubara H, Hirata Y, Yoshimi H et al (1987) Effects of steroid and thyroid hormones on synthesis of atrial natriuretic peptide by cultured atrial myocytes of rat. Biochem Biophys Res Commun 145:336-343

134. Mori Y, Nishikawa M, Matsubara H et al (1990) Stimulation of rat atrial natriuretic peptide (rANP) synthesis by triiodothyronine and thyroxine (T4): T4 as a prohormone in synthesizing rANP. Endocrinology 126:466-471

135. Liang F, Webb P, Marimuthu A et al (2003) Triiodothyronine increases brain natriuretic peptide (BNP) gene transcription and amplifies endothelin-dependent BNP gene transcription and hypertrophy in neonatal rat ventricular myocytes. J Biol Chem 278:15073-15083

136. Chang KC, Figueredo VM, Schreur JH et al (1997) Thyroid hormone improves function and Ca2+ handling in pressure overload hypertrophy. Association with increased sarcoplasmic reticulum Ca2+-ATPase and alpha-myosin heavy chain in rat hearts. J Clin Invest 100:1742-1749

137. Yegin E, Yigitoglu R, Ari Z et al (1997) Serum angiotensin-converting enzyme and plasma atrial natriuretic peptide levels in hyperthyroid and hypothyroid rabbits. Jpn Heart J 38:273-279

138. Woolf AS, Moult PJ (1988) Plasma concentrations of atrial natriuretic peptide in hypothyroidism. Br Med J 296:531

139. Yamaji T, Ishibashi M, Takaku F et al (1988) Plasma atrial natriuretic peptide in states of altered thyroid function. Endocrinol Jpn 35:343-348

140. Suzuki Y, Suzuki H, Ohtake R et al (1988) Changes in the plasma and urine alpha human atrial natriuretic peptide (alpha hANP) concentration in patients with thyroid disorders. Endocrinol Jpn 35:907-913

141. Shigematsu S, Iwasaki T, Aizawa T et al (1989) Plasma atrial natriuretic peptide, plasma renin activity and aldosterone during treatment of hyperthyroidism due to Graves' disease. Horm Metab Res 21:514-518

142. Tajiri J, Noguchi S, Naomi S et al (1990) Plasma atrial natriuretic peptide in patients with Graves' disease. Endocrinol Jpn 37:665-670

143. Widecka K, Krzyzanowska-Swiniarska B, Ciechanowski K et al (1993) Plasma concentrations of atrial natriuretic peptide and cyclic guanosine monophosphate in patients with hyperthyroidism before and after short-term treatment with methimazole. Endokrynol Pol 44:65-71

144. Schultz M, Faber J, Kistorp C et al (2004) N-terminal-pro-B-type natriuretic peptide (NT-pro-BNP) in different thyroid function states. Clin Endocrinol 60:54-59

145. Zimmerman RS, Gharib H, Zimmerman D et al (1987) Atrial natriuretic peptide in hypothyroidism. J Clin Endocrinol Metab 64:353-355

146. Widecka K, Gozdzik J, Dutkiewicz T et al (1990) Low plasma concentrations of atrial natriuretic peptide in untreated hypothyroid patients. J Intern Med 228:39-42

147. Wei T, Zeng C, Tian Y et al (2005) B-type natriuretic peptide in patients with clinical hyperthyroidism. J Endocrinol Invest 28:8-11

148. Faber J, Wiinberg N, Schifter S, Mehlsen J (2001) Haemodynamic changes following treatment of subclinical and overt hyperthyroidism. Eur J Endocrinol 145:391-396

149. Faber J, Petersen L, Wiinberg N et al (2002) Hemodynamic changes after levothyroxine treatment in subclinical hypothyroidism. Thyroid 12:319-324

150. Klein I (2005) Cardiovascular disease and disorders of other organ systems. In: Zipes DP, Libby P, Bonow RO, Braunwald E (eds) Braunwald's heart disease, Chapter 79, 7th edn. Elsevier Saunders, Philadelphia, pp 2051-2065

151. Franklyn JA, Gammage MD, Ramsden DB et al (1984) Thyroid status in patients after acute myocardial infarction. Clin Sci 67:585-590

152. Wiersinga WM, Lie KI, Toubler JL (1981) Thyroid hormones in acute myocardial infarction. Clin Endocrinol 14:367-374

153. Hamilton MA, Stevenson LW, Luu M, Walden JA (1990) Altered thyroid hormone metabolism in advanced heart failure. J Am Coll Cardiol 16:91-95

154. Klemperer JD, Klein I, Gomez M et al (1995) Thyroid hormone treatment after coronary artery bypass surgery. N Engl J Med 333:1522-1527

155. Murzi B, Iervasi G, Masini S et al (1995) Thyroid hormones homeostasis in pediatric patients during and after cardiopulmonary by-pass. Ann Thorac Surg 59:481-485

156. Holland FW 2nd, Brown PS Jr, Weintraub BD, Clark RE (1991) Cardiopulmonary bypass and thyroid function: a "euthyroid sick syndrome." Ann Thorac Surg 52:46-50

157. Utiger RD (1995) Altered thyroid function in nonthyroidal illness and surgery: to treat or not to treat? N Engl J Med 333:1562-1563

158. Chopra IJ (1997) Euthyroid sick syndrome: is it a misnomer? J Clin Endocrin Metab 82:329-334

159. De Groot LJ (1999) Dangerous dogmas in medicine: the nonthyroidal illness syndrome. J Clin Endocrin Metab 84:151-164

160. Moruzzi P, Doria E, Agostoni PG (1996) Medium-term effectiveness of L-thyroxine treatment in idiopathic dilated cardiomyopathy. Am J Med 101:461-467

161. Mullis-Jansson SL, Argenziano M, Corwin S et al (1999) A randomized double-blind study of the effect of triiodothyronine on cardiac function and morbidity after coronary bypass surgery. J Thorac Cardiovasc Surg 117:1128-1135

162. Bettendorf M, Schmidt KG, Grulich-Henn J et al (2000) Tri-iodothyronine treatment in children after cardiac surgery: a double-blind, randomised, placebo controlled study. Lancet 356:529-534

163. Hamilton MA, Stevenson LW, Fonarow GC (1998) Safety and hemodynamic effects of intravenous triiodothyronine in advanced congestive heart failure. Am J Cardiol 81:443-447

164. Malik FS, Mehra MR, Uber PA et al (1999) Intravenous thyroid hormone supplementation in heart failure with cardiogenic shock. J Card Fail 5:31-37

165. Spooner PH, Morkin E, Goldman S (1999) Thyroid hormone and thyroid hormone analogues in the treatment of heart failure. Coron Artery Dis 10:395-399

166. Iervasi G, Emdin M, Colzani RMP et al (2001) Beneficial effects of long-term triiodothyronine (T3) infusion in patients with advanced heart failure and low T3 syndrome. Washington, DC, Medimond Medical Publications, pp 549-553

167. Iervasi G, Pingitore A, Landi P et al (2003) Low-T3 syndrome: a strong prognostic predictor of death in patients with heart disease. Circulation 107:708-713

168. Pingitore A, Landi P, Taddei MC et al (2005) Triiodothyronine levels for risk stratification of patients with chronic heart failure. Am J Med 118:132-136

169. Cosson S (2004) Usefulness of B-type natriuretic peptide (BNP) as a screen for left ventricular abnormalities in diabetes mellitus. (Review) Diabetes Metab 30:381-386

170. Butler R, MacDonald TM, Struthers AD, Morris AD (1998) The clinical implications of diabetic heart disease. Eur Heart J 19:1617-1627

171. Devereux RB, Roman MJ, Paranicas M et al (2000) Impact of diabetes on cardiac structure and function: the strong heart study. Circulation 101:2271-2276

172. Matsubara H, Mori Y, Yamamoto J, Inada M (1990) Diabetes-induced alterations in atrial natriuretic peptide gene expression in Wistar-Kyoto and spontaneously hypertensive rats. Circ Res 67:803-813

173. Wu SQ, Kwan CY, Tang F (1998) Streptozotocin-induced diabetes has differential effects on atrial natriuretic peptide synthesis in the rat atrium and ventricle: a study by solution-hybridization-RNase protection assay. Diabetologia 41:660-665

174. Walther T, Heringer-Walther S, Tschope R et al (2000) Opposite regulation of brain and C-type natriuretic peptides in the streptozotocin-diabetic cardiopathy. J Mol Endocrinol 24:391-395

175. Christoffersen C, Goetze JP, Bartels ED et al (2002) Chamber-dependent expression of brain natriuretic peptide and its mRNA in normal and diabetic pig heart. Hypertension 40:54-60

176. Ruzicska E, Foldes G, Lako-Futo Z et al (2004) Cardiac gene expression of natriuretic substances is altered in streptozotocin-induced diabetes during angiotensin II-induced pressure overload. J Hypertens 22:1191-1200

177. Fredersdorf S, Thumann C, Ulucan C et al (2004) Myocardial hypertrophy and enhanced left ventricular contractility in Zucker diabetic fatty rats. Cardiovasc Pathol 13:11-19

178. Shin SJ, Lee YJ, Tan MS et al (1997) Increased atrial natriuretic peptide mRNA expression in the kidney of diabetic rats. Kidney Int 51:1100-1105

179. Lai FJ, Hsieh MC, Hsin SC et al (2002) The cellular localization of increased atrial natriuretic peptide mRNA and immunoreactivity in diabetic rat kidneys. J Histochem Cytochem 50:1501-1508

180. Ortola F, Ballermann BJ, Anderson S et al (1987) Elevated plasma atrial natriuretic peptide levels in diabetic rats. J Clin Invest 80:670-674

181. Obineche EN, Adeghate E, Chandranath IS et al (2004) Alterations in atrial natriuretic peptide and its receptors in streptozotocin-induced diabetic rat kidneys. Mol Cell Biochem 261:3-8

182. Vesely DL, Gower WR Jr, Dietz JR et al (1999) Elevated atrial natriuretic peptides and early renal failure in type 2 diabetic Goto-Kakizaki rats. Metabolism 48:771-778

183. Yegen E, Akcay F, Yigitoglu MR et al (1995) Plasma atrial natriuretic peptide levels in rabbits with alloxan monohydrate-induced diabetes mellitus. Jpn Heart J 36:789-795

184. Mulay S, Conliffe PR, Varma DR (1995) Increased natriuretic peptides in fetal hearts of diabetic rats. J Endocrinol 146:255-259

185. Bojestig M, Nystrom FH, Arnqvist HJ et al (2000) The renin-angiotensin-aldosterone system is suppressed in adults with Type 1 diabetes. J Renin Angiotensin Aldosterone Syst 1:353-356

186. Bayerle-Eder M, Zangeneh M, Kreiner G et al (2003) NP but not BNP reflects early left diastolic dysfunction in type 1 diabetics with myocardial dysinnervation. Horm Metab Res 35:301-307

187. Yano Y, Katsuki A, Gabazza EC et al (1999) Plasma brain natriuretic peptide levels in normotensive noninsulin-dependent diabetic patients with microalbuminuria. J Clin Endocrinol Metab 84:2353-2356

188. Nagai T, Imamura M, Mori M (2001) Brain natriuretic polypeptide in type 2 NIDDM patients with albuminuria. J Med 32:169-180
189. Magnusson M, Melander O, Israelsson B et al (2004) Elevated plasma levels of Nt-proB-NP in patients with type 2 diabetes without overt cardiovascular disease. Diab Care 27:1929-1935
190. Asakawa H, Fukui T, Tokunaga K, Kawakami F (2002) Plasma brain natriuretic peptide levels in normotensive type 2 diabetic patients without cardiac disease and macroalbuminuria. J Diabetes Complications 16:209-213
191. Igarashi M, Jimbu Y, Hirata A, Tominaga M (2005) Characterization of plasma brain natriuretic peptide level in patients with type 2 diabetes. Endocr J 52:353-362
192. Tokudome T, Horio T, Yoshihara F et al (2004) Direct effects of high glucose and insulin on protein synthesis in cultured cardiac myocytes and DNA and collagen synthesis in cardiac fibroblasts. Metabolism 53:710-715
193. Abel ED (2004) Insulin signaling in heart muscle: lessons from genetically engineered mouse models. Curr Hypertens Rep 6:416-423
194. Latronico MV, Costinean S, Lavitrano ML et al (2004) Regulation of cell size and contractile function by AKT in cardiomyocytes. Ann NY Acad Sci 1015:250-260
195. Tanabe A, Naruse M, Wasada T et al (1995) Effects of acute hyperinsulinemia on plasma atrial and brain natriuretic peptide concentrations. Eur J Endocrinol 132:693-698
196. Dawson A, Jeyaseelan S, Morris AD, Struthers AD (2005) B-type natriuretic peptide as an alternative way of assessing total cardiovascular risk in patients with diabetes mellitus. Am J Cardiol 96:933-934
197. Roussel R, Tregouet DA, Hadjadj S et al (2004) Investigation of the human ANP gene in type 1 diabetic nephropathy. Diabetes 53:1394-1398
198. Perico N, Benigni A, Gabanelli M et al (1992) Atrial natriuretide peptide and prostacyclin synergistically mediate hyperfiltration and hyperperfusion of diabetic rats. Diabetes 41:533-538
199. Kikkawa R, Haneda M, Sakamoto K et al (1993) Antagonist for atrial natriuretic peptide receptors ameliorates glomerular hyperfiltration in diabetic rats. Biochem Biophys Res Commun 193:700-705
200. Mau Pedersen M, Christiansen JS, Pedersen EB, Mogensen CE (1992) Determinants of intra-individual variation in kidney function in normoalbuminuric insulin-dependent diabetic patients: importance of atrial natriuretic peptide and glycaemic control. Clin Sci 83:445-451
201. Jacobs E, Vervoort G, Branten AJ et al (1999) Atrial natriuretic peptide increases albuminuria in type 1 diabetic patients: evidence for blockade of tubular protein reabsorption. Eur J Clin Invest 2:109-115
202. Nannipieri M, Penno G, Pucci L et al (1999) Pronatriodilatin gene polymorphisms, microvascular permeability, and diabetic nephropathy in type 1 diabetes mellitus. J Am Soc Nephrol 10:1530-1541
203. Nannipieri M, Posadas R, Williams K et al (2003) Association between polymorphisms of the atrial natriuretic peptide gene and proteinuria: a population-based study. Diabetologia 46:429-432
204. Schmidt S, Bluthner M, Giessel R et al (1998) A polymorphism in the gene for the atrial natriuretic peptide and diabetic nephropathy: Diabetic Nephropathy Study Group. Nephrol Dial Transplant 13:1807-1810
205. Ramasawmy R, Kotea N, Lu C et al (1992) Investigation of the polymorphic ScaI site by a PCR-based assay at the human atrial natriuretic peptides (hANP) gene locus. Hum Genet 90:323-324
206. Kato N, Sugiyama T, Morita H et al (2000) Genetic analysis of the atrial natriuretic peptide gene in essential hypertension. Clin Sci 98:251-258
207. Fang ZY, Schull-Meade R, Leano R et al (2005) Screening for heart disease in diabetic subjects. Am Heart J 149:349-354
208. Hall JE (2003) The kidney, hypertension, and obesity. Hypertension 41:625-633
209. Lauer MS, Anderson KM, Kannel WB et al (1991) The impact of obesity on left ventricular mass and geometry: the Framingham Heart Study. JAMA 266:231-236

210. Rocchini AP, Key J, Bondie D et al (1989) The effect of weight loss on the sensitivity of blood pressure to sodium in obese adolescents. N Engl J Med 321:580-585

211. Landsberg L (1992) Obesity and hypertension: experimental data. J Hypertens (Suppl 10):S195-201

212. Dessi-Fulgheri P, Sarzani R, Tamburrini P et al (1997) Plasma atrial natriuretic peptide and natriuretic peptide receptor gene expression in adipose tissue of normotensive and hypertensive obese patients. J Hypertens 15:1695-1699

213. Licata G, Volpe M, Scaglione R, Rubattu S (1994) Salt-regulating hormones in young normotensive obese subjects: effects of saline load. Hypertension 23:120-124

214. McCord J, Mundy BJ, Hudson MP et al (2004) Breathing Not Properly Multinational Study Investigators. Relationship between obesity and B-type natriuretic peptide levels. Arch Intern Med 164:2247-2252

215. Mehra MR, Uber PA, Park MH et al (2004) Obesity and suppressed B-type natriuretic peptide levels in heart failure. J Am Coll Cardiol 43:1590-1595

216. Wang TJ, Larson MG, Levy D et al (2004) Impact of obesity on plasma natriuretic peptide levels. Circulation 109:594-600

217. Messerli FH, Ventura HO, Reisin E et al (1982) Borderline hypertension and obesity: two pre-hypertensive states with elevated cardiac output. Circulation 66:55-60

218. Sarzani R, Paci VM, Dessi-Fulgheri P et al (1993) Comparative analysis of atrial natriuretic peptide receptor expression in rat tissues. J Hypertens 11(suppl 5):S214-15

219. Sarzani R, Dessi-Fulgheri P, Paci VM et al (1996) Expression of natriuretic peptide receptors in human adipose and other tissues. J Endocrinol Invest 19:581-585

220. Crandall DL, Ferraro GD, Cervoni P (1989) Effect of experimental obesity and subsequent weight reduction upon circulating atrial natriuretic peptide. Proc Soc Exp Biol Med 191:352-356

221. Sarzani R, Dessi-Fulgheri P, Salvi F et al (1999) A novel promoter variant of the natriuretic peptide clearance receptor gene is associated with lower atrial natriuretic peptide and higher blood pressure in obese hypertensives. J Hypertens 17:1301-1305

222. Grandi AM, Laurita E, Selva E et al (2004) Natriuretic peptides as markers of preclinical cardiac disease in obesity. Eur J Clin Invest 34:342-348

223. Krauser DG, Lloyd-Jones DM, Chae CU et al (2005) Effect of body mass index on natriuretic peptide levels in patients with acute congestive heart failure: a ProBNP Investigation of Dyspnea in the Emergency Department (PRIDE) substudy. Am Heart J 149:744-750

224. Das SR, Drazner MH, Dries DL et al (2005) Impact of body mass and body composition on circulating levels of natriuretic peptides. Results from the Dallas Heart Study. Circulation 112:2163-2168

225. Dessi-Fulgheri P, Sarzani R, Rappelli A (2003) Role of the natriuretic peptide system in lipogenesis/lipolysis. (Review) Nutr Metab Cardiovasc Dis 13:244-249

226. Johnston CI, Hodsman PG, Kohzuki M et al (1989) Interaction between atrial natriuretic peptide and the renin angiotensin aldosterone system. Endogenous antagonista. Am J Med 87(6B):S24-28

227. Gardner DG, Hane S, Trachewsky D et al (1986) Atrial natriuretic peptide mRNA is regulated by glucocorticoids in vivo. Biochem Biophys Res Commun 139:1047-1054

228. Matsubara H, Hirata Y, Yoshimi H et al (1987) Effects of steroid and thyroid hormones on synthesis of atrial natriuretic peptide by cultured atrial myocytes of rat. Biochem Biophys Res Commun 145:336-343

229. Gardner DG, Gertz BJ, Deschepper CF, Kim DY (1988) Gene for the rat atrial natriuretic peptide is regulated by glucocorticoids in vitro. J Clin Invest 82:1275-1281

230. Kanda K, Ogawa K, Miyamoto N et al (1989) Potentiation of atrial natriuretic peptide-stimulated cyclic guanosine monophosphate formation by glucocorticoids in cultured rat renal cells. Br J Pharmacol 96:795-800

231. Hong M, Liu JK, Bao T, Yang SN (1992) Effect of gluco- and mineralocorticoids on gene expression of atrial natriuretic peptide by rat atria in vivo. Chin Med J (Engl) 105:549-552

232. Vollmar AM, Colbatzky F, Schulz R (1992) Expression of atrial natriuretic peptide in thymic macrophages after dexamethasone treatment of rats. Cell Tissue Res 268:397-399

233. Nishimori T, Tsujino M, Sato K et al (1997) Dexamethasone-induced up-regulation of

adrenomedullin and atrial natriuretic peptide genes in cultured rat ventricular myocytes. J Mol Cell Cardiol 29:2125-2130

234. Zeidel ML (2000) Physiological responses to natriuretic hormones. In: Fray JCS, Goodman HM (eds) Handbook of physiology, Section 7, The endocrine system, Volume III: Endocrine regulation of water and electrolyte balance. New York, Oxford University Press, pp 410-435

235. De Bold AJ, Bruneau BG, Kuroski de Bold ML (1996) Mechanical and neuroendocrine regulation of the endocrine heart. Cardiovasc Res 31:7-18

236. Soualmia H, Barthelemy C, Masson F et al (1997) Angiotensin II-induced phosphoinositide production and atrial natriuretic peptide release in rat atrial tissue. J Cardiovasc Pharmacol 29: 605-611

237. Ma KK, Banas K, de Bold AJ (2005) Determinants of inducible brain natriuretic peptide promoter activity. (Review) Regul Pept 128:169-176

238. Kuroski de Bold ML (1999) Estrogen, natriuretic peptides and the renin-angiotensin system. Cardiovasc Res 41:524-531

239. Maffei S, Del Ry S, Prontera C, Clerico A (2001) Increase in circulating levels of cardiac natriuretic peptides after hormone replacement therapy in postmenopausal women. Clin Sci 101:447-453

240. Nuglozeh E, Mbikay M, Stewart DJ, Legault L (1997) Rat natriuretic peptide receptor genes are regulated by glucocorticoids *in vitro*. Life Sci 61:2143-2155

241. Ardaillou N, Blaise V, Placier S et al (1996) Dexamethasone upregulates ANP C-receptor protein in human mesangial cells without affecting mRNA. Am J Physiol 270:F440-446

242. Hashiguchi T, Higuchi K, Ohashi M et al (1989) Effect of porcine brain natriuretic peptide (pBNP) on human adrenocortical steroidogenesis. Clin Endocrinol 31:623-630

243. Defaye G, Lecomte S, Chambaz EM, Bottari SP (1995) Stimulation of cortisol production through angiotensin AT2 receptors in bovine fasciculata cells. Endocr Res 21:183-187

244. Denker PS, Vesely DL, Gomez-Sanchez CE (1990) Effect of pro-atrial natriuretic peptides 1-30, 31-67 and 99-126 on angiotensin II-stimulated aldosterone production in calf adrenal cells. J Steroid Biochem Mol Biol 37:617-619

245. Izumi Y, Honda M, Fukuda N et al (1990) Effect of atrial natriuretic peptide on adrenal renin and aldosterone. Endocrinol Jpn 37:47-52

246. Olson LJ, Lowe DG, Drewett JG (1996) Novel natriuretic peptide receptor/guanylyl cyclase A-selective agonist inhibits angiotensin II- and forskolin-evoked aldosterone synthesis in a human zona glomerulosa cell line. Mol Pharmacol 50:430-435

247. Szalay KS, Beck M, Toth M, de Chatel R (1998) Interactions between ouabain, atrial natriuretic peptide, angiotensin-II and potassium: effects on rat zona glomerulosa aldosterone production. Life Sci 62:1845-1852

248. Cherradi N, Brandenburger Y, Rossier MF et al (1998) Atrial natriuretic peptide inhibits calcium-induced steroidogenic acute regulatory protein gene transcription in adrenal glomerulosa cells. Mol Endocrinol 12:962-972

249. Ito T, Yoshimura M, Nakamura S et al (2003) Inhibitory effect of natriuretic peptides on aldosterone synthase gene expression in cultured neonatal rat cardiocytes. Circulation 107:807-810

250. Hayashi D, Kudoh S, Shiojima I et al (2004) Atrial natriuretic peptide inhibits cardiomyocyte hypertrophy through mitogen-activated protein kinase phosphatase-1. Biochem Biophys Res Commun 322:310-319

251. Heisler S, Tallerico-Melnyk T, Yip C, Schimmer BP (1989) Y-1 adrenocortical tumor cells contain atrial natriuretic peptide receptors which regulate cyclic nucleotide metabolism and steroidogenesis. Endocrinology 125:2235-2243

252. Chien CH, Tsai JH, Lee YJ (1990) Atrial natriuretic polypeptide in human adrenal pheochromocytoma: immunohistochemical and immunoelectron microscopical localization. Endocrinol Jpn 37:121-130

253. Lee YJ, Lin SR, Shin SJ, Tsai JH (1993) Increased adrenal medullary atrial natriuretic polypeptide synthesis in patients with primary aldosteronism. J Clin Endocrinol Metab 76:1357-1362

254. Lee YJ, Lin SR, Shin SJ et al (1994) Brain natriuretic peptide is synthesized in the human adrenal medulla and its messenger ribonucleic acid expression along with that of atrial natri-

uretic peptide are enhanced in patients with primary aldosteronism. J Clin Endocrinol Metab 79:1476-1482

255. Totsune K, Takahashi K, Murakami O et al (1994) Immunoreactive C-type natriuretic peptide in human adrenal glands and adrenal tumors. Peptides 15:287-290

256. Shionoiri H, Hirawa N, Takasaki I et al (1989) Functional atrial natriuretic peptide receptor in human adrenal tumor. J Cardiovasc Pharmacol 13(suppl 6):S9-12

257. Bodart V, Rainey WE, Fournier A et al (1996) The H295R human adrenocortical cell line contains functional atrial natriuretic peptide receptors that inhibit aldosterone biosynthesis. Mol Cell Endocrinol 118:137-144

258. Sarzani R, Opocher G, Paci MV et al (1999) Natriuretic peptide receptors in human aldosterone-secreting adenomas. J Endocrinol Invest 22:514-518

259. Marala RB, Sharma RK (1992) Three immunologically similar atrial natriuretic factor receptors. Mol Cell Biochem 109:71-75

260. Konrad EM, Thibault G, Schiffrin EL (1992) Autoradiographic visualization of the natriuretic peptide receptor-B in rat tissues. Regul Pept 39:177-189

261. Grandclement B, Ronsin B, Morel G (1997) The three subtypes of atrial natriuretic peptide (ANP) receptors are expressed in the rat adrenal gland. Biol Cell 89:29-41

262. Nagase M, Katafuchi T, Hirose S, Fujita T (1997) Tissue distribution and localization of natriuretic peptide receptor subtypes in stroke-prone spontaneously hypertensive rats. J Hypertens 15:1235-1243

263. Sugawara A, Nakao K, Morii N et al (1988) Atrial natriuretic factor in essential hypertension and adrenal disorders. Hypertension 11:1212-1216

264. Yamaji T, Ishibashi M, Yamada A et al (1988) Plasma levels of atrial natriuretic hormone in Cushing's syndrome. J Clin Endocrinol Metab 67:348-352

265. Sergev O, Racz K, Varga I et al (1991) Dissociation of plasma atrial natriuretic peptide responses to upright posture and furosemide administration in patients with normal-low renin, essential hypertension and primary aldosteronism. Clin Exp Hypert A 13:409-423

266. Opocher G, Rocco S, Carpene G et al (1992) Usefulness of atrial natriuretic peptide assay in primary aldosteronism. Am J Hypertens 5:811-816

267. Sala C, Ambrosi B, Morganti A (2001) Blunted vascular and renal effects of exogenous atrial natriuretic peptide in patients with Cushing's disease. J Clin Endocrinol Metab 86:1957-1961

268. Kato J, Etoh T, Kitamura K, Eto T (2005) Atrial and brain natriuretic peptides as marker of cardiac load and volume retention in primary aldosteronism Am J Hypertens 18:354-357

269. Stepniakowski K, Januszewicz A, Lapinski M et al. Plasma atrial natriuretic peptide (ANP) concentration in patients with pheochromocytoma

270. Clerico A, Recchia FA, Passino C, Emdin M (2006) Cardiac endocrine function is an essential component of the homeostatic regulation network: physiological and clinical implications. Am J Physiol Heart Circ Physiol 290:H17-29

271. Cappuccio FP, Markandu ND, Buckley MG et al (1989) Raised plasma levels of atrial natriuretic peptides in Addison's disease. J Endocrinol Invest 12:205-207

272. Cohen N, Gilbert R, Wirth A et al (1996) Atrial natriuretic peptide and plasma renin levels in assessment of mineralcorticoid replacement in Addison's disease. J Clin Endocrinol Metab 81:1411-1415

Chapter 7

Cardiac Natriuretic Hormone System as Target for Cardiovascular Therapy

Michele Emdin • Aldo Clerico

7.1 Background

Heart failure is a life-threatening cardiovascular disease that is increasing in prevalence in North America and Europe [1-3]. It is a common cause of death and is accompanied by high direct and indirect costs for treatment. The current situation faced by patients and the medical community with regard to this problem is one of high mortality, repeated hospitalizations, and combination therapies. The different classes of pharmacological agents that are currently used for patients suffering from heart failure include angiotensin-converting enzyme (ACE) inhibitors, angiotensin-receptor blockers, aldosterone antagonists, β-blockers, digitalis, diuretics, inotropic agents, nitrates, and vasodilators [1-3]. While these agents are all important therapeutic tools, the prognosis for patients with heart failure remains poor [1-3].

In this chapter we will review all the therapeutic implications of the CNH system. From a theoretical point of view, there are three ways in which the CNH system could be considered a possible target for therapeutic strategies in patients with cardiovascular diseases. At the present time, the standard pharmacological treatment for heart failure is based on drugs that counteract the neuro-endocrine system [1-3]. These drugs indirectly enhance the action of the CNH system by decreasing the counteracting system [4-8] and also by reducing the resistance to biological effects of endogenously produced natriuretic peptides [9, 10]. The second, more direct way is to administer biologically active peptides of the CNH family (especially synthetically produced BNP) to patients. The third approach is to enhance the activity of the CNH system by inhibiting their enzymatic degradation and therefore increasing their circulating levels. In the following sections, we will consider these aspects and discuss in detail the pathophysiological and clinical implications of these different therapeutic approaches.

7.2 Effects of Antagonists of Neuro-Hormonal Activation on CNH System

Drugs that counteract the detrimental effects of activation of the neuro-hormonal system have a key role in the current pharmacological treatment of heart failure, inducing amelioration of quality of life and life expectancy [1-3]. Some of these, such as ACE inhibitors, angiotensin II blockers, β-blockers, and spironolactone decrease the circulating levels of CNH [4-8], "normalize" their kinetics, and increase their biological activity [9], probably decreasing the systemic resistance to the biological effects of CNH [10].

After treatment with either enalapril or candesartan, the decrease in plasma levels of NT-proANP and NT-proBNP matches indices of reverse ventricular remodeling, such as reduction in ventricular volumes, and with clinical and prognostic improvement [11]. Valsartan, another angiotensin-receptor blocker, and perindopril, an ACE inhibitor, improve left ventricular function and ^{123}I-MIBG scintigraphic parameters in patients with heart failure, reducing plasma BNP concentration, too, after 6 months of treatment [12, 13].

As concerns the effect of β-blockers in congestive heart failure on the BNP plasma level, it has been claimed as heterogeneous, namely after metoprolol or carvedilol treatment [14]. Actually, carvedilol therapy is associated with a sustained decline in both CNH levels and left ventricular ejection fraction after 12 months of treatment [15, 16], with a dose-effect relationship [17]. If the effect on natriuretic peptide concentration is sustained, the same is not true for plasma renin activity [18-20]. Moreover, the best effect of carvedilol is predicted by higher levels of NT-proBNP [20]. As a matter of fact, whereas data on bisoprolol treatment in heart failure patients are lacking, its chronic administration in hypertensive patients increases the levels of natriuretic peptides [21-23]. The same seems true for carvedilol, which enhances the hypotensive action of ANP by increasing plasma ANP levels and enhancing the vascular response to ANP; these effects may be related to the down-regulation of the NPR-C receptor [24].

These observations may indicate that the overall effect of β-blockade depends on various factors, including the clinical model studied and the different pharmacological characteristics of drugs [5]. The paradoxical opposite behavior in heart failure and hypertensive patients, or in patients with cardiac insufficiency with different degrees of clinical severity, may be explained by a) the different level of overactivity of the counter-regulatory system (especially the adrenergic system), the main target of therapy, whose abolition tends to decrease plasma level of natriuretic peptides, and b) a stimulatory effect on plasma natriuretic peptide production/secretion or an inhibitory action on their clearance (or both). An important corollary of this interpretation is that the pathophysiological interpretation of this plasma concentration derives from the background level of activity of the counter-regulatory neuro-hormonal systems. It is theoretically conceivable that the effective balance between the activities of the two counter-regulatory systems is the most important pathophysiological mechanism responsible for disease progression. This balance can be only approximately estimated by circulating levels of neuro-hormones because autocrine and paracrine effects (better estimated by local tissue levels rather than circulating ones) have predominant effects. Evidently, further studies are necessary to clarify this important point.

Spironolactone improves vascular function (endothelial function, vascular ACE activity) and other markers of prognosis (BNP, collagen markers, and QT interval length) in patients with mild heart failure when added to optimal treatment including β-blockade [25]. Spironolactone administration in patients with severe chronic heart failure has opposite effects on circulating levels of natriuretic peptides (which decrease) and aldosterone and angiotensin II (which increase) [26, 27].

Levosimendan, an inotropic/vasodilator drug, without stimulating effects on adrenergic and dopaminergic systems, has been introduced recently for the treatment of acute heart failure [28, 29]. This drug shows a favorable hemodynamic and prognostic profile with a rapid clinical improvement in responding patients, similar to that obtained with inotropic drugs [28, 29]. The beneficial pharmacological effects could be related to decrease in BNP as well as in cytokine secretion [28, 29].

From a clinical point of view, it is important to note that the beneficial effects of different types of drugs as well as of non-pharmacological treatments (such as physical training, and mechanical assist or resynchronization therapies) are additive on CNH levels, as suggested by the case report illustrated in Figure 7.1.

In conclusion, the increased natriuresis and the other beneficial effects induced by drugs inhibiting the action of counter-regulatory systems in patients with heart failure suggest that the overwhelming activation of these systems should be considered as the predominant pathophysiological mechanism of disease progression. This implies a resistance to the biological action of CNH systems in patients with heart failure, probably at post-receptorial level [10] (see also Sect. 5.1.3 for more details). Unfortunately, the effects of the counter-regulatory system on down-regulation and/or desensitization of natriuretic peptide receptors are presently not well understood [10].

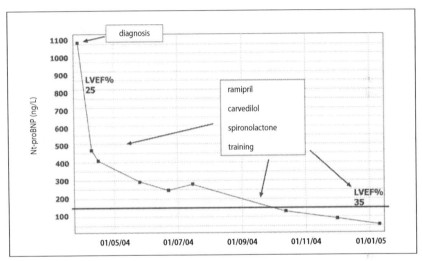

Fig. 7.1. Case report of a 51-year-old male with a presentation of class IV dyspnea associated with dilative cardiomyopathy. Over a 1-year period, optimization of pharmacological treatment and aerobic exercise training was able only partially to ameliorate systolic dysfunction. On the other hand, symptoms disappeared and plasma assay of NT-proBNP progressively ameliorated toward normal values. LVEF = left ventricular ejection fraction

7.3 Treatments Targeting the Increase of Circulating Levels of CNH

More recently, research has focused on the enhancement of the activity of the CNH system itself as an alternative target for improving the therapeutic approach in heart failure patients. In other words, if the heart's natural response to myocardial dysfunction is increased CNH production in order to increase vasodilatation, natriuresis, and diuresis, to decrease neuro-hormonal concentration, and also to improve diastolic function and ventriculoarterial coupling (as recently demonstrated [30]), therapeutic administration of CNH should theoretically mirror these beneficial effects. From a clinical point of view, this specific approach should present a safer profile as concerns arrhythmia occurrence, than the usual inotropic approach to decompensated heart failure patients [1].

This goal has been attempted by administering exogenous natriuretic peptides, either ANP [31], urodilatin [32] or BNP [33]. The latter, used in the USA with the trade name Natrecor (Scios), is a 32 amino acid peptide synthetic product and has been demonstrated to be chemically and structurally identical to endogenous human BNP [34, 35]. Alternatively, the scope of increasing ANP and BNP concentration has been attained by blocking the degradation pathways of the drug, e.g. using some neutral endopeptidase inhibitors [36, 37]. However, only preliminary pathophysiological studies have investigated the use of CNH both in healthy subjects and in heart failure patients with a favorable effect on endothelial function [38].

7.3.1 Natriuretic Peptides: Pharmacological Actions

The reported hemodynamic and renal effects of CNH in man differ largely between studies, because of differences in design and doses of peptide administered. Both ANP and BNP should theoretically show a favorable pharmacological profile in heart failure [40, 41].

Unlike other vasodilator agents, administration of ANP does not lead to reflex tachycardia and may be associated with bradycardia, indicating that ANP inhibits sympathetic nerve activity [42]. ANP has been found to exert a sympatho-inhibitory action in heart failure: this was most evident in response to reductions in atrial pressure that do not affect systemic blood pressure [43]. However, studies of ANP infusion in patients with congestive heart failure have demonstrated variable but largely attenuated hemodynamic and renal excretory effects, particularly in patients with advanced heart failure [44-46]. Moreover, trials with ANP did not confirm the expected efficacy [32]; indeed, its short half-life, the possible presence of a peripheral resistance, and the development of pharmacological tolerance may affect its favorable pharmacological profile.

In the pharmacological range, BNP has clear blood pressure and afterload lowering effects, and the kidney blood flow and filtration is increased with concomitant natriuresis and diuresis [39]. In the physiological range, BNP does not affect blood pressure and reduces preload only, and induces natriuresis/diuresis without changes in renal blood flow and filtration. There is increasing evidence from vascular studies that BNP preferentially acts on the venous system, resulting in preload reduction, in contrast to ANP, which acts preferentially on the arterial system to reduce afterload [39].

The direct vascular action of CNH is probably mediated by activation of the guanylyl cyclase-coupled natriuretic peptide receptor-A (NPR-A) on the membrane surface of vascular smooth muscle cells [39, 42, 45, 46] (see Sects. 3.4 and 3.5 for more details). Decreased cardiac filling pressures also may be partly attributable to other known actions of natriuretic peptides, i.e. inhibition of activation of the rennin-angiotensin system, inhibition of sympathetic neurotransmission, reduction in intravascular volume through natriuresis and diuresis, and reduction in intravascular volume secondary to changes in capillary permeability [39, 40, 42].

7.3.2 Use of Synthetic Natriuretic Peptides: Clinical Trials

At the present time, nesiritide is the most used synthetic analog of BNP. This peptide drug has been recommended to be administered as a fixed-dose infusion at a dose of 0.015 micrograms per kilogram per minute, without a loading bolus [34]. However, the doses of nesiritide administered were 0.003, 0.01, 0.03, and 0.1 µg/kg/min in the preliminary studies [34]. At the lowest dose tested, minimal or no effect on various hemodynamic parameters was observed. As the dose of nesiritide was increased, dose- and concentration-related effects on hemodynamics were seen [34]. These included [34]:

1. Reductions in preload, as measured by reductions in pulmonary capillary wedge pressure, and mean right atrial pressure.
2. Reductions in afterload, as characterized by decrease in systemic vascular resistance, and dose-related increases in cardiac index were seen.
3. These were accompanied by modest dose-related reductions in blood pressure; no effect on heart rate was seen at any but the highest dose.

At the highest dose, very potent hemodynamic effects were observed, characterized by the frequent development of symptomatic hypotension. In conclusion, nesiritide administration results in dose-related hemodynamic effects, and doses in the range of 0.01-0.03 µg/kg/min are considered the likely optimal dose range for patients with heart failure [34].

When compared with standard therapy consisting primarily of dobutamine [51, 52] or milrinone [52], nesiritide was found to result in similar improvements in global clinical status, in the symptoms and prognosis of decompensated congestive heart failure. From the retrospective analysis of 65,180 patient episodes of acute heart failure from the Acute Decompensated Heart Failure National Registry (ADHERE) [52], a multicenter registry designed prospectively to collect data on each episode of hospitalization for acute decompensated heart failure and its clinical outcomes, therapy with either a natriuretic peptide or vasodilator was associated with significantly lower in-hospital mortality than positive inotropic therapy in patients hospitalized with acute decompensated heart failure. The risk of in-hospital mortality was similar for nesiritide and nitroglycerin [52]. Furosemide associated with BNP has more profound diuretic and natriuretic responses than furosemide alone and also increases glomerular filtration rate without activation of aldosterone [53]. A summary of prominent therapeutic trials to date is reported in Table 7.1 [33, 51, 54-56].

Alternative use of BNP includes subcutaneous and oral administration. One study has suggested that subcutaneous delivery of hBNP may be a viable therapeutic alternative to intravenous modes of delivery [57]. Another study has recently reported for the first time that a novel conjugated oral preparation of BNP (CONJ-hBNP, Fig. 7.2) activates cGMP and significantly reduces MAP in dogs, thus implying an efficacious coupling of CONJ-hBNP to the natriuretic receptor-A [58]. However, BNP has a very short half-life in circulation (about 15-20 min in humans), which limits its application to acute heart failure and requires continuous i.v. infusion. In order to provide superior pharmacological benefits of endogenous peptide hormone to other stages of chronic congestive heart failure and to eliminate problems associated with drug delivery via continuous i.v. infusion, a long-acting form of BNP (AlbuBNP) was designed by recombinant fusion to human serum albumin [59]. The elimination half-life in mice was dramatically increased from 3 minutes for BNP to 12-19 hours for AlbuBNP [59]. This drug was suggested for use in chronic congestive heart failure, post-acute follow-up, and post-myocardial infarction [59].

Table 7.1. Prominent heart failure clinical trials conducted with nesiritide

Study	No. of Subjects	Study design	hBNP Dosing
FUSION[22]	210	Multi-center, randomized, open-label, 12-week, 3 arm-parallel group (1:1:1 ratio), pilot study comparing patients receiving standard care plus nesiritide (inotropes excluded; 2 arms), or standard care only (1 arm), which may include inotropes	Low-dose nesiritide Week 1: 0.5 µg/kg bolus with 0.0025 µg/kg/min 4-h infusion Weeks 2–12: one half to 2 times week 1 dose High-dose nesiritide: Week 1: 1.0 µg/kg bolus with 0.005 µg/kg/min 4-h infusion Weeks 2–12: one half to 2 times week 1 dose
PROACTION[23]	250	PMulti-center, randomized, double-blind, placebo-controlled pilot study in emergency departments	2 µg/kg IV bolus, followed by a fixed-dose infusion of 0.01 µg/kg/min for a minimum of 12 h, in addition to standard care
VMAC[24]	489	Randomized, double-blind, placebo- and nitroglycerin-controlled, parallel design for first 3 hours, then crossover of placebo patients for double-blind active-control period	2 µg/kg IV bolus, followed by a fixed-dose infusion of 0.01 µg/kg/min. An adjustable dose treatment arm permitted dose increases every 3 h up to a maximum infusion dose of 0.03 µg/kg/min
PRECEDENT[17]	246	Randomized, open-label, parallel, active controlled (dobutamine) study	0.015 or 0.030 µg/kg/min as a fixed-dose IV infusion (not preceded by a bolus)
Comparative trial[3]	305	Randomized, open-label, active controlled, parallel design	0.015 or 0.03 µg/kg/min as a fixed-dose IV infusion (preceded by a small bolus) for up to 7 days
Efficacy trial[3]	127	Randomized, double-blind, placebo-controlled, parallel design for first 6 hours, then active controlled, open-label study thereafter	0.015 or 0.03 µg/kg/min as a fixed-dose IV infusion (preceded by a small bolus) for up to 5 days

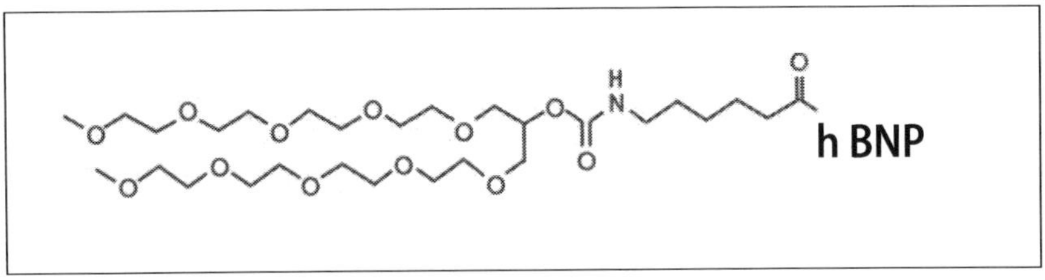

Fig. 7.2. Structure of CONJ-hBNP-021. The structure of CONJ-hBNP includes the human peptide chain of BNP covalently linked to a short amphiphilic oligomer. Proprietary technology (Nobex) has been developed in which short, amphiphilic oligomers are covalently attached to peptides, such as BNP. In contrast to standard PEGylation technology, this technique uses comparatively small, amphiphilic oligomers that are monodispersed and comprise both a hydrophobic (alkyl) moiety and a hydrophilic polyethylene glycol (PEG) moiety. The oligomers are intended to improve the pharmacokinetic and pharmacodynamic profiles of the peptide and potentially to enable oral administration

Nevertheless, evidence of resistance to the natriuretic effects of BNP was shown in half the subjects studied by Abraham et al. [60], and very recently its increasing and widespread use in the USA (600,000 patients treated), after the Food and Drug Administration approval in 2001, has been challenged [61]. Compared with non-inotropic-based control therapy, nesiritide has been associated with an increased risk of death after treatment for acutely decompensated heart failure [62]. The possibility of an increased risk of death should be investigated in a large-scale, adequately powered, controlled trial before routine use of nesiritide for acutely decompensated heart failure [61]. Moreover, according to Topol's definition, the benefit of nesiritide infusion should actually be considered "not verified" [61].

Recently, ularitide, a synthetic version of the renal natriuretic peptide urodilatin, was also found to be hemodynamically active, producing beneficial clinical effects in patients with acute heart failure. It is well tolerated at doses up to 30 ng/kg/min, according to a phase IIb clinical study. In SIRIUS II trial, ularitide was reported to have no effect on renal function, nor did it increase mortality during the 30 days after administration.

7.4 Pharmacological Blockade of Degradation and Receptor Antagonism

The short half-life of natriuretic peptides and lack of an oral formulation limit the option of an exogenous application of the peptide as a long-term therapeutic strategy. Therefore, pharmacological inhibition of the enzymatic degradation of CNH has been considered as an attractive alternative therapeutic target.

The two main mechanisms for CNH inactivation and removal are the specific receptor-mediated clearance and the degradation by some enzymes, such as the zinc metallopeptidase neutral endopeptidase (NEP) (Fig. 7.3). NEP is an endothelial, membrane-bound metallopeptidase with zinc at its active site, which cleaves endogenous peptides at the amino side of hydrophilic residues [63]. The membrane-bound metallopeptidase has a similar catalytic unit to ACE. NEP is widely distributed in endothelial cells, vascular smooth muscle cells, cardiac myocytes, renal epithelial cells, and fibroblasts [64-66]. NEP is also found within the lung, gut, adrenal glands, brain, and heart. It catalyzes the degradation of a number of endogenous vasodilator peptides, including ANP, BNP, CNP, substance P, and bradykinin, as well as vasoconstrictor peptides, including endothelin-1 (ET-1) and angiotensin II [65, 69].

Selective NEP inhibitors prevent the degradation of natriuretic peptides, both *in vitro* and *in vivo*, and thus increase their biological activity. In addition to degrading vasoactive peptides to inactive breakdown products, NEP is also involved in the enzymatic conversion of big ET-1 to its active form, the vasoconstrictor peptide ET-1. However, ET-1 is also activated by the endothelin-converting enzyme-1 (ECE-1) [70]; hence, the balance of effects of NEP inhibition on vascular tone will depend on the extent of NEP involvement in the processing of big ET-1 [71]. In the human forearm circulation, certain NEP inhibitors cause vasoconstriction rather than vasodilatation, indicating that under physiological conditions, vasoconstrictor peptides, such as angiotensin II and endothelins, can be important substrates for vascular NEP [72]. This explains why NEP inhibitors such as candoxatril, thiorphan and phosphoramidon increase circulat-

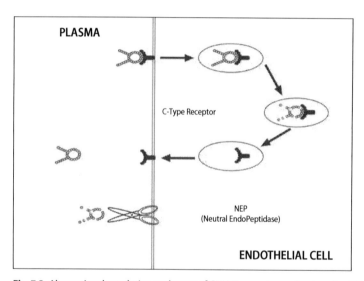

Fig. 7.3. Alternative degradation pathways of CNH. Two main mechanisms for CNH inactivation and removal are known: the specific receptor-mediated clearance and the degradation by some plasma and tissue enzymes, such as the zinc metallopeptidase neutral endopeptidase (NEP)

ing ANP concentrations in humans and induce natriuresis, but do not lower [73-79] or even increase blood pressure in normotensive subjects [80]. In patients with essential hypertension, certain NEP inhibitors lower blood pressure [81-83]; whereas others increase it [84]. Chronic treatment with NEP inhibitors augments the effects of ANP and lowers blood pressure in patients with hypertension, but these effects may be blunted by an increased activity of the renin-angiotensin-aldosterone and sympathetic nervous system or by down-regulation of ANP receptors.

The blood pressure response to endopeptidase inhibition in hypertensive patients depends on the relative effects on vasodilator (including ANP) and vasoconstrictor (including the renin-angiotensin-aldosterone and sympathetic systems) [85]. NEP antagonists induce ANP level increase and natriuresis with little change in potassium excretion in heart failure patients, but have shown little efficacy in the experimental setting [63].

Accordingly, in patients with congestive heart failure, NEP inhibitors do not reduce afterload although they decrease pulmonary capillary wedge pressure, presumably due to their natriuretic effect [86-88]. In patients with moderate to severe heart failure, NEP inhibitors given acutely induce a dose-dependent diuresis [88], while chronic treatment does not provide this clinical benefit. Other possible explanations for the limited beneficial effect of NEP inhibitors in heart failure are tolerance to ANP, most likely due to down-regulation of ANP receptors and/or activation of the renin-angiotensin-aldosterone system (Fig. 7.4).

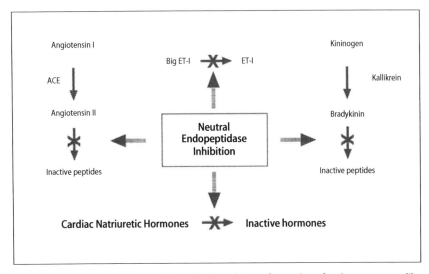

Fig. 7.4. Action sites of NEP. NEP catalyses the degradation of a number of endogenous vasodilator peptides, including ANP, BNP, CNP, and bradykinin, as well as vasoconstrictor hormones, including endothelin-1 (ET-1) and angiotensin II

7.5 Combined ACE and NEP Inhibition

The renin-angiotensin-aldosterone system, endothelin system, kallikrein-kinin system and the natriuretic peptides are important modulators of cardiovascular homeostasis. These systems are altered in conditions such as hypertension and chronic heart failure, leading to the rationale of simultaneously blocking these systems (regulated through similar endothelial, membrane-bound enzymes, the ACE and NEP). Actually, the combination of an ACE with a NEP inhibitor (vasopeptidase inhibitors) has been shown to result in a more potent natriuretic effect than NEP antagonist alone, in experimental models, because of the effect on both angiotensin II and bradykinin degradation [36]. These drugs exert some beneficial effects in patients with arterial hypertension, heart failure and/or angina pectoris (Fig. 7.5) [76, 89-92].

Though natriuresis and decrease in renin response to the NEP/ACE inhibitor omapatrilat are superior to ACE inhibition alone [93], its prognostic value, as concerns the reduction of the risk of death and hospitalization in chronic heart failure, is not greater than ACE inhibition alone, as shown by a large clinical trial that compared the effects of omapatrilat to enalapril [93].

These results are not encouraging for these new pharmaceutical agents. Not only is there no additive benefit in NEP inhibition on top of ACE inhibition in hypertension or chronic heart failure, these agents also have an increase in the potentially life-threatening side-effect of angioedema. It remains to be seen whether this is specific to omapatrilat or common to all vasopeptidase inhibitors. Perhaps the combination of an angiotensin receptor antagonist with a NEP inhibitor may potentially enable inhibition of both these neuro-humoral systems without the unwanted bradykinin side-effects.

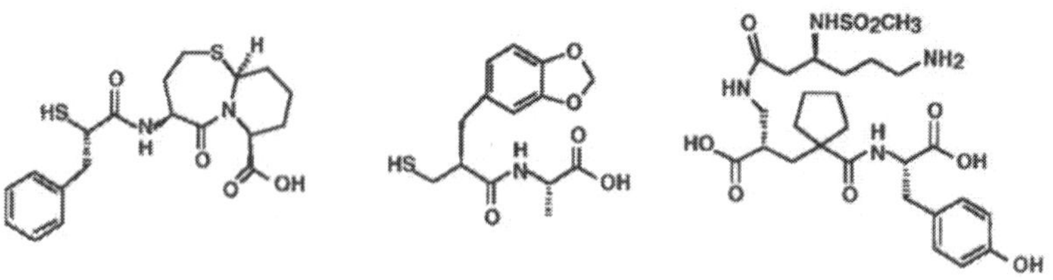

Fig. 7.5. Chemical structure of drugs with vasopeptidase activity

7.6 Conclusive Remarks

The positive hemodynamic and prognostic effect of neuro-hormonal antagonists is accompanied by a decrease in natriuretic hormone plasma concentration, likely reflecting a re-balancing of the counter-regulatory systems, modulating vasomotion and salt-water homeostasis. This finding points out the potential of the follow-up of the BNP/NT-proBNP value as an index of the effectiveness of conventional treatment.

On the other hand, up-to-date evidence on the pharmacological agonism of the cardiac natriuretic system is contradictory: a pathophysiological basis for the lack of superior efficacy and prognostic value of drugs acting on plasma concentrations of cardiac natriuretic hormones lies in the phenomenon of peripheral resistance [10], still not well understood or clinically characterizable in individual patients.

From a clinical point of view, it is important to underline that the marked resistance to CNH action may also explain the fact that administration of CNH analogs (such as nesiritide) may be no more effective than conventional treatment in patients with decompensated congestive heart failure [61]. Indeed, according to the hypothesis of CNH resistance [10], an increase in circulating levels of biologically active hormones (obtained by the inhibition of NEP or by nesiritide infusion) can be useful only if there is a significant decrease in the activation of the counter-regulatory system induced by the concomitant administration of drugs inhibiting this system (such as ACE inhibitors, angiotensin II receptor antagonists, and β-blocker agents). Future research should address this topic to go a step further in the comprehension of the actual relevance of BNP overexpression in heart failure, and possibly to define novel therapeutic targets, at the receptor and post-receptor processing of hormone signaling.

References

1. The Task Force on Acute Heart Failure of the European Society of Cardiology (2005) Guidelines on the diagnosis and treatment of acute heart failure, pp 1-36
2. The Task Force for the diagnosis and treatment of chronic heart failure of the European Society of Cardiology (2005) Guidelines for the diagnosis and the treatment of chronic heart failure. Updated, pp 1-45
3. ACC/AHA 2005 guideline update for the diagnosis and treatment of chronic heart failure in the adult (2005) A report of the American College of Cardiology/American Heart Association Task Force on Practice Guidelines (writing committee to update the 2001 guidelines for the evaluation and management of heart failure). American College of Cardiology Foundation and the American Heart Association, Inc, pp 1-82
4. Richards AM, Lainchbury JG, Nicholls MG et al (2002) BNP in hormone-guided treatment of heart failure. Trends Endocrinol Metab 13:151-155
5. Latini R, Masson S, De Angelis N, Anand I (2002) Role of brain natriuretic peptide in the diagnosis and management of heart failure: current concepts. J Card Fail 8:288-299
6. Richards M, Troughton RW (2004) NT-proBNP in heart failure: therapy decisions and monitoring. Eur J Heart Fail 6:351-354
7. Bettencourt P (2004) NT-proBNP and BNP: biomarkers for heart failure management. Eur J Heart Fail 6:359-363
8. Cowie MR, Mendez GF (2002) BNP and congestive heart failure. Prog Cardiovasc Dis 44:293-321
9. Clerico A, Iervasi G, Pilo A (2000) Turnover studies on cardiac natriuretic peptides: methodological, pathophysiological and therapeutical considerations. Curr Drug Metab 1:85-105
10. Clerico A, Recchia FA, Passino C, Emdin M (2005) Cardiac endocrine function is an essential component of the homeostatic regulation network: physiological and clinical implications. Am J Physiol Heart Circ Physiol
11. Yan RT, White M, Yan AT et al (2005) Randomized Evaluation of Strategies for Left Ventricular Dysfunction (RESOLVD) Investigators. Usefulness of temporal changes in neurohormones as markers of ventricular remodeling and prognosis in patients with left ventricular systolic dysfunction and heart failure receiving either candesartan or enalapril or both. Am J Cardiol 96:698-704
12. Kasama S, Toyama T, Hatori T et al (2005) Comparative effects of valsartan and enalapril on cardiac sympathetic nerve activity and plasma brain natriuretic peptide in patients with congestive heart failure. Heart 92:625-630
13. Kasama S, Toyama T, Kumakura H et al (2005) Effects of perindopril on cardiac sympathetic nerve activity in patients with congestive heart failure: comparison with enalapril. Eur J Nucl Med Mol Imaging 32:964-971

14. Yoshizawa A, Yoshikawa T, Nakamura I et al (2004) Brain natriuretic peptide response is heterogeneous during beta-blocker therapy for congestive heart failure. J Card Fail 10:310-315
15. Frantz RP, Olson LJ, Grill D et al (2005) Carvedilol therapy is associated with a sustained decline in brain natriuretic peptide levels in patients with congestive heart failure. Am Heart J 149:541-547
16. Takeda Y, Fukutomi T, Suzuki S et al (2004) Effects of carvedilol on plasma B-type natriuretic peptide concentration and symptoms in patients with heart failure and preserved ejection fraction. Am J Cardiol 94:448-453
17. Konishi H, Nishio S, Tsutamoto T et al (2003) Serum carvedilol concentration and its relation to change in plasma brain natriuretic peptide level in the treatment of heart failure: a preliminary study. Int J Clin Pharmacol Ther 41:578-586
18. Fung JW, Yu CM, Yip G et al (2003) Effect of beta blockade (carvedilol or metoprolol) on activation of the renin-angiotensin-aldosterone system and natriuretic peptides in chronic heart failure. Am J Cardiol 92:406-410
19. Hirooka K, Yasumura Y, Ishida Y et al (2001) Comparative left ventricular functional and neurohumoral effects of chronic treatment with carvedilol versus metoprolol in patients with dilated cardiomyopathy. Jpn Circ J 65:931-936
20. Richards AM, Doughty R, Nicholls MG et al (2001) (Australia-New Zealand Heart Failure Group). Plasma N-terminal pro-brain natriuretic peptide and adrenomedullin: prognostic utility and prediction of benefit from carvedilol in chronic ischemic left ventricular dysfunction. J Am Coll Cardiol 37:1781-1787
21. Van den Meiracker AH, Lameris TW, van de Ven LL, Boomsma F (2003) Increased plasma concentration of natriuretic peptides by selective beta1-blocker bisoprolol. J Cardiovasc Pharmacol 42:462-468
22. Deary AJ, Schumann AL, Murfet H et al (2002) Influence of drugs and gender on the arterial pulse wave and natriuretic peptide secretion in untreated patients with essential hypertension. Clin Sci 103:493-499
23. Tanaka M, Ishizaka Y, Ishiyama Y et al (1996) Chronic effect of beta-adrenoceptor blockade on plasma levels of brain natriuretic peptide during exercise in essential hypertension. Hypertens Res 19:239-245
24. Yoshimoto T, Naruse M, Tanabe A et al (1998) Potentiation of natriuretic peptide action by the beta-adrenergic blocker carvedilol in hypertensive rats: a new antihypertensive mechanism. Endocrinology 139:81-88
25. MacDonald JE, Kennedy N, Struthers AD (2004) Effects of spironolactone on endothelial function, vascular angiotensin converting enzyme activity, and other prognostic markers in patients with mild heart failure already taking optimal treatment. Heart 90:765-770
26. Rousseau MF, Gurne O, Duprez D et al (2002) Belgian RALES Investigators. Beneficial neurohormonal profile of spironolactone in severe congestive heart failure: results from the RALES neurohormonal substudy. J Am Coll Cardiol 40:1596-1601
27. Tsutamoto T, Wada A, Maeda K et al (2001) Effect of spironolactone on plasma brain natriuretic peptide and left ventricular remodeling in patients with congestive heart failure. J Am Coll Cardiol 37:1228-1233
28. Avgeropoulou C, Andreadou I, Markantonis-Kyroudis S et al (2005) The Ca2+-sensitizer levosimendan improves oxidative damage, BNP and pro-inflammatory cytokine levels in patients with advanced decompensated heart failure in comparison to dobutamine. Eur J Heart Fail 7:882-887
29. Kyrzopoulos S, Adamopoulos S, Parissis JT et al (2005) Levosimendan reduces plasma B-type natriuretic peptide and interleukin 6, and improves central hemodynamics in severe heart failure patients. Int J Cardiol 99:409-413
30. Nakajima K, Onishi K, Dohi K et al (2005) Effects of human atrial natriuretic peptide on cardiac function and hemodynamics in patients with high plasma BNP levels. Int J Cardiol 104:332-337
31. Connelly TP, Francis GS, Williams KJ et al (1994) Interaction of intravenous atrial natriuretic factor with furosemide in patients with heart failure. Am Heart J 127:392-399

32. Mitrovic V, Seferovic P, Simeunovic D et al (2005) A randomized, double-blind, placebo-controlled phase II study of ularitide in patients with acute decompensated congestive heart failure. J Card Fail 11(6 suppl):S151. Abstract 227

33. Colucci WS, Elkayam U, Horton DP et al (2000) Intravenous nesiritide, a natriuretic peptide, in the treatment of decompensated congestive heart failure. Nesiritide Study Group. N Engl J Med 343:246-253

34. Report from the United States Food and Drug Administration Center for drug evaluation and research division of cardio-renal products (1999) Cardiovascular and Renal Drugs Advisory Committee, 87th meeting, January 29 (available on the web site: *http://www.fda.gov/ohrms/dockets/ac/99/transcpt/3490t2.rtf*)

35. Silver MA, Maisel A, Yancy CW et al (2004) BNP Consensus Panel 2004: A clinical approach for the diagnostic, prognostic, screening, treatment monitoring, and therapeutic roles of natriuretic peptides in cardiovascular diseases. Congest Heart Fail 10(5 suppl 3):1-30

36. Kentsch M, Otter W (1999) Novel neurohormonal modulators in cardiovascular disorders. The therapeutic potential of endopeptidase inhibitors. Drugs R D 1:331-338

37. Kostis JB, Klapholz M, Delaney C et al (2001) Pharmacodynamics and pharmacokinetics of omapatrilat in heart failure. J Clin Pharmacol 41:1280-1290

38. Schmitt M, Gunaruwan P, Payne N et al (2004) Effects of exogenous and endogenous natriuretic peptides on forearm vascular function in chronic heart failure. Arterioscler Thromb Vasc Biol 24:911-917

39. Houben AJ, van der Zander K, de Leeuw PW (2005) Vascular and renal actions of brain natriuretic peptide in man: physiology and pharmacology. Fundam Clin Pharmacol 19:411-419

40. Koller KJ, Goeddel DV (1992) Molecular biology of the natriuretic peptides and their receptors. Circulation 86:1081-1088

41. Deutsch A, Frishman WH, Sukenik D et al (1994) Atrial natriuretic peptide and its potential role in pharmacotherapy. J Clin Pharmacol 34:1133-1147

42. Zeidel ML (2000) Physiological responses to natriuretic hormones. In: Fray JCS, Goodman HM (eds) Handbook of physiology, Section 7, The endocrine system, Volume III: Endocrine regulation of water and electrolyte balance. New York, Oxford University Press, pp 410-435

43. Abramson BL, Ando S, Notarius CF et al (1999) Effect of atrial natriuretic peptide on muscle sympathetic activity and its reflex control in human heart failure. Circulation 99:1810-1815

44. Cody RJ, Atlas SA, Laragh JH et al (1986) Atrial natriuretic factor in normal subjects and heart failure patients. J Clin Invest 78:1362-1374

45. Fifer MA, Molina CR, Quiroz AC et al (1990) Hemodynamic and renal effects of atrial natriuretic peptide in congestive heart failure. Am J Cardiol 65:211-216

46. Crozier IG, Nicholls MG, Ikram H et al (1986) Haemodynamic effects of atrial peptide infusion in heart failure. Lancet 2:1242-1245

47. Saito H, Ogihara T, Nakamaru M et al (1987) Hemodynamic, renal, and hormonal responses to alpha-human atrial natriuretic peptide in patients with congestive heart failure. Clin Pharmacol Ther 42:142-147

48. Molina CR, Fowler MB, McCrory S et al (1988) Hemodynamic, renal and endocrine effects of atrial natriuretic peptide infusion in severe heart failure. J Am Coll Cardiol 12:175-186

49. Zhou HL, Fiscus RR (1989) Brain natriuretic peptide (BNP) causes endothelium independent relaxation and elevation of cyclic GMP in rat thoracic aorta. Neuropeptides 14:161-169

50. Wong SKF, Garbers DL (1992) Receptor guanylyl cyclases. J Clin Invest 90:299-305

51. Burger AJ et al (2002) Effect of nesiritide (B-type natriuretic peptide) and dobutamine on ventricular arrhythmias in the treatment of patients with acutely decompensated CHF: the PRECEDENT study. Am Heart J 144:1102-1108

52. Abraham WT, Adams KF, Fonarow GC et al (2005) ADHERE Scientific Advisory Committee and Investigators; ADHERE Study Group. In-hospital mortality in patients with acute decompensated heart failure requiring intravenous vasoactive medications: an analysis from the Acute Decompensated Heart Failure National Registry (ADHERE). J Am Coll Cardiol 46:57-64

53. Cataliotti A, Boerrigter G, Costello-Boerrigter LC et al (2004) Brain natriuretic peptide enhances

renal actions of furosemide and suppresses furosemide-induced aldosterone activation in experimental heart failure. Circulation 109:1680-1685

54. Yancy CW, Saltzberg MT, Berkowitz RL et al (2004) Safety and feasibility of using serial infusions of nesiritide for heart failure in an outpatient setting (from the FUSION I trial). Am J Cardiol 94:595-601

55. Peacock WF (2003) Clinical and economic impact of nesiritide. Am J Health Syst Pharm 60(suppl 4):S21-26

56. Publication Committee for the VMAC Investigators (2002) Intravenous nesiritide vs. nitroglycerin for treatment of decompensated heart failure. JAMA 287:1531-1540

57. Clemens LE, Almirez RG, Baudouin KA et al (1998) Pharmacokinetics and biological actions of subcutaneously administered human brain natriuretic peptide. J Pharmacol Exp Ther 287:67-71

58. Cataliotti A, Schirger JA, Martin FL et al (2005) Oral human brain natriuretic peptide activates cyclic guanosine 3',5'-monophosphate and decreases mean arterial pressure. Circulation 112:836-840

59. Wang W, Ou Y, Shi Y (2004) AlbuBNP, a recombinant B-type natriuretic peptide and human serum albumin fusion hormone, as a long-term therapy of congestive heart failure. Pharm Res 21:2105-2111

60. Abraham WT, Lowes BD, Ferguson DA et al (1998) Systemic hemodynamic, neurohormonal, and renal effects of a steady-state infusion of human brain natriuretic peptide in patients with hemodynamically decompensated heart failure. J Card Fail 4:37-44

61. Topol EJ (2005) Nesiritide - not verified. N Engl J Med 353:113-116

62. Sackner-Bernstein JD, Kowalski M, Fox M, Aaronson K (2005) Short-term risk of death after treatment with nesiritide for decompensated heart failure: a pooled analysis of randomized controlled trials. JAMA 293:1900-1905

63. Margulies KB, Barclay PL, Burnett JC Jr (1995) The role of neutral endopeptidase in dogs with evolving congestive heart failure. Circulation 91:2036-2042

64. Graf K, Koehne P, Grafe M et al (1995) Regulation and differential expression of neutral endopeptidases 24.11 in human endothelial cells. Hypertension 26:230-235

65. Erdos EG, Skidgel RA (1989) Neutral endopeptidase 24.11 (enkephalinase) and related regulators of peptide hormones. Faseb J 3:145-151

66. Dussaule JC, Stefanski A, Bea ML et al (1993) Characterization of neutral endopeptidase in vascular smooth muscle cells of rabbit renal cortex. Am J Physiol 264:F45-52

67. Lang CC, Motwani JG, Coutie WJ, Struthers AD (1992) Clearance of brain natriuretic peptide in patients with chronic heart failure: indirect evidence for a neutral endopeptidase mechanism but against an atrial natriuretic peptide clearance receptor mechanism. Clin Sci 82:619-623

68. Kenny AJ, Bourne A, Ingram J (1993) Hydrolysis of human and pig brain natriuretic peptides, urodilatin, C-type natriuretic peptide and some C-receptor ligands by endopeptidase-24.11. Biochem J 291:83-88

69. Skidgel RA, Engelbrecht S, Johnson AR, Erdos EG (1984) Hydrolysis of substance P and neurotensin by converting enzyme and neutral endopeptidase. Peptides 5:769-776

70. Berger Y, Dehmlow H, Blum-Kaelin D et al (2005) Endothelin-converting enzyme-1 inhibition and growth of human glioblastoma cells. J Med Chem 48:483-498

71. Murphy LJ, Corder R, Mallet AI, Turner AJ (1994) Generation by the phosphoramidon-sensitive peptidases, endopeptidase-24.11 and thermolysin, of endothelin-1 and c-terminal fragment from big endothelin-1. Br J Pharmacol 113:137-142

72. Ferro CJ, Spratt JC, Haynes WG, Webb DJ (1998) Inhibition of neutral endopeptidase causes vasoconstriction of human resistance vessels *in vivo*. Circulation 97:2323-2330

73. Danilewicz JC, Barclay PL, Barnish IT et al (1989) UK-69,578, a novel inhibitor of EC 3.4.24.11 which increases endogenous ANF levels and is natriuretic and diuretic. Biochem Biophys Res Commun 164:58-65

74. Gros C, Souque A, Schwartz JC et al (1989) Protection of atrial natriuretic factor against degradation. Diuretic and natriuretic responses after *in vivo* inhibition of enkephalinase (EC 3.4.24.11) by acetorphan. Proc Natl Acad Sci USA 86:7580-7584

75. Schwartz JC, Gros C, Lecomte JM, Bralet J (1990) Enkephalinase (EC 3.4.24. 11) inhibitors: protection of endogenous ANF against inactivation and potential therapeutic applications. Life Sci 47:1279-1297

76. Northridge DB, Jardine AG, Alabaster CT et al (1989) Effects of UK 69,578: a novel atriopeptidase inhibitor. Lancet 2:591-593

77. Richards AM, Wittert G, Espiner EA et al (1991) Prolonged inhibition of endopeptidase 24.11 in normal man: renal, endocrine and haemodynamic effects. J Hypertens 9:955-962

78. O'Connell JE, Jardine AG, Davies DL et al (1993) Renal and hormonal effects of chronic inhibition of neutral endopeptidase (EC 3.4.24.11) in normal man. Clin Sci 85:19-26

79. Bevan EG, Connell JM, Doyle J et al (1992) Candoxatril, a neutral endopeptidases inhibitor: efficacy and tolerability in essential hypertension. J Hypertens 10:607-613

80. Ando S, Rahman MA, Butler GC et al (1995) Comparison of candoxatril and atrial natriuretic factor in healthy men. Effects on hemodynamics, sympathetic activity, heart rate variability, and endothelin. Hypertension 26:1160-1166

81. Richards AM, Crozier IG, Espiner EA et al (1993) Plasma brain natriuretic peptide and endopeptidases 24.11 inhibition in hypertension. Hypertension 22:231-236

82. Ogihara T, Rakugi H, Masuo K et al (1994) Antihypertensive effects of the neutral endopeptidase inhibitor SCH 42495 in essential hypertension. Am J Hypertens 7:943-947

83. Fettner SH, Pai S, Zhu GR et al (1995) Pharmacokinetic-pharmacodynamic (PK-PD) modeling for a new antihypertensive agent (neutral metalloendopeptidase inhibitor SCH 42354) in patients with mild to moderate hypertension. Eur J Clin Pharmacol 48:351-359

84. Singer DR, Markandu ND, Buckley MG et al (1991) Dietary sodium and inhibition of neutral endopeptidase 24.11 in essential hypertension. Hypertension 18:798-804

85. Richards AM, Wittert GA, Crozier IG et al (1993) Chronic inhibition of endopeptidases 24.11 in essential hypertension: evidence for enhanced atrial natriuretic peptide and angiotensin II. J Hypertens 11:407-416

86. Kahn JC, Patey M, Dubois-Rande JL et al (1990) Effect of sinorphan on plasma atrial natriuretic factor in congestive heart failure. Lancet 335:118-119

87. Good JM, Peters M, Wilkins M et al (1995) Renal response to candoxatrilat in patients with heart failure. J Am Coll Cardiol 25:1273-1281

88. Trindade PT, Rouleau JL (2001) Vasopeptidase inhibitors: potential role in the treatment of heart failure. Heart Fail Monit 2:2-7

89. Sagnella GA (2002) Vasopeptidase inhibitors. J Renin Angiotensin Aldosterone Syst 3:90-95

90. Dawson A, Struthers AD (2002) Vasopeptidase inhibitors in heart failure. J Renin Angiotensin Aldosterone Syst 3:156-159

91. Floras JS (2002) Vasopeptidase inhibition: a novel approach to cardiovascular therapy. Can J Cardiol 18:177-182

92. Chaitman BR, Ivleva AY, Ujda M et al (2005) Antianginal efficacy of omapatrilat in patients with chronic angina pectoris. Am J Cardiol 95:1283-1289

93. Packer M, Califf RM, Konstam MA et al (2002) Comparison of omapatrilat and enalapril in patients with chronic heart failure: the Omapatrilat Versus Enalapril Randomized Trial of Utility in Reducing Events (OVERTURE). Circulation 106:920-926

Chapter 8

"Inconclusive" Remarks:
Past, Present and Future of Natriuretic Peptides

"Deep in my heart" something different from contractile proteins and equally fundamental for the biology of human beings has been described.

Heart has a brain: it senses the changes in its "milieu interieur" and this kind of perception has an efferent arm, i.e. the synthesis and secretion of "brain peptides", the B-type natriuretic hormones.

Though the actual origin of this definition comes from the tissue where the peptides were originally identified, we might say that these agents act as heart's brain transmitters, able to re-establish the lost homeostasis of salt–water equilibrium or to positively influence vasomotion and vital tissue perfusion.

These molecules are probably as old as life on our planet, present in vegetal and animal beings. Prokaryotes and eukaryotes share them and complex organisms present with slightly different peptides secreted with different biological activities by different tissues and organs. The cardiovascular, immune, renal, reproductive, and nervous systems all recognize a role for one or more "natriuretic" peptides. They are not only natriuretic, but show multiple physiological actions, regulating arterial pressure, plasma volume in response to physical activity posture changes, and so on.

And they might be considered not only as an index of the physiological heart's response to stress, but also as the "tears" of a "broken heart". When the disease hits the myocardium, this is its signal for the whole body, and for the doctor, too.

Physicians now have a unique opportunity to add this new powerful humoral sign, which will help to clarify the diagnosis when it is doubtful in the emergency setting. It will help to follow-up the effect of treatment and to quantify clinical improvement. It will tell "more" truth than the usual markers about the patient's outcome. It will discover undiagnosed silent disease, when symptoms are not present or are underestimated, even by the patient himself.

It will push the physician to think in a "physiological" fashion, which is the best way to care for the patient. This heart is "lonely" no more, even when it suffers: these peptides act as a golden shield against other molecules, such as catecholamines, angiotensin, aldosterone, and endothelins, which, after a brief transient compensatory effect, act in a detrimental way on the clinical course and outcome.

The natriuretic peptides augment the blood supply in diseased patients, reduce fluid overload, and are effective in blunting the process of vascular/myocardial fibrosis hypertrophy.

Twenty years after their discovery by de Bold, these musketeers are still very young, and much remains to be understood of their individual differential profiles and their extra-cardiovascular actions.

We feel that the chapters of this book update us, but only temporarily. This saga is continuing and we hope to add what will follow in the future.

Subject Index

Made in the USA
Lexington, KY
02 January 2016